WN

MCQs in
Clinical Radiology

Gastrointestinal
and Hepatobiliary
Radiology

D1549713

VOLUME 3

MCQs in Clinical Radiology

Gastrointestinal and Hepatobiliary Radiology

(Question Bank for FRCR)

Prabhakar Rajiah
MBBS MD FRCR
Senior Registrar in Radiology
Manchester
United Kingdom

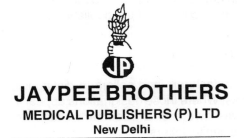

JAYPEE BROTHERS
MEDICAL PUBLISHERS (P) LTD
New Delhi

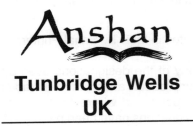

**Tunbridge Wells
UK**

First published in the UK by

Anshan Ltd
in 2006
6 Newlands Road
Tunbridge Wells
Kent TN4 9AT, UK

Tel/Fax: +44 (0)1892 557767
E-mail: info@anshan.co.uk
www.anshan.co.uk

ISBN 1 904798 551

British Library Cataloguing in Publication Data
A catalogue record for this book is available from the British Library

Printed in India by Sanat Printers, Kundli, Haryana

Foreword

Radiology is not just X-rays anymore. The rapid strides made in imaging technology has revolutionised radiology with advent of Ultrasound, Computed Tomography, Magnetic Resonance Imaging, PET Scanning and Interventional Radiology. Integration of these recent advances into the syllabus has increased the burden placed on radiology trainees facing Fellowship Exams. There is a burning need for simple and accurate resource to make the process of facing examinations a less daunting task.

In preparing this book, Dr Prabhakar Rajiah has been successful in developing a comprehensive practice resource for the Fellowship Exams. This book is in the same format to the Fellowship Exams and has been written using up-to-date and accurate information. This is easily the most extensive and largest collection of MCQs in radiology available today. The main strength of the book the categorisation of questions into related subtopics and the thorough,detailed explanation provided with the answers at the end of each section. The questions are of varying difficulty, covering amongst others, differential diagnosis, epidemiology, which is the staple of any Fellowship Exam and recent imaging techniques. The questions cover the three key components, anatomy, techniques and pathology. This should benefit everyone from the beginner to the more accomplished.

I am in no doubt, that this book is an ideal way of revising for the exams. It is also a good companion for self-assessment and would be of interest for senior radiologists who would like to update their knowledge and stay informed about current practices and imaging methods. This book is an ideal combination of information and revision resource.

Dr Biswaranjan Banerjee MBBS FRCS FRCR
Consultant Radiologist
Tameside General Hospital
Manchester
United Kingdom

Preface

Multiple choice questions (MCQs) have now become the standard and the most preferred means of assessing knowledge in all medical specialities including radiology. Along with the tremendous advances made in the various subspecialities of radiology, the level of knowledge not just in depth but also in breadth and the skill required to sit MCQ exams has increased as well. The format of the Fellowship Exams over the recent years has been changed to reflect these advances.

There is no gain saying the fact that the best method of preparing for these exams is keeping abreast of recent advances reading the standard radiology textbooks and journals. However, there is a place for books such as these, which can be used to develop knowledge and hone skills necessary for success in these exams. This book has been written primarily as a revision tool for those sitting MCQ exams in Gastrointestinal Radiology. This book can be approached in two ways. The best way is to read a particular topic in a recognised textbook or journal and subsequently test the knowledge gained using the questions in the corresponding chapter of this book. Alternatively, the book can be used first to identify lacunae in the knowledge base, which can then be corrected using journals and textbooks. It is imperative to realise that while this book cannot be a substitute for textbooks or journals, it can be a valuable revision tool prior to exams. It can also be used by those in an advanced stage, who do not have to stick to any particular format as an informal and fun way of gaining and self-testing radiological knowledge.

The format in this book is the same as used in the Fellowship Exams of the Royal Colleges of UK, Ireland, Hong Kong, Australia and New Zealand. The Royal College of UK Exam has 30 questions to be answered in one and half hours. Each question has five stems with true or false answers. The book has more than 1000 questions, each with five statements. Detailed explanations have been provided for the questions at the end of each chapter. The book has been divided into individual chapters, which will enable the reader to assess his strength and weakness, and correct deficiencies in knowledge. Due emphasis has been given to Anatomy, Techniques and Pathology, which are the important components of the Fellowship Exam. A detailed bibliography is provided at the end of this book for further reading.

Prabhakar Rajiah

Contents

Contents

1 Pharynx and Esophagus

1. **Gastrointestinal tract:**
   A. The hindgut extends from the hepatic flexure to rectum
   B. The proximal esophagus is supplied by inferior thyroid artery
   C. The midgut is supplied by celiac artery
   D. The hindgut is supplied by inferior mesenteric artery
   E. The mid third of esophagus is supplied by aorta

2. **Normal anatomy of the gastrointestinal tract:**
   A. The stomach folds normally measure 10 mm
   B. The areae gastricae measure less than 3 mm
   C. Valvulae conniventes measure 3 mm in jejunum
   D. Valvulae conniventes are 1 mm thick in ileum
   E. Maximum diameter of jejunal loops is 4 cm

3. **Esophagus:**
   A. The esophagus extends from C6 till D12
   B. The cervical esophagus runs slightly to the right of midline
   C. The thoracic esophagus is located slightly to the left of midline
   D. The esophagus is in direct contact with the posterior aspect of the left atrium
   E. The esophageal hiatus is surrounded by fibres of right crus of diaphragm

4. **The esophageal hiatus transmits the following:**
   A. The left vagus   B. The right vagus
   C. Lymphatics   D. Left gastric artery branches
   E. Phrenic nerve

5. **Esophagus:**
   A. The right wall of the esophagus is seen in chest X-rays
   B. Pleuroesophageal line is seen above the level of D4
   C. Motility studies of esophagus are performed in the erect position
   D. The three anatomical narrowings in esophagus are seen anteriorly and on the right side
   E. The lower esophagus drains into the posterior mediastinal nodes

6. **Esophagus:**
   A. The lower esophageal vestibule is seen only when there is a stricture in the lower end of esophagus
   B. The B ring is usually seen above the diaphragm
   C. The Z line is the mucosal esophagogastric junction
   D. 'A' ring is seen at the upper end of vestibule
   E. Aberrant left main pulmonary artery produces an indentation on the posterior aspect of the upper esophagus

7. **Barium examination:**
   A. The mortality of barium perforation is 100%
   B. Use of barium is not a contraindication to CT examination within two days
   C. Coating with water-soluble contrast is almost the same as that of barium
   D. Complications of aspiration is more with barium than with water-soluble contrast media
   E. When perforation of esophagus is suspected and water-soluble contrast study is normal, barium examination should be performed

8. **Concentrations of barium used for the different examinations:**
   A. Enema—150% w/v   B. Meal—250%
   C. Swallow—150%   D. Small bowel enema—100%
   E. Follow through—150%

9. **Radionuclide gastroesophageal reflux study:**
   A. Milk is used in infants
   B. Tc DTPA is used with orange juice is used in adults
   C. If no reflux is demonstrated in routine images, compression should be applied till a pressure of 100 mm Hg is obtained
   D. Imaging has to be carried for 60 minutes
   E. In infants reflux is more common in the supine position

10. **Buscopan is contraindicated in:**
    A. Cardiac failure   B. Asthma
    C. Glaucoma   D. Prostatism
    E. Cardiac arrhythmias   F. Myasthenia gravis

11. **Swallow and meal:**
    A. Varices are best demonstrated in the erect RAO position
    B. Pharyngeal pouch is a traction diverticulum
    C. Areae gastricae in the gastric antrum should be visualized satisfactorily to assess good coating
    D. Buscopan increases the risk of aspiration
    E. Barium can cause appendicitis

12. Dilatation of esophageal strictures:
A. Esophageal tumors are a contraindication
B. A stiff guide wire is required for crossing the stricture
C. Tracheoesophageal fistula is a contraindication
D. Angioplasty balloons are contraindicated
E. 22 mm balloon is used for dilatation of strictures

13. Pharynx:
A. Nodularity at the base of the tongue is due to lingual thyroid
B. Vallecula is situated between median and lateral aryepiglottic fold
C. Lower end of hypopharynx is collapsed except during passage of bolus
D. Aspiration cannot occur before swallowing
E. Aspiration always induces coughing reflux

14. The following are considered protective mechanisms for airway during swallowing:
A. Depression of larynx
B. Coughing
C. Anterior tilt of epiglottis
D. Abduction of true and false vocal cords
E. Approximation of thyroid and cricoid cartilage

15. Innervation of pharyngeal muscles:
A. All the soft palate muscles are supplied by the X nerve
B. All the pharyngeal muscles, except stylopharyngeus are supplied by the IX nerve
C. All the laryngeal muscles are supplied by the recurrent laryngeal nerve
D. All the tongue muscles are supplied by the XII nerve
E. Pharyngeal plexus contains the superior cervical ganglion

16. Stages of swallowing:
A. In the oral phase, the back of tongue and soft palate form a seal to prevent premature leakage of bolus into pharynx
B. Nasal regurgitation is prevented by the apposition of the soft palate and passavants cushion
C. The bolus is compressed by the pharyngeal contraction at the tail of the bolus
D. Larynx moves upwards and forwards when the bolus enters the oropharynx
E. Elevation of epiglottis is due to contraction of thyroepiglotticus

17. **Pharyngeal pouch:**
    A. Pharyngeal pouch can cause obstruction of esophagus
    B. Incidence of carcinoma in pharyngeal pouch is 5%
    C. The pouch usually extends posteriorly and to the right of the esophagus
    D. Associated with gastric ulcer
    E. Seen at C4 level

18. **Pharynx:**
    A. Chronic gastroesophageal reflux is a predisposing factor for formation of pharyngeal pouch
    B. Prominent cricopharyngeus is associated with gastroesophageal reflux
    C. Pronouncing long vowels during examination makes the pharynx narrow and is useful for motility studies
    D. The distal hypopharynx is best visualised only during swallowing
    E. Barium is instilled through nose for better visualisaton of soft palate

19. **Pharynx:**
    A. Pharynx manipulates a thin barium better than barium paste
    B. Thin barium is used for demonstrating laryngeal penetration
    C. Stop procedure if penetration occurs to carina
    D. Physiological bolus is better manipulated than non-physiological bolus
    E. Functional studies are avoided in sitting posture

20. **Examination of pharynx:**
    A. Pharyngeal mucosa should not be dry as the findings will be spurious
    B. Insulin should be avoided on the morning of examinations
    C. The mouth and oropharyngeal phase of swallowing should be done in all cases
    D. For double contrast of pharynx, 250% w/v of barium has to be used
    E. Modified Valsalva's maneuver is necessary for better visualisation of valleculae

21. **Video swallow:**
    A. Aspiration is common with the neck in flexed position
    B. Aspiration is common with thick fluid than thin fluid
    C. Aspiration is more due to CNS causes
    D. Sedation is necessary
    E. CNS cause affects voluntary than involuntary swallowing

22. **Endoscopic ultrasound of gastrointestinal tract:**
    A. The frequency of the probe used is 3.5-7 MHz
    B. All the five bowel layers are seen
    C. Endoscopic ultrasound is better than CT at local T staging for esophageal carcinoma
    D. Malignant nodes are hyperechoic
    E. Oval shapes are definitive for malignant nodes

23. **Recognised causes of dysphagia:**
    A. Botulism
    B. Syphilis
    C. Meningitis
    D. Streptomycin
    E. Azathioprine

24. **Esophagus:**
    A. At the level of D7 the esophagus is situated on the right side
    B. At the level of T10, the esophagus is situated in the midline
    C. The crossing of aortic arch is usually 35 cm from the incisor
    D. The diaphragm is situated 60 cm from the incisor
    E. In the mid third of esophagus, both striated and nonstriated muscles are present

25. **Esophageal motility:**
    A. Motility studies should be done in the RAO erect position
    B. The patient should swallow the barium at least twice for a satisfactory motility study
    C. The peristaltic wave is faster in thoracic esophagus than cervical esophagus
    D. The cricopharyngeus causes a posterior indentation in the barium column
    E. The normal peristaltic wave is always lumen obliterating

26. **Esophageal motility:**
    A. A mild reflux at the level of aortic arch is a normal phenomenon
    B. Tertiary contractions are not lumen obliterating
    C. Rosary bead and corkscrew appearance are forceful nonlumen obliterating contractions
    D. Administration of mecholyl results in sustained lumen obliterating contraction in the distal third of the esophagus
    E. Both peristaltic and nonperistaltic contractions in esophagus can move only in the aboral direction

27. **Esophageal motility:**
    A. Gastroesophageal reflux initiates secondary peristalsis
    B. Primary and secondary peristalsis is essentially the same except for the mode of initiation
    C. In a wet swallow, a primary peristalsis is initiated in 95% of cases
    D. Nonperistaltic contraction is limited to the smooth muscle segment only
    E. In adult, 1 nonperistaltic contraction is seen in 20% of patients

28. **Esophageal motility:**
    A. The velocity of peristalsis in the pharynx is 10-25 cm/sec
    B. In esophagus, the peristalsis takes 1.5 seconds in total
    C. Lower esophageal sphincter will open for a period for 8 seconds only when the bolus comes through
    D. Both the striated and smooth muscles are stimulated in the same way during peristaltic wave
    E. During peristalsis only the transverse muscle contracts

29. **Esophagus:**
    A. In presbyesophagus, there is decreased incidence of complete peristalsis sequences
    B. In hypertensive lower esophageal sphincter, the resting pressure is more than 40 mm Hg
    C. In chalasia, there is gross reflux
    D. Nonperistaltic contractions are seen in intestinal pseudo-obstruction
    E. Hiatus hernia is associated with scleroderma

30. **Diffuse esophageal spasm:**
    A. The contractions are nonlumen obliterating
    B. Esophageal wall is thickened
    C. The pain is increased by stress and relieved by nitroglycerine
    D. Nonperistaltic contractions seen in the skeletal portion of esophagus
    E. Abnormal contractions should be seen in at least 10% of swallows

31. **The following are complications of gastroesophageal reflux disease:**
    A. Prominent cricopharyngeus
    B. Pharyngeal pouch
    C. Asthma
    D. Laryngitis
    E. Tachycardia

32. Barrett's esophagus:
- A. An ulcer is necessary for diagnosis
- B. Seen in scleroderma
- C. Is premalignant
- D. Associated with a high esophageal stricture
- E. Associated with diffuse esophageal spasm

33. Corkscrew esophagus:
- A. Associated with epiphrenic diverticula
- B. Epiphrenic diverticulum are common near the gastroesophageal junction
- C. Primary and secondary waves are absent
- D. Antidepressants are used for treatment
- E. Predisposes for development of esophageal cancer

34. Stricture of esophagus is seen in:
- A. Scleroderma
- B. Achalasia
- C. Peptic ulcer
- D. Fundoplication
- E. Mediastinal lymph nodes

35. Caustic strictures:
- A. Acids produce more damage than alkalis
- B. Most commonly seen at the site of crossing of left main bronchus
- C. Stricture may be seen immediately after the acute phase
- D. Loss of mucosal pattern is seen immediately after alkali ingestion
- E. The stricture is irregular

36. Caustic stricture:
- A. The stricture is short segmental
- B. The appearance of alkali and acid stricture is different
- C. Stricture caused by prolonged intubation is long and irregular
- D. Strictures are irregular in all carcinomas of esophagus
- E. Predisposes to development of carcinoma

37. Causes of double barrel esophagus:
- A. Intramural diverticulum
- B. Mallory-Weiss tear
- C. Esophageal duplication
- D. Squamous cell carcinoma
- E. Kaposi's sarcoma

38. Causes of long smooth esophageal narrowing:
- A. Adenocarcinoma
- B. Reflux
- C. Alendronate
- D. Radiation
- E. Candidiasis

39. **Stricture of esophagus is seen in:**
    A. Pemphigus
    B. Epidermolysis bullosa
    C. Herpes
    D. Leiomyoma
    E. Behçet's disease

40. **Causes of failure of relaxation of lower esophageal sphincter:**
    A. Presbyesophagus   B. Scleroderma
    C. Carcinoma   D. Haematoma
    E. Candida esophagitis

41. **Giant esophageal ulcers (>1 cm) are seen in:**
    A. Cytomegalovirus   B. Herpes simplex
    C. Iron sulphate tablets D. Ibuprofen
    E. Reflux esophagitis

42. **Candida esophagitis:**
    A. Odynophagia is characteristic
    B. Associated with scleroderma
    C. Shaggy esophagus is characteristic
    D. Intramural pseudodiverticulosis
    E. Associated with oral thrush

43. **Candida esophagus:**
    A. Predisposes to gastric bezoar
    B. Peristalsis is increased
    C. Cobblestone appearance
    D. Polypoidal mass
    E. Plaques are oriented transversely

44. **Herpes:**
    A. Most common opportunistic infection in esophagus
    B. Associated herpetic lesions seen in lips and oral mucosa
    C. Common in upper esophagus above the level of left main bronchus
    D. Multiple plaques are the most common radiological presentation
    E. Superficial punctate ulcers are common than plaques

45. **Hiatal hernia:**
    A. 60% of hiatal hernias are sliding and 40% are rolling
    B. The gastroesophageal junction is at its normal position in sliding hiatal hernia
    C. Ovarian cysts are recognised causes
    D. Erect position is the best for demonstrating hiatal hernia
    E. Pneumonitis is a complication of hiatal hernia

46. **The following findings indicate presence of hiatal hernia:**
    A. More than 5 folds extending more than 2 cm above diaphragm
    B. Presence of areae gastricae within herniated fundus
    C. B ring situated more than 1 cm from the diaphragmatic hiatus
    D. Semilunar defect in medial wall of fundus
    E. Notch in the superior and left lateral aspect of hernia

47. **Mallory-Weiss tear:**
    A. Common near the gastroesophageal junction
    B. Seen in cirrhotic patients
    C. History of vomiting is always present
    D. The tear is multiple in majority
    E. Transverse orientation

48. **Differential diagnosis of lesions which expand the esophagus:**
    A. Squamous cell carcinoma
    B. Adenocarcinoma
    C. Spindle cell carcinoma
    D. Leiomyosarcoma
    E. Fibrovascular polyp

49. **Esophageal ulcer:**
    A. Pemphigus is associated with esophageal ulcer
    B. Gastroesophageal reflux leads to transverse folds in esophagus
    C. Barrett's esophagus is lined by squamous epithelium
    D. Columnar lined esophagus is usually narrowed
    E. It is very uncommon for squamous cell carcinoma to present as a solitary esophageal ulcer

50. **Common indications of esophageal dilatation:**
    A. Peptic stricture
    B. Corrosive stricture
    C. Stricture caused by mediastinal nodes
    D. Achalasia
    E. Prior to radiation therapy in malignancy

51. **Esophageal varices are seen in:**
    A. IVC web
    B. Hepatic adenoma
    C. Constrictive pericarditis
    D. Schistosomiasis
    E. Umbilical sepsis

52. **Causes of lower esophageal narrowing:**
    A. Drugs
    B. Achalasia
    C. Diffuse esophageal spasm
    D. Esophagitis
    E. Presbyesophagus

53. **TB of esophagus:**
    A. May resemble the appearance of candidiasis
    B. Usually secondary to mediastinal lymph nodes
    C. Associated with TB spine
    D. Associated with caseating mediastinal lymph node
    E. Causes giant esophageal ulcer

54. **Esophagus:**
    A. Carcinosarcoma produces characteristic widening of lumen at the site of the tumour
    B. Mucosal lesions make an angle of more than 90 degrees with the esophageal wall
    C. Papilloma is the most common benign tumour of esophagus
    D. Adenomas can arise only from Barrett's esophagus
    E. Adenomas are premalignant, but smaller than inflammatory polyps

55. **Esophagitis:**
    A. HIV produces giant diamond ulcer similar to cytomegalovirus
    B. CMV produces ulcer near the gastroesophageal junction
    C. Multiple small ulcers exclude CMV and are likely to be herpetic
    D. Diffuse mucosal abnormality in CMV
    E. The area between ulcers is normal without any plaque in herpes

56. **Esophagus:**
    A. Inflammatory esophagogastric polyp is premalignant
    B. Glycogen acanthosis produces severe symptoms and are common in the upper third
    C. Acanthosis nigricans produces only endoscopic lesions, but radiological visualisation is difficult
    D. All leiomyomas are resected for fear of leiomyosarcoma
    E. Leiomyomas are multiple in 40% of cases

57. **Leiomyoma:**
    A. Most common in the middle esophagus
    B. Premalignant
    C. Can present as marked thickening of esophagus
    D. Sharply outlined by barium on both sides
    E. The epicenter of the lesion lies outside the projected contour of the esophagus

58. **Esophageal tuberculosis:**
    A. The mucosa is normal in majority of cases
    B. Pulsion diverticula is commonly seen
    C. Fistula formation in an AIDS patient is suggestive of tuberculosis
    D. The most common site of primary tuberculosis in esophagus is at the level of tracheal bifurcation
    E. The narrowing of esophagus is irregular

59. **Fibrovascular polyp of esophagus:**
    A. Invariably sessile
    B. Originates in the distal esophagus near the esophagogastric junction
    C. Progressive growth of the mass indicates malignant conversion
    D. Bleeding caused by patient biting the tumour
    E. The position of the tumour varies with deglutition

60. **Achalasia cardia:**
    A. Diagnosis not made in the absence of a dilated esophagus
    B. Mimics malignancy
    C. Carcinoma is a complication
    D. Candida esophagitis is associated
    E. Recurrent chest infections are common

61. **Achalasia cardia:**
    A. The resting lower esophageal sphincter is normal in early achalasia
    B. High amplitude, simultaneous repetitive contractions can be seen in achalasia
    C. Peristaltic wave is not seen in cervical esophagus
    D. Decreased cell bodies in the dorsal motor nucleus of vagus is a cause of the disease
    E. There is a high female preponderance

62. **Differential diagnosis of multiple submucosal masses in esophagus:**
    A. Retention cysts
    B. Leukemia
    C. Kaposi's sarcoma
    D. Epidermolysis bullosa
    E. Glycogenic acanthosis

63. **Esophagus:**
    A. An extraluminal mass is effaced when the esophagus is maximally distended with barium
    B. Granular cell tumours are lined by squamous epithelium
    C. Multiple hemangiomas indicate Osler-Rendu-Weber syndrome
    D. Duplication cysts are common in the right side of the esophagus
    E. Retention cyst is due to dilatation of mucous glands in the submucous layer

64. **Esophageal cancer:**
    A. 10% of esophageal malignancies
    B. Common in males
    C. 70% of adenocarcinomas rise from Barrett's esophagus
    D. Common in the lower than upper part of esophagus
    E. Ulcerative type is the most common type of tumour

65. **Esophageal cancer risk factors:**
    A. Asbestos
    B. Celiac disease
    C. Smoking
    D. Tylosis
    E. History of pharyngeal cancer

66. **Esophageal cancer in plain X-ray:**
    A. Mediastinal widening
    B. Right paratracheal stripe widening
    C. Widened azygoesophageal recess
    D. Air fluid level
    E. Aspiration pneumonia

67. **Esophageal cancer:**
    A. Celiac nodes involved in the lower esophageal tumours
    B. Supraclavicular nodules are involved in the middle third tumours
    C. Varicoid form resembles candida esophagitis
    D. Presence of celiac nodes implies survival of only three months
    E. T2 tumour involves the muscularis propria

68. **Staging of esophageal cancer:**
    A. Wall thickness less than 10 mm is not significant
    B. Mass in contact with aorta more than 90 degrees is not resectable
    C. High frequency of esophageal spread with tumours more than 3 cm
    D. Failure of bowing of the trachea during expiration is a sensitive indicator of invasion
    E. Tracheoesophageal fistula is the only accurate indicator of tracheal invasion

69. **Esophageal nodules are seen in:**
    A. Glycogenic acanthosis
    B. Barrett's
    C. Reflux
    D. Candida
    E. Leiomyoma

70. **Scleroderma esophagus:**
    A. Esophagus is involved before any other organ
    B. It is the second GI location to be involved after small intestine
    C. Hypotonia is seen involving the whole length of esophagus
    D. There is narrowing of the lower esophageal sphincter
    E. Stricture is commonly seen at the level of aortic arch

71. **Achalasia cardia:**
    A. The incidence of carcinoma is around 2%
    B. Absent gastric bubble in X-ray abdomen is a reliable sign
    C. Mycobacterial infections are common in achalasia
    D. Drinking Coke increases the esophageal emptying
    E. Amyl nitrate inhalation worsens the achalasia

72. **Achalasia cardia:**
    A. The dilated esophagus in achalasia is usually seen in the left side in the chest X-ray film
    B. Achalasia causes lateral displacement of trachea rather than anteroposterior displacement
    C. Trypanosoma infection is a recognized cause of achalasia
    D. Achalasia cannot be diagnosed if there are esophageal contractions
    E. Barium swallow can open the sphincter in achalasia

73. **Causes of esophageal rings:**
    A. Transverse mucosal fold
    B. Epidermolysis bullosa
    C. Leiomyoma
    D. Peptic stricture
    E. Aberrant subclavian artery

74. **Causes of esophageal webs:**
    A. Graft-versus-host disease
    B. Heterotopic gastric mucosa
    C. Esophagitis
    D. Epidermolysis bullosa
    E. Plummer-Vinson syndrome

75. **Esophageal perforation:**
    A. Most common location is in the upper esophagus at the site of aortic arch crossing
    B. Associated with left-sided pleural effusion if the perforation is in the upper third
    C. Causes obstruction of superior vena cava
    D. In the upper esophagus, the cricopharynx is the most common level of damage
    E. Widening of mediastinum is seen only in upper esophageal perforation

76. **Esophageal perforation:**
    A. Subcutaneous emphysema is seen
    B. Pneumothorax
    C. Contrast studies are positive in 90%
    D. Barium is absolutely contraindicated for diagnosing perforation
    E. CT shows periesophageal fluid collection

77. **Causes of esophageal perforation:**
    A. Esophageal carcinoma
    B. Barrett's esophagus
    C. Emesis
    D. Intubation
    E. Candida

78. **Aortoesophageal fistula:**
    A. Infected aortic aneurysm is a recognized cause
    B. Foreign body impaction is a recognized cause
    C. Water-soluble contrast hardly demonstrates the leak
    D. Haemetemesis in a patient with aortic aneurysm is pathogno-monic
    E. Barium is preferred for satisfactory examination

79. **Esophagitis:**
    A. Odynophagia is a feature seen in infectious esophagitis and uncommon in reflux esophagitis
    B. Infections are most common in the distal third of esophagus
    C. Esophageal stasis is a predisposing factor for candida
    D. Snakeskin pattern of involvement indicates diffuse infiltration by large plaques in candida
    E. Polypoid appearance in candida indicates development of carcinoma

80. **Recognised presentations of candida:**
    A. Aortoesophageal fistula
    B. Tracheoesophageal fistula
    C. Perforation
    D. Pseudodiverticulosis
    E. Carcinoma

81. **Esophageal webs:**
    A. May be asymptomatic
    B. Well seen in endoscopy
    C. AP views of barium are best for diagnosis
    D. Associated with clubbing
    E. Can occur in absence of iron deficiency

82. **Endoscopic ultrasound:**
    A. Varix is seen in layer four
    B. Leiomyoma arises in layer three or two
    C. Smooth muscle tumour > 3 cm will be considered leiomyosarcoma regardless of appearance
    D. Majority of benign intramural tumours arise from the third layer
    E. Carcinoid arises from layer 1

83. **Esophagus:**
    A. In candida, ulcers are more commonly seen than plaques
    B. In herpes, the mucosa is normal in between superficial ulcers
    C. HIV and CMV ulcers cannot be differentiated radiologically
    D. Sinus tracts are often associated with tuberculous esophagitis
    E. Bougie should be used in caustic strictures only after three weeks

84. **Common drugs producing esophagitis:**
    A. Clindamycin
    B. Cimetidine
    C. Indomethacin
    D. Theophylline
    E. Ciprofloxacin

85. **Esophagus:**
    A. Potassium tablets usually cause ulcers in distal esophagus, when used in mitral stenosis and cardiac failure
    B. Crohn's esophagitis always have small bowel involvement
    C. Apthous ulcers are seen in Crohn's
    D. In epidermolysis bullosa, strictures are most common in lower esophagus, near the GE junction
    E. In epidermolysis and pemphigus vulgaris, the webs are seen in midthoracic esophagus

86. **Esophageal varices:**
    A. Valsalva maneuver is essential for demonstrating
    B. Swallowing makes the varices clear
    C. LAO is a good position for diagnosing varices
    D. The barium should be given in generous amounts so that the varices are seen as huge serpiginous filling defects
    E. The esophagus should be in relaxed phase

87. **Causes of uphill varices in esophagus:**
    A. IVC obstruction below hepatic veins
    B. Splenomegaly
    C. Budd-Chiari syndrome
    D. Splenic vein thrombosis
    E. Cirrhosis

88. **Esophageal varices:**
    A. Downhill varices are always due to superior vena caval obstruction
    B. Downhill varices are seen throughout the length of esophagus
    C. Esophageal carcinoma cannot be confused with varices
    D. The veins enhance in CT scans
    E. The descending aorta will be silhouetted in plain film

89. Varices:
   A. Isolated gastric varices are seen in splenic vein obstruction
   B. Administration of buscopan makes visualisation of varices difficult
   C. Plain X-ray shows posterior mediastinal mass in erect views
   D. Dysphagia is as frequent as seen in varicoid carcinoma
   E. Sclerosed veins show laminated appearance in contrast enhanced CT

90. Postoperative esophagus:
   A. Nissen's fundoplication produces an irregular fundal filling defect
   B. Perforation after esophageal dilatation is most common in the left posterolateral wall just below diaphragm
   C. In post op period, if no leak is demonstrated in water-soluble contrast, barium should be used
   D. If aspiration is suspected, water-soluble contrast is the first agent to be used
   E. Eccentric ballooning of esophagus is common after Heller's cardiomyotomy

91. Esophageal web:
   A. Associated with macrocytic anemia
   B. Most common in cervical esophagus
   C. Visualised in partial distension
   D. Thickness > 3 mm
   E. Right angle to the anterior esophageal wall

92. Recognised causes of aortoesophageal fistula:
   A. Esophageal carcinoma   B. Syphilis
   C. Foreign body ingestion   D. Barrett's esophagus
   E. Sarcoidosis

93. Candida esophagitis:
   A. AIDS defining illness
   B. Steroid intake is a high risk factor
   C. Foamy esophagus, is usually due to artifacts
   D. Bubbles seen in candida are uniform in size and mobile
   E. Shaggy esophagus is more common AIDS-associated candida than other causes of candida

94. Associations of Plummer-Vinson syndrome:
   A. Iron deficiency anemia
   B. Thyroid disorder
   C. Koilonychia
   D. Glossitis
   E. Cricopharyngeal carcinoma

95. Increased esophageal transit time is seen in:
  A. Diffuse esophageal spasm
  B. Gastroesophageal reflux
  C. Scleroderma
  D. Achalasia
  E. Presbyesophagus

96. Intramural pseudodiverticulosis:
  A. Associated with esophageal strictures
  B. Barium shows these diverticula communicating with the lumen
  C. They are arranged perpendicular to the long axis of esophagus
  D. Herniation of mucosa through the muscularis propria
  E. Reflux is the most common cause

97. Reflux esophagitis:
  A. The gastroesophageal junction is always involved
  B. Nonperistaltic waves are seen in distal esophagus
  C. Transverse folds are seen
  D. Granular folds are seen
  E. Abnormal motility with alkaline barium

98. Factors preventing reflux:
  A. Diaphragmatic crus
  B. Rossette folds of gastric mucous membrane at cardia
  C. Intra-abdominal esophagus
  D. Phrenoesophageal membrane
  E. Gastroesophageal angle

99. Associations of gastroesophageal reflux:
  A. Rolling hiatal hernia
  B. Scleroderma
  C. Gastroesophageal polyp
  D. Peptic ulcer
  E. Intubation

100. Complications of reflux:
  A. Iron deficiency anemia B. Pulmonary fibrosis
  C. Carcinoma   D. Schatzki ring
  E. Perforation

101. Reflux:
  A. LPO position is the best position for diagnosis
  B. Water siphon test has 20% false negative rate
  C. In radionuclide study, the esophageal activity is more than 4% of stomach activity
  D. Provocative manoeuvres have 75% accuracy
  E. High activity will be seen in pertechnate scan

ANSWERS

1. **A-F, B-T, C-F, D-T, E-T**

   The foregut extends from the esophagus to the 2nd part of duodenum, midgut from 2nd part of duodenum to the junction of mid and distal third of transverse colon and the hindgut from distal transverse colon to rectum. The foregut is supplied by branches of celiac artery, the midgut by superior mesenteric artery and hindgut by inferior mesenteric artery. The upper 1/3rd of esophagus gets blood supply from inferior thyroid artery, mid 1/3rd from aorta and distal 1/3rd from celiac artery.

2. **A-F, B-T, C-F, D-T, E-T**

   Stomach folds—3-5 mm; areae gastricae—2-3 mm; jejunum—4 cm with valvulae—2 mm thick; ileum—3 cm with valvulae 1 mm thick.

3. **A-F, B-F, C-T, D-F, E-T**

   The esophagus extends for a distance of 25 cm from C6 till D10. The cervical esophagus is slightly to the left and although, it is in midline, when entering thorax, it is slightly towards the left, in the thorax. The esophagus is separated from the left atrium by the pericardium. The esophageal hiatus is situated at level of D10, surrounded by the right crus of diaphragm and runs for a distance of 3 cm in the abdomen.

4. **A-T, B-T, C-T, D-T, E-F**

   Esophageal hiatus at level of D 10, transmits the vagus nerves, lymphatics and esophageal branches of left gastric artery.

5. **A-T, B-T, C-F, D-F, E-F**

   The right wall of esophagus and azygos (azygoesophageal line) are seen in chest X-rays.

   Pleuroesophageal line is seen above level of D4, where the pleura is in direct contact with the esophagus. Motility studies are performed in the prone position to eliminate the influence of gravity. The narrowings are seen in the anterior and the left side. The first is at the junction of cricopharynx and esophagus (15 cm) the second where the aortic arch and left main bronchus cross (25 cm) and the third is at entry into diaphragm (40 cm).

   The upper esophagus drains into deep cervical nodes, midportion into posterior mediastinal nodes and lower esophagus drains into the celiac nodes.

6. **A-F, B-F, C-T, D-T, E-F**

   The vestibule is the normal dilatation seen in the lower end of esophagus. 'A' ring is seen at the upper end of the vestibule and the B ring is the lower end. The B ring is usually seen below the diaphragm and well visualized only in hiatal hernia. The Z line is the mucosal junction between stomach and esophagus. Aberrant left main pulmonary artery produces an anterior impression, whereas the more common aberrant right subclavian artery produces impression in the posterior aspect.

7. **A-F, B-F, C-F, D-F, E-T**
   Mortality is 50%. Barium will produce extensive artifacts, if CT is done within two weeks. Coating with water-soluble contrast is very poor and is mainly to diagnose perforation or obstruction. Aspiration of barium produces only mild pneumonitis but aspiration of water-soluble contrast produces pulmonary edema.

8. **A-F, B-T, C-F, D-F, E-F**
   Enema—115% w/v. Meal—250, swallow—250, follow through—60-100, small bowel enema—60

9. **A-T, B-T, C-T, D-T, E-T**
   Tc DTPA or Tc colloid is mixed with either milk or acidified orange juice and patient placed in recumbent position. Images are acquired every 5 sec till 60 minutes to demonstrate reflux and terminated once it is demonstrated. Rapid images every 0,5 sec can be used for demonstrating esophageal transit.

10. **A-T, B-F, C-T, D-T, E-T, F-T**
    Also contraindicated in mechanical bowel obstruction, megacolon, thyrotoxicosis and allergy.

11. **A-F, B-F, C-T, D-T, E-T**
    Varices are best demonstrated in the supine RPO position. Normal views are obtained in the RAO position. Buscopan relaxes the lower esophageal sphincter, increasing reflux of gastric contents. There are two types of diverticula—pulsion and traction. Pulsion diverticula occurs proximal to obstruction and is due to herniation of mucosa through the wall. Traction divertcula are caused due to traction by extrinsic lesions.

12. **A-F, B-F, C-T, D-F, E-T**
    Esophageal tumours are not contraindication. The tip should be floppy, to traverse the stricture. Good relief is obtained by dilating between 40 and 54 F. Strictures are not dilated more than 60 F.

13. **A-T, B-F, C-T, D-F, E-F**
    Aspiration can occur during swallowing, or before swallowing due to premature leakage from mouth or after swallowing due to overflow of retained or regurgitated bolus. Aspiration need not necessarily induce coughing, especially in those with neuromuscular weakness. In these patients, the laryngeal epithelium is not

sensitive to aspiration, producing a silent aspiration without coughing. Valleculae are situtated between the median and lateral glossoepiglottic folds.

14. **A-F, B-T, C-F, D-F, E-F**
Transient suspension of respiration, posterior tilt of epiglottis, elevation of larynx, closure of laryngeal aperture, adduction of true and false vocal cords, apposition of thyroid and hyoid cartilages and contraction of constrictor compressing epiglottis against laryngeal aperture are other protective mechanisms.

15. **A-F, B-F, C-F, D-F, E-T**
All the soft palate muscles X, except tensor veli palatini V
All pharyngeal muscles X, except stylopharyngeus IX
All laryngeal muscles, Rec Laryng N, except cricothyroid, superior laryng N.
All tongue muscles XII, except palatoglossus, X nerve.
Pharyngeal plexus comprises IX, X, sympathetic trunk, superior cervical ganglion.

16. **A-T, B-T, C-T, D-T, E-T**

17. **A-T, B-T, C-F, D-T, E-F**
Pharyngeal pouch, is due to outpouching of posterior pharyngeal wall through the oblique and transverse muscle fibres of crico-pharyngeus, at the level of C5/6. It is commonly seen posteriorly and to the left and can cause compression of esophagus. Associations include gastric ulcer, hiatus hernia, achalasia and esophageal spasm. Carcinoma incidence in between 0.4 and 8%.

18. **A-T, B-T, C-F, D-T, E-T**
Pronouncing long vowels such as OOO and EEE, makes the pharynx larger and visualisation is better. For soft palate, 1-2 ml of barium is instilled through a tube into the nose and high density barium is swallowed.

19. **A-F, B-T, C-T, D-F, E-F**
Pharynx manipulates cohesive bolus better than liquid, hence barium paste is better tolerated than thick barium which is better tolerated than thin barium.
Small nonphysiological bolus, i.e. 2-5 ml is manipulated safer than large physiological bolus 5-10 ml. Functional studies are usually done with erect lateral views. But if it not possible, it can be done in the sitting lateral views.

20. **A-F, B-T, C-T, D-T, E-T**
Modified Valsalva's manoeuvre is done to expand pharynx and obtain better visualisation of structures. Dry pharyngeal mucosa

is essential for good coating. Hence, smoking and chewing are avoided on the day of examination and the patient is nil oral from the night before.

21. **A-T, B-F, C-T, D-F, E-T**

22. **A-F, B-T, C-T, D-F, E-F**
    Higher frequency probes, more than 10 MHz are used for endoscopic ultrasound. The bowel layers are seen as alternating hyper- and hypoechoic layers. The mucosa and muscularis mucosa junction is hyperechoic, musclaris mucosa—hypoechoic, sub-mucosa—hyperechoic, muscularis propria—hypoechoic, serosa—hyperechoic. Endoscopic ultrasound has very high accuracy for assessing the exact involvement of the different layers of the bowel. Normal lymph nodes are hypoechoic with hyperechoic fatty hilum. Malignant nodes are hypoechoic. Normal lymph nodes are oval but malignant nodes are round.

23. **A-T, B-T, C-T, D-T, E-T**
    Other drugs that can produce dysphagia include tetracycline, neomycin, ACTH, prednisone, antidepressants, antipsychotics, sedatives and tryptophan.

24. **A-F, B-T, C-F, D-F, E-T**
    The esophagus starts in the median plane. It is on the left side till the root of the neck. At level of T5, it is median, at level of T7, it is on left side and in T10 it is midline. There are at least four narrowings seen. Cricopharynx—15 cm from incisor, crossing of aortic arch—22.5 cm, crossing of left main bronchus—27 cm and diaphragm—40 cm in the upper third of esophagus, only striated muscle is present, in lower third only smooth muscle is present, in the middle third, the striated muscle is gradually replaced by smooth muscle.

25. **A-T, B-F, C-F, D-T, E-T**
    Motility studies are performed ideally in the prone RAO position to eliminate the influence of gravity. The patient swallows about 5-10 ml of barium and should make only one swallow. If a second swallow is made before the first peristaltic sequence ends, the peristaltic wave will be inhibited and this will cause spurious abnormal appearance. The normal peristaltic wave is inverted V-shaped and is lumen obliterating. This is progressive stripping, fastest in cervical esophagus and slow in thoracic esophagus, due to high intra-abdominal pressure.

26. **A-T, B-T, C-F, D-T, E-F**
    There is a mild proximal escape of contrast at the level of aortic arch, which is more pronounced in elderly. This is due to low

amplitute pressure trough seen at the junction of skeletal muscle and smooth muscle. Unlike normal peristaltic wave, a tertiary contraction is a feeble, repetitive, nonlumen obliterating, nonperistaltic contraction. Corkscrew contraction is a forceful nonlumen obliterating contraction. But a rosary bead or kebab appearance is a nonperistaltic lumen obliterating contraction. A normal peristaltic wave can move only in the aboral direction, but a nonperistaltic wave can move in both directions.

27. A-T, B-T, C-T, D-T, E-T

Primary peristalsis is a rapid wave of inhibition followed by a slower wave of contraction. It is initiated in the brainstem, medulla. Secondary peristalsis is initiated by local esophageal stimulation by distension from either reflux or barium or remnant bolus. Hence, only the mode of initiation differs after which both propagate distally in the same way. Primary peristalsis is initiated in 70-90% of dry swallows and 95% of wet swallows, but secondary peristalsis is initiated only in 40-65% of swallows. Nonperistaltic waves are limited to the smooth muscle segment. In elderly, repetitive spontaneous nonperistaltic contraction is seen in up to 10%.

28. A-T, B-F, C-T, D-F, E-F

In pharynx, the peristaltic wave moves at the rate of 10-25 cm/sec and it takes 1.5 seconds. In esophagus, it moves at the rate of 2-4 cm/sec and it takes 6-8.5 seconds. Upper esophageal sphincter relaxes for 0.5 seconds in 0.2-0.3 sec after initiation of swallowing. Lower esophageal sphincter opens only when there is bolus and remains open for 6-8 seconds. The sphincter relaxes in 100% of young adults. During peristalsis both the longitudinal and transverse muscles contract, but the longitudinal muscle contractions which produces esophageal shortening is not commonly visible. It is visible with movement of B ring above hiatus and by noting markers such as diverticula or rings.

29. A-T, B-T, C-T, D-T, E-T

In scleroderma, there is patulous lower esophageal sphincter, producing gross gastroesophageal reflux. Esophagus is dilated and there are teritary contractions. SLE and Raynaud's disease produce similar changes. In presbyesophagus, the motility is affected in 20% of those above 70 years. There is decreased incidence of complete peristalsis, increased prevalence of nonperistaltic contractions and incomplete lower esophageal sphincter relaxation. Chalasia is seen in neonates and is characterised by intermittent relaxation of lower esophageal sphincter producing copious reflux and vomiting. This is believed to be due to delay in development of neuromuscular control in the lower esophageal control. Intestinal pseudo-obstruction is characterised by gross distension of gastrointesintal tract without mechanical obstruction or paralytic ileus. They are associated with nonperistaltic contractions or aperistalsis.

30. **A-F, B-T, C-T, D-F, E-T**
Diffuse esophageal spasm is characterised by simultaneous, repetitive, forceful, nonperistaltic lumen obliterating contractions in the distal smooth muscle part of esophagus. The proximal one-third is normal. The esophagus is thickened and this is best seen in the right wall, measuring more than 2 cm. The patient has intermittent chest pain that mimicks angina. The pain is increased by stress or large bolus, relieved by nitroglycerine and can radiate to shoulders and left arm.

31. **A-T, B-T, C-T, D-T, E-T**
Foreign body sensation in throat, pain, lateral pharyngeal pouch, cough, hoarseness of voice, granuloma, ulcer and spasm of larynx, aspiration pneumonia, chronic lung disease, sleep apnoea, bradycardia and syncope are other recognised complications of gastroesophageal reflux.

32. **A-F, B-T, C-T, D-F**
Seen in 37% of scleroderma patients. Associated with low or mid-esophageal stricture.
Predisposing factor for adenocarcinoma of esophagus. The stricture is seen close to the gastroesophageal junction in the lower third of esophagus.

33. **A-T, B-T, C-T, D-T, E-F**
Corkscrew esophagus is produced due to abnormal tertiary peristaltic waves, which are not associated with normal primary and secondary peristaltic waves.
Epiphrenic diverticulum is a pulsion diverticulum due to the high pressure created by the waves. Right anterior oblique views are essential for eliminating the effect of gravity.

34. **A-T, B-T, C-T, D-T, E-T**

35. **A-F, B-F, C-T, D-T, E-F**
Alkalis produce more damage than acids. Most common site is the distal end followed by crossing of left main bronchus. Stricture may be seen immediately or it may take months to years, depending on the severity of the injury. Loss of mucosal pattern and spasm are seen immediately after the ingestion due to oedema. The stricture is long segmental and smooth.

36. **A-F, B-F, C-F, D-F, E-T**
Caustic Stricture is long segmental. The appearances of both acid and alkalis strictures are similar and cannot be distinguished. Stricture caused by prolonged intubation is long and smooth, similar to that of caustic strictures. Strictures can be smooth in squamous cell carcinoma. There is increased risk of squamous cell carcinoma in caustic strictures.

37. **A-T, B-T, C-T, D-F, E-F**
Also seen in dissecting intramural haematoma and intramural abscess.

38. **A-F, B-T, C-T, D-T, E-T**
Caustic stricutre and prolonged intubation are the most common causes.
Other causes are congenital esophageal stenosis and surgical repair of congenital atresia.

39. **A-T, B-T, C-F, D-T, E-F**
Inflammatory—reflux, Crohn's, scleroderma, corrosives, iatrogenic—prolonged nasogastric intubation, radiotherapy, fundoplication. Neoplastic—carcinoma, leiomyoma, leiomyosarcoma, carcinosarcoma, lymphoma, mediastinal lymph nodes. Miscellaneous—epidermolysis bullosa, pemphigus.

40. **A-T, B-F, C-T, D-T, E-F**
Achalasia is the most common cause of failure of relaxation of LES. Other causes include hypertensive sphincter, diffuse esophageal spasm and fibrotic strictures.

41. **A-T, B-T,C-F, D-F, E-F**
Cytomegalovirus, HIV, TB, actinomycosis, caustics, potassium chloride, quinidine and radiation are causes of giant ulcer.

42. **A-T, B-T, C-T, D-T, E-T**
Scleroderma and other diseases which delay esophageal emptying are predisposing causes. Shaggy esophagus is a serrated appearance due to coalescence of ulcers, erosions and pseudo-membranes.

43. **A-T, B-F, C-T, D-T, E-F**
Peristalsis is sluggish.
Polypoidal mass is due to occasional presence of a mycetoma.
Plaques are oriented longitudinally.

44. **A-F, B-T, C-F, D-F, E-T**
Candida is the most common opportunistic infection in esophagus. Herpes infection is by HSV-1 virus. Common in midesophagus at

level of left main bronchus. Multiple superficial punctate, linear, stellate ulcers are the most common lesions. Superfical plaques are uncommon.

45. **A-F, B-F, C-T, D-F, E-T**
About 99% are sliding and only 1% is rolling or paraesophageal. In sliding type, the OG junction herniates along with stomach. In rolling type, the stomach herniates but OG junction is in normal position. The hernia reduces and is difficult to distend in erect position. Prone RAO is the best position for diagnosing hiatal hernia. Obstruction and reflux are other complications. Obesity, pregnancy, giant ovarian cysts and ascites are recognised causes.

46. **A-T, B-T, C-F, D-T, E-T**
B ring should be situated more than 1 cm from the diaphragmatic hiatus. The diaphragmatic hiatus has to be identified indirectly, by noting the diaphragmatic impression or by asking the patient to sniff, when the diaphragmatic impression becomes prominent and by noting stopping of peristalsis abruptly. Intraluminal polypoid mass can be seen due to prolapsed mucosa. Occasionally, a riding ulcer can be seen at the hiatal orifice due to gastric mucosa. The notch is due to gastric sling fibers.

47. **A-T, B-T, C-T, D-F, E-F**
The tear is longitudinal and involves the mucosa and submucosa. It is due to raised pressure secondary to vomiting.

48. **A-F, B-T, C-T, D-T, E-T**
Spindle cell carcinoma is also called carcinosarcoma.

49. **A-T, B-T, C-F, D-F, E-T**
Barrett's esophagus is lined by at least 2 cm of columnar epithelium. This segment is dilated and usually bell/tent-shaped.

50. **A-T, B-T, C-F, D-T, E-T**
Mediastinal nodes cause extrinsic compression.

51. **A-T, B-F, C-T, D-T, E-T**
Schistosomiasis and umbilical sepsis are recognised causes of portal hypertension which result in esophageal varices.

52. **A-F, B-T, C-T, D-T, E-T**
Drugs more commonly affect the upper part at the site of crossing left main bronchus.
Scleroderma is another well-known cause.

53. **A-T, B-T, C-T, D-T, E-T**
TB is secondary to mediastinal nodal spread or ingestion of organisms. Usually an active pulmonary infection is not seen.

54. **A-T, B-F, C-F, D-F, E-F**
    Carcinosarcoma has both epithelial and mesenchymal elements. It is common in the midesophagus. But unlike other tumours, this produces dilatation of the lumen at the level of tumour. Mucosal lesions usually make an angle <90 degrees with the lumen. Submucosal lesions make 90 degrees and extrinsic lesions more than 90 degrees. Leiomyoma is the most common benign tumour in the esophagus accounting for 50% of all benign tumours. Papilloma constitutes less than 5% of esophageal tumours. Adenomas can also arise from ectopic gastric mucosa. Adenomas are larger, lobulated and nodular than benign inflammatory polyps.

55. **A-T, B-T, C-F, D-F, E-T**
    In CMV a single large ulcer or multiple small superficial ulcers are seen.
    The intervening mucosa is usually normal. In herpes, the mucosa between ulcers is without plaques.

56. **A-F, B-F, C-F, D-F, E-F**
    Inflammatory esophagogastric polyp is a giant thickened gastric fold extending into the distal esophagus, seen in reflux esophagitis. It is not premalignant and is made of inflammatory and granulation tissue. Glycogen acanthosis produces small nodular lesions throughout esophagus, which are common in the mid and lower third esophagus, because they are well-visualised here. They are not symptomatic unlike candida, which has similar appearance in early stages. Acanthosis nigricans produces a similar radiological appearance, as tiny nodules. Leiomyomas without dysphagia or bleeding are not resected. Leiomyomas are multiple in only less than 5% of cases.

57. **A-F, B-F, C-T, D-T, E-F**
    About 60% are seen in distal esophagus, 30% in midesophagus and 10% in proximal esophhagus. It is not premalignant. It is usually seen as a well-defined submucosal lesion which makes an angle of 90 degrees with the wall. A characteristic sign is forked stream sign, which indicates a round filling defect sharply outlined by barium on both sides. The main differentials are the extrinsic lesions. The extrinsic lesions make an obtuse angle, the epicenter lies outside the projected contour of esophagus, move with esophagus on respiration and deglutition. But a submucosal lesion, makes a right angle and the epicenter is within the projected contour of the esophagus.

58. **A-T, B-F, C-T, D-T, E-F**
    Esophageal tuberculosis is usually secondary to mediastinal lymphadenopathy, producing a smooth narrowing, with intact

mucosa. There is a traction diverticula, not a pulsion diverticula. Less than 60% of lumen is affected.

59. **A-F, B-F, D-F, D-T, E-T**
Fibrovascular polyp is a giant pedunculated intraluminal mass, which arises from the cervical esophagus close to the cricopharynx and extends downwards and progressively elongates due to continuous peristalsis and traction of food. It is made of fibrovascular and fatty elements and covered by squamous epithelium. It is not premalignant. It can occupy the entire esophagus. The tumour can regurgitate as a fleshy sausage-shaped mass into the mouth and the patient can bite the tumour to produce bleeding. It can occlude the larynx. Barium shows a smooth, sausage-shaped mass, which is completely surrounded by a layer of barium and which varies with deglutition. Fat value can be seen in CT.

60. **A-F, B-T, C-T, D-T, E-T**
Typical achalasia is characterised by triad of elevated resting lower esophageal sphincter pressure, incomplete relaxation of sphincter and absence of primary peristalsis in most or all of esophageal body. The esophagus may not be dilated in early achalasia and in a subtype of achalasia called the vigorous achalasia.

61. **A-F, B-T, C-F, D-T, E-F**
Early achalasia—The resting lower esophageal sphincter pressure is elevated. Normal LES relaxation. Aperistalsis. Lesser esophageal dilatation. Younger patients.
Vigorous achalasia—Elevated resting lower esophageal sphincter pressure. Absent LES relaxation and high amplitude simultaneous repetitive contractions. These present with chest pain and less esophageal dilatation. There is no sexual predilection in achalasia. The above two variants can represent a part of the spectrum of achalasia or transitional motility disorders evolving eventually into the classical achalasia. Peristaltic wave is seen in cervical esophagus and up to the aortic arch level, since it affects only the smooth muscle portion of esophagus. There are many theories for the formation of achalasia, most common including absence of ganglion cells of Auerbachs plexus or decreased cell bodies in dorsal motor nucleus of vagus.

62. **A-T, B-T, C-T, D-F, E-F**
Other causes include multiple leiomyomas, lymphomas and melanoma metastasis.

63. **A-T, B-T, C-T, D-T, E-T**
Common benign submucosal tumours include leiomyoma, hemangioma, lipoma, granular cell tumour, fibroma and retention cysts. These are common in the distal third or middle third.

64. **A-T, B-T, C-T, D-T, E-F**
Squamous cell carcinomas are the most common type.
There are four types, polypoid, ulcerative, varicoid and infiltrating, of which polypoid is the most common.

65. **A-T, B-T, C-T, D-T, E-T**
Achalasia, Barrett's esophagus, radiation and caustic strictures are other recognised risk factors.

66. **A-T, B-T, C-T, D-T, E-T,**
Tracheal deviation/indentation, azygoesophageal recess convex to the lung and mass extending into gastric bubble are other suggestive findings.

67. **A-T, B-T, C-T, D-T, E-T**
T1-submucosa, T2-muscularis propria, T3-adventitia, T4-adjacent structures. Varicoid tumours can resemble varices and candida esophagitis. Unlike varices, these are fixed and do not change in appearance with posture or deglutition.

68. **A-F, B-F, C-T, D-F, E-T**
Wall thickening more than 5 mm is significant. Mass in contact with aorta more than 90 degrees was considered unresectable. But still 20-70% of these tumours in absence of metastasis are resected.

69. **A-T, B-T, C-T, D-T, E-F**
Superficial spreading carcinoma and artefacts are other causes.

70. **A-T, B-F, C-F, D-F, E-F**
Esophagus is often the first organ to be involved. It is the first GI organ to be involved.
Hypotonia affects only the smooth muscle portion of the distal third of the esophagus.
The lower esophageal sphincter is patulous and causes gastroesophageal reflux in 70%.
Stricture is due to reflux and seen 3-4 cm above the gastroesophageal junction.

71. **A-T, B-T, C-T, D-T, E-F**
There is 2-7% incidence of carcinoma. The risk of carcinoma is 2. 7-14 times that of a normal person. Dilated esophagus with absent gastric bubble is reliable. Mycobacterial infections (Fortuitum-cheiloni) are seen in lung due to chronic aspiration. The lower esophageal sphincter is opened by carbonated drinks and amylnitrate.

72. **A-F, B-F, C-T, D-F, E-T**
Achalasia is characterized by dilated esophagus, absence peristalsis and incomplete relaxation of lower esophageal sphincter. Vigorous

contractions, however, are seen in the early stages. Chagas' disease caused by *Trypanosoma* is a recognized cause. Achalasia causes anterior bowing of trachea. Initial swallows fail to open the lower esophageal sphincter. But when the hydrostatic pressure of the barium exceeds that of sphincter, it opens and is called Hurst phenomenon. The barium then squirts through the narrow lumen. Chest X-ray shows right-sided convex opacity.

73. **A-T, B-T, C-T, D-T, E-T**
Schatzki ring, annular peptic stricture, annular carcinoma/ leiomyoma, pemphigus, caustics, congenital stenosis and muscular ring are other causes.

74. **A-T, B-T, C-T, D-T, E-T**
The most common cause is idiopathic which is seen within a few cm of cricopharynx and common above 50 years. It is characterized by plication of normal squamous mucosa with inflammation.

75. **A-F, B-F, C-T, D-T, E-T**
The most common location is the lower esophagus. In the upper esophagus, cricopharynx is the most common level. Upper esophageal perforation- associated with right pleural effusion and widened mediastinum. Lower esophageal perforation-associated with left pleural effusion and minimal changes in mediastinum. The associated mediastinal collection can be associated with compression of SVC.

76. **A-T, B-T, C-T, D-F, E-T**
If water-soluble contrast study is negative and the clinical suspicion is high, barium should be administered for evaluating small perforation.

77. **A-T, B-T, C-T, D-T, E-F**
Iatrogenic injuries are the most common causes of perforation. Boerhaave syndrome is spontaneous perforation due to raised intra-abdominal pressure and relaxed esophageal sphincter, as it happens in vomiting.

78. **A-T, B-T, C-T, D-T, E-F**
Ruptured aortic aneurysm is the most common cause. Esophageal carcinoma is a rare cause. Barium is avoided. The typical clinical history is several small episodes of hematemesis, followed by a latent period (probably due to vasoconstriction) and then fatal haematemesis.

79. **A-T, B-F, C-T, D-T, E-F**
Infections are most common in the proximal third of esophagus. Snakeskin or cobblestone pattern is due to confluent involvement

by large plaques. Polypoid appearance can be seen in candida due to coalescent mass of mycelia or necrotic debri.

80. **A-T, B-T, C-T, D-T, E-F**
Double barrelled esophagus is caused due to intramural track beneath the plaques or due to pseudomembranes.

81. **A-T, B-F, C-F, D-T, E-T**
Webs are best seen in lateral view. Endoscopy, often, misses the web. In Plummer-Vinson/Paterson-Kelly syndrome, webs, koilonychia, clubbing and anemia are seen.

82. **A-F, B-F, C-T, D-T, E-T**
Most of the intramural benign tumours such as lipoma, carcinoid, fibroma, lipoma, granular cell tumour, varix and cyst are seen in the submucosa, which is layer 3. Leiomyoma, rising from smooth muscle, can be seen either in 2nd layer (M. mucosa) or fourth layer (M. propria). Carcinoid arises from the epithelial layer but lies in the third layer.

83. **A-T, B-T, C-T, D-T, E-T**
Giant ulcers are seen both in CMV and HIV, and these can often be differentiated only by endoscopy and demonstration of intranuclear inclusions. Tuberculosis is often associated with extrinsic caesating nodes.

84. **A-T, B-T, C-T, D-T, E-F**
Cromolin sodium, 5 FU, ascorbic acid, quinidine, aspirin, alprenalol, doxycycline, tetracycline, lincomycin and phenylbutazone are other drugs causing esophagitis.

85. **A-T, B-T, C-T, D-F,E-F**
KCl is used with digoxin in cardiac failure, including those caused by mitral heart disease. Usually, the drugs cause stricture in the midesophagus. In mitral stenosis, the left atrial hypertrophy, indents and compresses the distal esophagus, thus predisposing it to ulcer at this location. Crohn's disease involves the esophagus the least. It is always associated with ileocolitis. Cobblestone pattern, thick folds, intramural tracking, strictures, perforation and filiform polyps are other features of Crohn's. Epidermolysis bullosa produces multiple bullae, which are broken by trauma of food particles, which heal with scarring and producing strictures and webs in later stages. The strictures are the most common in the upper esophagus close to the aortic arch. Webs are the most common in the cervical esophagus close to cricopharynx.

86. **A-T, B-F, C-T, D-F, E-T**
Swallowing will produce peristaltic wave which will obliterate the varices. Hence, the images should be acquired in between

peristalsis. The patient can be asked to spit, to avoid peristaltic waves. Recumbent RAO is the optimal position. The esophagus should be in a relaxed state for optimal visualisation of varices. Barium should be given only sufficient to coat the mucosa, so that the varices can be visualised.

87. **A-T, B-T, C-T, D-T, E-T**
Uphill varices are due to collateral formation from portal vein via azygos vein and esophageal collaterals to the SVC. These varices are seen in the lower part of esophagus.

88. **A-T, B-F, C-F, D-T, E-T**
Downhill varices are seen only in the upper part of esophagus and is due to SVC obstruction, the blood being diverted via the azygos veins to the IVC or the portal venous system. The varicoid form of esophageal carcinoma can be easily confused with the varices, but they do not change configuration when the esophagus contracts.

89. **A-T, B-F, C-F, D-F, E-T**
Isolated gastric varices are also seen in portal hypertension. Buscopan relaxes the esophagus and makes visualisation easier. Plain X-ray occasionally shows a posterior mediastinal mass. This is seen only in recumbent view since the flow may be diverted in erect view. It is common when esophageal and paraesophageal veins are dilated and less common when azygos and hemiazygos veins are dilated. Dysphagia is very common in varicoid carcinoma, but uncommon in varices. The appearance is rigid and fixed in varicoid and variable in varices. There is a sharp demarcation in varicoid carcinoma; but in varices, there is a gradual tapering. Sclerosed veins show an outer high density and inner low density due to inflammation and edema.

90. **A-F, B-F, C-T, D-F, E-T**
Fundoplication is done for hiatus hernia and it produces a smooth filling defect in fundus. Perforation after balloon dilatation is the most common from the left posterolateral wall just above the dome of the diaphragm. If aspiration or airway fistula is suspected, water-soluble contrast is avoided to prevent pulmonary edema and barium is the first choice.

91. **A-F, B-T, C-F, D-F, E-T**
Associated with iron deficiency anemia. Most common near cricopharyngeus.
Best visualised in full distension. Thickness is less than 3 mm.

92. **A-T, B-T, C-T, D-F, E-F**
Rupture of thoracic aortic aneurysm is the most common cause.

Clinically seen as Chiari triad, which has chest pain or dysphagia, a herald bleed followed by massive upper GI bleed.

93. **A-T, B-T, C-F, D-T, E-T**
Foamy esophagus, is presence of uniform, mottled, mobile lucencies in esophagus, which is due to production of gas by the organism.

94. **A-T, B-T, C-T, D-T, E-F**
Cricopharyngeal carcinoma is not a part of this syndrome, which is also called Paterson-Kelly syndrome. This syndrome is a predisposing cause for cricopharyngeal carcinoma.

95. **A-T, B- F, C-T, D-T, E-T**
Normal transit time is 15 seconds. 500 mCi of sulphur colloid is given in 10 ml of water.
Esophageal stricture/tumour and pharyngeal pouch are other causes of increased transit time.

96. **A-T, B-F, C-F, D-F, E-T**
This is not due to herniation of mucosa, but accumulation of barium in dilated ducts of esophageal mucosal glands.
They are arranged parallel to the long axis of the esophagus and they will be seen lying outside the esophagus not communicating with it. Reflux, candida and caustic strictures are recognised causes.

97. **A-T, B-T, C-T, D-T, E-F**
The disease always extends into esophagus from the gastroeso-phageal junction.
Transverse folds are called feline patterns. Granular or nodular folds, ulceration and stricture are recognised radiological findings. Abnormal motility is seen with acid barium.

98. **A-T, B-T, C-T, D-T, E-T**
The gastroesophageal angle is usually 70-100 degrees. Phrenico-esophageal membrane is a firm, elastic structure that tethers the distal esophagus to diaphragm. The gastroesophgeal angle has a valvular effect. The esophagus extends for 2 cm into the abdomen. There is a band of muscle on the fundus of stomach, which acts as a sling, accentuating the gastroesophageal angle and reduced reflux.

99. **A-F, B-T, C-T, D-F, E-T**
Sliding hiatal hernia is associated. Gastroesophageal polyp is a prominent mucosal fold which extends across the GE junction into esophagus.

100. A-T, B-T, C-T, D-T, E-F
Barrett's esophagus, acute aspiration, and esophagitis are the other complications.

101. A-F, B-F, C-T, D-F, E-T
RPO position is the best position for diagnosing reflux. Water siphon test has 5% false negative rate. Provocative manoeuvres such as coughing, sneezing, swallowing have 50% accuracy. High activity in pertechnate scan is due to ectopic gastric mucosa in Barrett's mucosa. Measuring esophageal pH has high accuracy.

2 Stomach

1. Stomach:
A. Stomach has a volume of 1500 ml
B. Obese individuals have a J-shaped stomach
C. The stomach is completely covered by peritoneum
D. The fundus is the portion of stomach above the cardiac orifice
E. Incisura is a constant notch at the lower end of the greater curvature

2. Stomach:
A. The stomach has three layers
B. The muscular layer has two groups of muscles
C. The oblique muscles are parallel to the lesser curvature
D. The pylorus is situated 2.5 cm to the right of the midline
E. Stomach is supplied by all the branches of the celiac artery

3. Right gastric artery can arise from the following arteries:
A. Left hepatic artery
B. Gastroduodenal artery
C. Middle hepatic A
D. Right hepatic A
E. Aorta

4. Gastroduodenal A originates from the following arteries:
A. Superior mesenteric A
B. Aorta
C. Right hepatic artery
D. Left hepatic artery
E. Middle hepatic artery

5. Stomach:
A. The folds are arranged with good regularity
B. Rugae are in mosaic pattern in the pylorus
C. 111 Indium DTPA is used to assess gastric emptying
D. The stomach lymph nodes drain into the celiac nodes
E. Areae gastricae are most prominent in the fundus

6. **Gastric emptying studies:**
   A. A combined liquid and solid meal should never be used
   B. In 111 labelled resin breads are used for assessing emptying of solids
   C. Dynamic images should be acquired if there is dumping syndrome
   D. Images are acquired every five minutes
   E. Solid emptying studies are carried on till 90 minutes

7. **Gastric arteries:**
   A. The smallest branch of celiac artery is the right gastric artery
   B. Aberrant left hepatic artery arising from the left gastric artery is seen in 25% of individuals
   C. The left gastric artery arises from the aorta in 0.25% of individuals
   D. The left gastric artery does not have any branches
   E. The left gastric anastomoses with only the right gastric artery

8. **Endoscopic ultrasound:**
   A. Stomach filled with degassed water before scanning
   B. Endoscopic ultrasound is the best view for fundus
   C. Inflated bag of water can be used to create a better acoustic window
   D. Prepyloric region of lesser curvature is a blind area for endoscopic scans
   E. Scanning plane should be parallel to the bowel wall

9. **Arteries supplying the stomach originate from the corresponding arteries:**
   A. Left gastric artery—celiac artery
   B. Right gastric artery—common hepatic artery
   C. Short gastric arteries—left gastric artery
   D. Accessory left gastric artery—splenic artery
   E. Right gastroepiploic artery—supraduodenal artery

10. **The stomach bed has the following structures:**
    A. Pancreas   B. Splenic flexure
    C. Spleen   D. Diaphragm
    E. Left kidney

11. **The following are the best views for visualising the corresponding portion of stomach:**
    A. Duodenal cap—RAO
    B. Antrum—LAO
    C. Body—RAO
    D. Left lateral, with head up—fundus
    E. LAO—lesser curvature

12. **Glucagon:**
    A. Acts longer than buscopan
    B. Onset of action is more delayed than buscopan
    C. Higher dose is required for barium enema than meal
    D. Allergic reactions are seen
    E. Prolongs small intestinal transit

13. **Drugs used in barium:**
    A. Metoclopramide decreases the gastric emptying time, but does not affect the small intestinal transit
    B. 50 mg is the normal oral dose of Metoclopramide
    C. Open angle glaucoma is an absolute contraindication for buscopan use
    D. Buscopan is a relaxant and works for two hours
    E. Gastric dilatation is a complication of buscopan use

14. **Thickened folds in stomach are seen in:**
    A. Pancreatic tumours
    B. Metastasis
    C. Eosinophilic enteritis
    D. Pernicious anemia
    E. Ménètrier's disease

15. **Menetriers disease:**
    A. Associated with increased acid production
    B. Associated with hypoproteinemia
    C. Premalignant
    D. Spares the antrum
    E. Thickening of fold is maximal at the lesser curvature

16. **Stomach:**
    A. Antrum is spared in type II eosinophilic gastritis
    B. Peripheral eosinophil level in blood is normal in eosinophilic gastritis
    C. Rams horn sign (narrowed funnel-shaped antrum) indicates carcinoma
    D. Pseudo Billroth sign—indicates Crohn's disease
    E. Tuberculous ulcers are more common in the lesser curvature

17. **Causes of Linitis plastica appearance of stomach:**
    A. Crohn's disease
    B. Treatment of hepatic tumours
    C. Amyloidosis
    D. Sarcoidosis
    E. Duplication cyst

18. **Common causes of mucosal lesion in stomach:**
    A. Villous tumour
    B. Ectopic pancreas
    C. Hemangioma
    D. Leiomyoma
    E. Hamartomatous polyp

19. **Stomach:**
    A. Lead pipe stomach is seen in Crohn's disease
    B. Gastric volvulus is a recognised cause of emphysematous gastritis
    C. The air enters through ischemic wall in gastric emphysema
    D. Mottled pattern of gas in stomach indicates gastric emphysema than emphysematous gastritis
    E. Helicobacter pylori produces thickening of folds in the antrum and body

20. **Bowel duplication:**
    A. In esophagus, associated with multiple spinal abnormalities
    B. Duplicated segment may extend on either side of the diaphragm
    C. May contain gastric mucosa and develop peptic ulcers
    D. Never communicates with bowel lumen
    E. Esophagus and ileum are the most common sites

21. **Causes of antral narrowing:**
    A. Crohn's disease
    B. Eosinophilic granuloma
    C. Pancreatic rest
    D. Radiation
    E. Sarcoidosis

22. **Gastrocolic fistulas are seen in:**
    A. Carcinoma pancreas
    B. Crohn's disease
    C. Pancreatitis
    D. Actinomycosis
    E. Ischemic colitis

23. **Gastric diverticulum:**
    A. Associated with ectopic pancreatic rest
    B. Commonly seen in the greater curvature
    C. Traction diverticulum is more common than pulsion diverticulum
    D. Associated with mass effect in the adjacent folds
    E. Least common site of diverticulum in the GI tract

24. **Causes of chronic gastric dilatation:**
    A. Dermatomyositis
    B. Lead poisoning
    C. Porphyria
    D. Muscular dystrophy
    E. Cholecystitis

25. **Stomach:**
    A. 50% of those with hypertrophic pyloric stenosis (adults) have gastric ulcers
    B. Antral mucosal diaphragm is parallel to the gastric wall and is situated within 3 cm of pyloric canal
    C. 65% of gastric outlet obstruction is caused by antral carcinoma
    D. Adult onset hypertrophic pyloric stenosis produces high grade obstruction in majority
    E. All the antral mucosal diaphragms produce symptoms

26. **Common causes of submucosal lesions in stomach wall:**
    A. Inflammatory fibroid polyp
    B. Varices
    C. Duplication cyst
    D. Neurofibromatosis
    E. Carcinoid

27. **CT scan for gastric cancer:**
    A. In CT, stomach wall is considered thickened only when it is at least 2 cm, in fully distended state
    B. In contrast enhanced scans, all the layers of normal stomach show good contrast enhancement
    C. Esophagogastric junction lesions are best seen in prone position
    D. The proximal cancers are best seen in the left lateral decubitus position
    E. Diagnosing N1 nodes is not critical for clinical management

28. **CT scan for gastric cancer staging:**
    A. Helical CT scan can detect 75% of early gastric cancers
    B. Loss of the multilayered pattern of enhancement is seen in 95% of elevated type of gastric cancers
    C. Metastasis is uncommon in lymph nodes less than 1.5 cm
    D. If lymph nodal enhancement is more than 100 HU, it is considered metastatic, even if it is not enlarged
    E. A short to long axis ratio of 0.7 is indicative of metastasis, even if the lymph node is less than 1 cm

29. **Stomach and duodenum:**
    A. Most common location of intraluminal diverticula is in the greater curvature
    B. Duodenal varices are always associated with esophageal varices
    C. Duodenal web is commonly located in the bulb
    D. Gastric outlet obstruction caused by antral carcinoma is painless
    E. Superior mesenteric syndrome is commonly due to duodenal compression at level of L2-3

30. **Predisposing factors for gastric carcinoma:**
    A. Blood group O   B. Low socio-economic status
    C. Smoked food   D. Adenomatous polyps
    E. Gastrinomas

31. **Endoscopic ultrasound:**
    A. Perigastric lymph nodes can be seen with endoscopic ultrasound
    B. In linitis plastica the normal stratification of the gastric wall is lost
    C. Has 85% sensitivity for T staging
    D. Homogeneously hypoechoic nodes are benign
    E. Endoscopic ultrasound cannot differentiate benign and malignant ulcer

32. **Gastric carcinoma:**
    A. 95% are adenocarcinomas
    B. Involvement of perigastric nodes within 3 cm is N1
    C. Para-aortic nodes are N2
    D. Invasion of diaphragm is T4a
    E. Most common location is the cardia

33. **Gastric carcinoma:**
    A. Majority are polypoidal fungating mass
    B. The superficial spreading carcinoma is confined to mucosa only
    C. Scirrhous carcioma is characterised by rigidity of stomach
    D. 70% of ulcers in lesser curvature are likely to be malignant
    E. 90% of ulcer in the fundus is likely to be benign

34. **Gastric carcinoma:**
    A. Wall thickness more than 5 mm in fully distended state is abnormal
    B. Increased density is seen in the soft tissue around stomach
    C. Lymphadenopathy below the level of renal pedicle indicates lymphoma more than carcinoma
    D. Linitis plastica shows enhancement
    E. Serosal surface nodules indicate peritoneal metatasis

35. **Gastric carcinoma:**
    A. Metastasis to ovarian surface is Krukenberg's tumour
    B. Blumer shelf metastasis occurs in the rectal wall
    C. Metastasis to the bone is sclerotic
    D. Type I early cancer is excavated
    E. Type III early cancer is flat

36. **Ulcers:**
    A. Ulceration is rarely found in early gastric carcinoma
    B. Haematemesis is due to peptic ulcer in 1/3rd of cirrhotic patients
    C. Esophageal ulceration is a recognized complication of potassium ingestion
    D. Solitary rectal ulcer syndrome is associated with occult rectal prolapse
    E. Malignancy is a recognized complication of Hunner's ulcer

37. **The following are risk factors for gastric carcinoma:**
    A. Chronic atrophic gastritis
    B. Hypertrophic gastritis
    C. Nitrites
    D. Gastrojejunostomy
    E. Peutz-Jeghers syndrome

38. **Gastric cancer:**
    A. An ulcerated cancer, is classified as Type I in the advanced cancer classification
    B. Helicobacter pylori is a predisposing factor for gastric carcinoma
    C. High zinc and talc in food are predisposing factors for development of carcinoma
    D. More common in males
    E. There is 10% risk of cancer in pernicious anemia

39. **Gastric ulcer:**
    A. Any ulcer in fundus and proximal greater curvature is malignant unless proven otherwise
    B. Presence of fibrosis in the base of ulcer hastens the healing of ulcer
    C. Sump ulcers are most common in the distal part of the greater curvature
    D. Ulcer collar is parallel to the long axis of the ulcer
    E. Ulcer collar connects the crater to the lumen

40. Ulcer:
  A. Gastric ulcer is due to increased secretion of acid and duodenal ulcer is due to decreased resistance
  B. Dragstedt ulcers are those produced due to gastric stasis
  C. Lesser curve ulcers are best seen in erect compression views
  D. Ulcers are called giant only when they are more than 5 cm
  E. Barium cannot detect ulcers less than 1 cm

41. Gastric ulcer:
  A. Benign ulcer in greater curvature has malignant features
  B. 80% of multiple ulcers are benign
  C. Even round ulcers become linear after healing
  D. Hour glass stomach is produced due to badly scarred antral ulcer
  E. Unequivocally benign ulcers require follow-up only with barium

42. Stomach:
  A. There is increased risk of carcinoid tumours in those with pernicious anemia
  B. In hypertrophic gastropathy, the associated hyperchlorhydria produces protein losing enteropathy
  C. The most common polyp in stomach is hamartomotous polyp
  D. Hyperplastic polyps are seen commonly in the fundus
  E. Adenomatous polyps are seen in Peutz-Jeghers syndrome

43. Stomach:
  A. Type A chronic gastritis affects the antrum
  B. Increased risk of cancer is seen in both Type A and B chronic atropic gastritis
  C. 10% of type B gastritis develop cancer in 10-20 years
  D. 10% of those with adenomatous polyps develop cancer in five years
  E. Carcinoma in stump of previous surgery has a latent period of 15-20 years

44. Malignancies producing an appearance similar to linitis plastica:
  A. Kaposi's sarcoma
  B. Breast cancer
  C. Direct invasion by colon cancer
  D. Direct invasion by cancer pancreas
  E. Ovarian cancer

45. Ulcer:
   A. Hamptons line is situated between the collar and the crater
   B. A niche is seen commonly in the lesser curvature
   C. Ulcer mound is caused due to mucosal edema
   D. In malignant ulcer, the convex border of the meniscus is directed towards the lumen
   E. Malignant ulcer is highly unlikely to have meniscoid configuration

46. There is increased incidence of peptic ulcer in the following conditions:
   A. Hyperparathyroidism
   B. Gout
   C. Anticoagulants
   D. Cirrhosis
   E. Insulinoma

47. Common causes of acute dilatation of stomach:
   A. Spinal injury
   B. Diabetic ketoacidosis
   C. Hypoglycemia
   D. Vagotomy
   E. Ganglion blocking drugs

48. Gastric volvulus:
   A. Presents with vomiting
   B. Mesenteroaxial volvulus is around an axis extending from lesser to greater curvature
   C. Associated with phrenic nerve palsy
   D. Results in emphysema
   E. Nasogastric tube is passed into stomach for administering barium

49. Lesions involving stomach and duodenum:
   A. Lymphoma
   B. Crohn's
   C. Eosinophilic gastroenteritis
   D. Strongyloidosis
   E. Tuberculosis

50. Causes of widened retrogastric space:
   A. Acute pancreatitis
   B. Choledochal cyst
   C. Distended gallbladder
   D. Obesity
   E. Aortic aneurysm

51. Stomach lymphoma:
A. Most common site of extranodal Hodgkin's disease
B. Majority are Hodgkin's type
C. Predominantly seen in the antrum
D. Esophagus is the least common part of GIT involved
E. The gastric wall is rigid

52. The following are features of lymphoma which differentiate it from carcinoma:
A. Wall thickening is not as extensive as in carcinoma
B. Splenomegaly
C. Lymph nodes below the level of renal pedicle
D. Contrast enhancement
E. Ulceration

53. Features of stomach lymphoma:
A. Fold thickening
B. Ulceration
C. Linitis plastica
D. Hyperrugosity
E. Broad tortuous folds

54. Gastric leiomyoma:
A. Most common benign tumour of stomach
B. Majority are subserosal
C. Forms obtuse angle with the gastric wall
D. Haemorrhage is the most common clinical presentation
E. Surface is usually irregular

55. Stomach leiomyosarcoma:
A. Pathology alone can differentiate leiomyoma and leiomyosarcoma
B. Associated with pulmonary hamartomas
C. Contrast can be seen extending from the stomach into the tumour
D. 3% of stomach malignancies
E. Lymph nodal spread is common

56. GIST (gastrointestinal stromal tumour):
A. Arise from smooth muscle
B. Arise from mutation in tyrosine kinase gene
C. Makes obtuse angle with the stomach wall
D. Stomach capacity is reduced
E. Gleévec is the drug which is used for specific treatment of this disease

57. **Gastric surgery:**
    A. Gastric atony is seen in 20% of cases of highly selective vagotomy
    B. There is increased risk of bezoar formation after gastric surgery
    C. The pacemaker for the distal stomach is situated in the greater curvature
    D. Pneumothorax is a complication of gastric surgery
    E. In selective vagotomy, the motor and acid secretory activity of the entire stomach is denervated

58. **Postgastric surgery:**
    A. There is 25% incidence of diarrhoea after truncal vagotomy
    B. Increased incidence of gallstone formation
    C. Leak from the duodenal stump occurs in 2-5 days
    D. Pancreatitis is a cause of stomal obstruction in Billroth II surgery
    E. Afferent loop obstruction is a closed loop obstruction

59. **Endoscopic ultrasound of bowel wall:**
    A. The mucosa and submucosa are echogenic
    B. Muscle is always hypoechoic
    C. Serosa is not visualized
    D. Patient is in left lateral position for scanning
    E. Air is not a hindrance to scanning

60. **Endoscopic ultrasound:**
    A. The thickness of each layer seen in endoscopic ultrasound is not the same as in histological specimen
    B. The extent of lumen distension alters the thickness of layers
    C. Thickness increases with oblique scanning
    D. The mucosa, submucosa and muscularis propria are all of same thickness
    E. 9 layers are seen when miniprobe is used

61. **Endoscopic ultrasound:**
    A. Highest accuracy is obtained for gastric cancers
    B. A bleb is raised on the wall of stomach to localize lesion
    C. T1 tumours involve only the first layer
    D. T3 involves the fifth layer
    E. In linitis plastica, irregular layers 3 and 4 are seen with normal mucosa

62. **Features of malignant lymph nodes in endoscopic ultrasound:**
    A. 5 mm
    B. Oval contour
    C. Sharp demarcated border
    D. Hypoechoic
    E. Peripheral halo

63. **Gastric surgery:**
    A. Recurrence is more common in gastric rather than duodenal ulcer
    B. Hypercalcemia is a common cause of recurrent ulcer
    C. Vomiting of food mixed with bile and pain not relieved after vomiting is suggestive of afferent loop obstruction
    D. Chronic afferent loop obstruction is more common in Billroth II than I
    E. Gastrocolic fistula is best diagnosed with barium meal than enema

64. **Causes of acute delay in gastric emptying:**
    A. Stress
    B. Ileus
    C. Gastric surgery
    D. Duodenal ulcer
    E. Zollinger-Ellison syndrome

65. **Causes of rapid gastric emptying:**
    A. Hypothyroidism
    B. Uremia
    C. Celiac sprue
    D. Zollinger-Ellison syndrome
    E. Gastric ulcer

66. **Causes of chronically delayed gastric emptying:**
    A. Gastric ulcer
    B. Scleroderma
    C. Anorexia
    D. Intestinal pseudo-obstruction
    E. Amyloidosis

67. **Stomach:**
    A. 40% of FAP patients have fundal hyperplastic polyps
    B. 90% of polyps are hyperplastic
    C. Hyperplastic polyps are larger than adenomatous polyps
    D. Adenomatous polyps more than 2 cm—50% are malignant
    E. In duodenum, adenomatous polyps are more common than hyperplastic polyps

68. **Stomach:**
    A. A soap bubble pattern is indicative of villous adenoma
    B. 90% of benign submucosal lesions are leiomyomas
    C. 80% of villous adenomas more than 4 cm are malignant
    D. Leiomyoma produces distortion of areae gastricae
    E. Bulls eye lesion indicates malignant transformation in leiomyoma

69. **Widened retrogastric space is seen in:**
    A. Omental hernia
    B. Ascites
    C. Enlarged right lobe of liver
    D. Adrenal tumour
    E. Stromal tumour of stomach

70. Stomach:
A. Villous tumours are very prone for obstruction
B. Leiomyomas can be differentiated from leiomyosarcoma by size only
C. 95% of leiomyomas are exogastric, growing outside from the stomach
D. A submucosal lesion changing in size and appearance with fluoroscopy is leiomyoma
E. Ectopic pancreatic rest is always seen in the greater curvature within 6 cm of the pylorus

71. Ectopic pancreatic rest:
A. Duodenum is commonly affected than stomach
B. Only acini are seen but islet cells are not seen
C. A central umbilication is a charactersitic feature
D. Contrast will reflux into the duct in barium examination
E. Poorly differentiated lesions are called adenomyosis

72. The following are featuers of malignant gastric ulcer and are not common in benign ulcers:
A. Convergence of folds to the edge of the crater
B. Irregular shape of ulcer
C. Club-shaped thick folds
D. Deeper ulcers
E. No healing

73. The following are features of benign ulcer and are not common in malignant ulcer:
A. Crescent sign
B. Carman Meniscus sign
C. Hamptons line
D. Projecting beyond the wall
E. Eccentric ulcer collar

74. Gastritis:
A. Erosive gastritis does not extend beyond muscularis mucosa
B. Punctate collection of barium with surrounding halo is typical appearance of erosive gastritis
C. In hypertrophic gastritis, there is direct correlation between the degree of fold thickening and amount of acid produced
D. Hypertrophic gastritis is associated with protein losing enteropathy
E. Hypertrophic gastritis is the most common in the antrum

75. Causes of aphthous ulcers in stomach:
A. Crohn's
B. Burns
C. Cytomegalovirus
D. Stress ulcers
E. NSAIDs

ANSWERS

1. **A-T, B-F, C-T, D-T, E-F**
   Obese individuals have transverse steerhorn type of stomach and thin individuals have J-shaped stomach. The incisura is a constant notch seen at the lower end of the lesser curvature. This forms the boundary between the body and pylorus.

2. **A-F, B-F, C-T, D-T, E-T**
   Stomach has four layers, the adventitia, muscular layer, submucosa and mucosa
   There are longitudinal, circular and oblique muscles in the muscular layer.

3. **A-T, B-T, C-T, D-T, E-F**
   Proper hepatic A and left hepatic A (40%) are the common arteries of origin of the right gastric artery.

4. **A-T, B-F, C-T, D- T, E-F**
   About 75% arise from the hepatic artery proper.

5. **A-F, B-F, C-T, D-T, E-F**
   The folds are regular in the lesser curvature and not so in the remaining areas. It is parallel in the pylorus and mosaic in the greater curvature.
   Areae gastricae are most prominent in the antrum and measure 2-3 mm.

6. **A-F, B-T, C-T, D-T, E-T**
   For liquid—Tc labelled orange juice. For solids—Tc labelled scrambled eggs. For combination—In 111 labelled resin breads and Tc labelled orange juice are used.
   In dumping syndrome, the emptying can be very rapid and hence it is acquired dynamically. Images are acquired, with the patient standing, every five minutes for 60 min in case of liquids and 90 minutes for solids. Images are acquired in two planes.

7. **A-F, B-T, C-F, D-F, E-F**
   The smallest branch of celiac artery is the left gastric artery. This arises from the aorta in 2%. The left gastric artery has small cardioesophageal arteries. The left gastric artery anastomoses with right gastric A, short gastric A, cardioesophageal branches of inferior phrenic artery and gastric branches of gastroepiploic arteries.

8. **A-T, B-F, C-T, D-T, C-F**
   The fundus and prepyloric regions are blind areas in endoscopic ultrasound, especially because adequate water filling cannot be

obtained in these areas. Scanning plane is perpendicular to the bowel wall.

9. **A-T, B-T, C-F, D-T, D-F**
Short gastric arteries (4-10) arise from splenic artery. These are prominently seen in angiograms only if there is hiatal hernia, when they are pulled up.
Accessory left gastric artery is larger than the short gastric arteries.
Right gastroepiploic artery is a branch of gastroduodenal A and left gastroepiploic A is a branch of splenic A.

10. **A-T, B-F, C-T, D-T, E-T**
Splenic flexure is not involved. Pancreas, transverse colon and mesocolon, left kidney, left adrenal, spleen and diaphragm constitute the stomach bed.

11. **A-T, B-F, C-F, D-T, E-T**
RAO—duodenal cap, antrum, greater curvature. SUPINE—body, antrum. LAO—Lesser curvature. Left lateral and head up and erect—fundus.

12. **A-F, B-T, C-T, D-T, E-F**
Glucagon—onset of action after 1 min and lasts for 15 minutes. 0.3 mg required in barium meal and 1.0 mg for barium enema. Does not affect small bowel transit. Is also contraindicated in insulinoma and glucagonoma.

13. **A-F, B-F, C-F, D-F, E-T**
Metoclopramide is used in barium follow through to decrease the small bowel transit time. About 20 mg is the normal dose and extrapyramidal side effects are seen if the dose is high. Closed-angle glaucoma, angina and myasthenia gravis are contraindications of buscopan. Buscopan acts immediately after IV adminis-tration and the action lasts for 15 minutes. Gastric dilatation, urinary retention, blurred vision and dry mouth are side effects of buscopan.

14. **A-T, B-T, C-T, D-F, E-T**
Stomach fold thickening is caused by lymphoma, metastasis, amyloidosis, eosinophilic enteritis, Zollinger-Ellison syndrome and Menetriers disease.

15. **A-F, B-T, C-F, D-T, E-F**
In Menetriers disease, there is marked hypertrophy of glands, with hypertrophy of the gastric folds, but there is no increased acid secretion (hypochlorhydria). It is normal or decreased. Mucosal

secretion is increased. Protein losing enteropathy is characteristic. It is typically seen in the fundus and body, with antral sparing. Fold thickening is maximal at the greater curvature. Barium is diluted due to increased secretion.

16. **A-F, B-T, C-F, D-T, E-T**
Eosinophilic gastritis Type I—Antrum, II—body and antrum, III—antral sparing.
Crohn's disease produces apthous ulcers, cobblestone pattern, thick folds, filiform polyps, narrowing, gastrocolic fisula, Ram horns sign, Pseudo-Billroth I sign—contiguous narrowing of stomach and duodenum destroying all antral landmarks, mimicking the gastroduodenostomy of Billroth I. Stomach is the least common site of tuberculosis in GIT.

17. **A-T, B-T, C-T, D-T, E-F**
Linitis plastica refers to diffuse infiltration of stomach wall producing persistently narrowed, nondistensible stomach. The common causes are:
Tumours—scirrhous carcinoma, metastasis, lymphoma
Chronic ulcer—chronic gastritis, Crohn's, eosinophilic gastritis, PAN, sarcoid, amyloid.
Tuberculosis, syphilis, actinomycosis, strongyloidosis, toxoplasmosis, histoplasmosis, cryptosporidiosis, cytomegalovirus
Radiotherapy, chemotherapy, corrosives, pancreatitis.

18. **A-T, B-T, C-F, D-F, E-T**
Leiomyoma and hemangioma are submucosal lesions.
Hyperplastic polyp and adenomatous polyp are other causes.

19. **A-F, B-T, C-F, D-F, E-T**
Lead pipe stomach indicates luminal narrowing with loss of fold pattern and is seen in strongyloides infection. Gastric emphysema is presence of air in the wall of stomach, which enters through a mucosal rent and is associated with gastric outlet obstruction or trauma. The bubbles are linear along the circumference of stomach. In emphysematous gastritis, infection with *E. coli, Proteus, Clostridium* and *Staphylococcus aureus* are the causative organisms. Volvulus, surgery and caustics are predisposing factors. The gas is seen as mottled or amorphous collections.

20. **A-T, B-T, C-T, D-F, E-T**
Usually, duplication cysts do not communicate with the bowel. But they can communicate.

21. **A-T, B-T, C-F, D-T, E-T**
Carcinoma, sarcoidosis and peptic ulcer are other causes.

22. **A-T, B-T, C-T, D-T, E-F**
    Gastrocolic fistulas are seen in tumours of stomach, colon and pancreas and inflammatory conditions such as peptic ulcer, Crohn's disease, tuberculosis, actinomycosis and chronic pancreatitis.

23. **A-F, B-F, C-T, D-F, E-T**
    It is associated with aberrant pancreas near the antrum. Commonly seen in the posterior wall adjacent to the cardia. Greater curvature is the least most common location. It is a traction diverticulum due to scarring. Pulsion diverticulum is uncommon in stomach.

24. **A-T, B-T, C-T, D-T, E-F**
    Polio, tabes dorsalis are other causes (syphilis), brain tumour, scleroderma and dermatomyositis are other causes.

25. **A-T, B-F, C-F, D-F, E-F**
    Adult onset hypertrophic pyloric stenosis is considered as a milder form of infantile pyloric stenosis. Usually, it is asymptomatic and rarely produces high grade obstruction. About 50% have associated gastric ulcers secondary to stasis. Antral mucosal diaphragm is a thin membranous septa located within 3 cm of pyloric canal and is perpendicular to the gastric long axis. If the aperture is less than 1 cm, severe gastric outlet obstruction is produced with projectile vomiting. A differential diagnosis is prominent transverse mucosal fold, but this will not extend the whole circumference across the lumen. About 65% of gastric outlet obstruction is caused by peptic ulcer and 35% is caused by cancer.

26. **A-T, B-T, C-T, D-T, E-T**
    Leiomyoma, leiomyoblastoma, leiomyosarcoma, lymphoma, metastasis, Kaposi's, leukemia, multiple myeloma, ectopic pancreatic rest, hemangioma, lymphangioma, lipoma and extramedullary hematopoiesis are other causes.

27. **A-F, B-F, C-T, D-F, E-T**
    Normal stomach wall is 5 mm. In fully distended stomach, the wall is considered thickened, if it is more than 1 cm. Water-filled stomach with IV contrast is a good method of assessing the gastric wall. After contrast, three layers of stomach can be identified. The inner mucosa and outer muscular and serosal layer show good enhancement. The middle submucosa does not enhance much. Proximal cancers are best seen in right lateral decubitus and antral cancers are best seen in left lateral decubitus. N1 nodes are those which are within 3 cm of the primary tumour, along the lesser or greater curvature. These are always removed at surgery. N2 nodes are more than 3 cm from primary tumour and include splenic, celiac and common hepatic nodes. Diagnosis of these nodes is essential

as removal of these will improve survival. N3 nodes are inoperable and include retropancreatic, mesenteric and para-aortic nodes.

28. A-F, B-T, C-T, D-T, E-T
Helical CT detects 92% of advanced gastric cancer and 50% of early gastric cancer. Wall thickening and loss of multilayered pattern is seen in almost all cases of advanced gastric cancer and elevated type of early gastric cancer. But it is seen only in 15% of depressed early gastric cancers. Usually, lymph nodes are considered enlarged if they are more than 10 mm. Portal nodes are enlarged if they are more than 8 mm itself.

29. A-T, B-T, C-F, D-T, E-T
The most common location of true diverticula is in the fundus. Intraluminal diverticula is seen proximal to obstruction and is the most common in the greater curvature of stomach. Isolated duodenal varices are very rare. Superior mesenteric artery syndrome is common in asthenic patients and is due to compression of third part of duodenum between the root of mesentery and aorta, at level of L2-3 spine.

30. A-T, B-T, C-T, D-T, E-F
Smoking, salted food, high fat, low fibers, H. pylori, chronic atrophic gastritis, partial gastrectomy, family history, polyposis syndromes are other causes.

31. A-T, B-F, C-T, D-F, E-T
Endoscopic ultrasound can predict accurate T stage, perigastric spread and perigastric lymph nodes. In linitis plastica, the normal stratification is preserved, but there is marked thickening, especially the fourth layer. Other cancers disrupt the architecture of the wall. T1 is confined to mucosa and submucosa, T2—involves the serosa, T3—penetrates the serosa without invasion of contiguous structures, T4—invation of contiguous structure. Endoscopic ultrasound is very good in predicting the exact stage. Lymph nodes which are homogeneously hypoechoic and which are round are suspicious for malignancy. N1 nodes can be assessed, but N2 nodes cannot be visualised using endoscopic ultrasound.

32. A-T, B-T, C-T, D-F, E-F
STAGING
T1—mucosa, submucosa, T2—muscularis, serosa, T3—through serosa, T4A—invasion of contiguous tissue, T4B—adjacent organs. N1—perigastric nodes within 3 cm, N2— perigastric nodes more than 3 cm from stomach, N3—para-aortic, mesenteric, hepato-duodenal, retropancreatic.
The most common location is the pylorus, followed by lesser curvature.

33. **A-F, B-F, C-T, D-F, E-F**
The types of cancers are polypoidal, ulcerating, infiltrating scirrhous and superficial spreading. The ulcerative type is the most common type of cancer. Scirrhous cancer is the linitis plastica type characterised by diffuse infiltration of the wall. 70% of greater curvature ulcers, 90% of fundus ulcers and 15% of lesser curvature ulcers are likely to be malignant.

34. **A-F, B-T, C-T, D-T, E-F**
Wall thickness more than 10 mm in a fully distended state is abnormal. Increased density indicates extension to the perigastric fat. Serosal nodules indicate lymphatic involvement.

35. **A-T, B-T, C-T, D-F, E-F**
Staging of early gastric cancer.
I—protruding type >0.5 cm, II—<0.5 cm, A—elevated, B—flat, C—depressed, III—excavation.

36. **A-F, B-T, C-T, D-T, E-F**
Ulceration is one of the subtypes of early gastric carcinoma. Hunner's ulcer is an interstitial inflammation of the bladder.

37. **A-T, B-F, C-T, D-T, E-T**

38. **A-F, B-T, C-T, D-T, E-T**
Advanced gastric cancers are classified as Type I—polypoidal fungating, II—ulcerated, III—infiltrative ulcerated and IV—linitis plastica. Highly salted food, smoked food, polycyclic hydrocarbons, high fat, contaminated oil, low consumption of fruits and vegetables, nitrates and nitrites, protein malnutrition, smoking, acidic soil, increased lead and zinc in water, talk, nitrate fertilisers, family history, Gardner's syndrome, familial adenomatous polyposis, Peutz-Jeghers syndrome, hereditary nonpolyposis colon cancer syndrome are a few other predisposing factors. The risk of cancer is 3-6 times higher in H. pylori infection.

39. **A-T, B-F, C-T, D-F, E-T**
Presence of fibrous tissue in the base of the ulcer delays healing of the ulcer. Sump ulcers are created due to NSAIDs and other drugs, which produce characteristic ulcers in the distal portion of the greater curvature. Ulcer collar connects the ulcer crater to the lumen and is parallel to the longitudinal axis of the stomach, not the ulcer.

40. **A-F, B-T, C-T, D-F, E-F**
Gastric ulcers are due to decreased resistance to acid and duodenal ulcers are formed due to increased secretion. Dragstedt ulcers are stasis ulcers and are typically seen in pyloric stenosis. Anterior wall

ulcers will be best seen in prone compression view. Anterior wall ulcers can be seen in prone Trendelenburg view with double contrast. Barium can visualise ulcers more than 5 mm. Gastric ulcers are called giant when they are more than 3 cm. Duodenal ulcers are giant when they are more than 2 cm.

41. **A-T, B-T, C-T, D-F, E-T**

Ulcers in greater curvature are malignant in majority of cases, and even benign ulcers have malignant appearances. Hence, endoscopy and biopsy are required in all these cases. Multiple ulcers are common in the antrum and body. NSAIDs, Zollinger-Ellison syndrome and hyperparathyroidism are some of the causes of multiple ulcers. Scarring results in decrease of size and linear shape of round and oval ulcers. Scarring may not be present in subsequent barium examination. Hour glass stomach is due to scarring of body. Scarring of antrum produces gastric outlet obstruction. Equivocal ulcers require endoscopy and if scopy is negative, follow-up barium and scopy are required.

42. **A-T, B-F, C-F, D-F, E-T**

In pernicious anemia there is increased risk of gastric cancer, because of bacterial overgrowth due to achlorhydria, gastrin, chronic inflammation and luminal pH changes. There is also risk of carcinoid, due to prolonged acid suppression, hypergastrinemia and neuroendocrine hyperplasia. Hyperplastic polyps are the most common in the stomach (75-95%) seen in the antrum. Hamartomatous polyps seen in 10% are common in the fundus. Adenomatous polyps large pedunculated and seen anywhere. Hyperplastic polyps are seen in 10% of patients with carcinoma. Hamartomatous polyps are not premalignant. Adenomatous polyps are associated with FAP and Peutz-Jeghers syndrome.

43. **A-F, B-T, C-T, D-T, E-T**

Type A gastritis affects the body and fundus, associated with high levels of antiparietal cell antibodies producing pernicious anemia. Type B is found in antrum and caused by mucosal injury due to H. pylori, or toxins. There is 2-3 times increased risk of gastric cancer with gastritis. Carcinoma in stump of previous surgery is due to achlorhydria, enterogastric reflux of bile and intenstinal metaplasia.

44. **A-T, B-T, C-T, D-T, E-F**

non-Hodgkin's lymphoma, omental metastasis are other malignant causes for this imaging appearance.

45. **A-T, B-T, C-T, D-T, E-F**

Hampton's line is the mucosa at the entrance to the ulcer and is seen between the ulcer collar and the ulcer crater. This is seen in all benign ulcers. One of the characteristic features of a malignant ulcer is the Carman-Kirklin meniscus sign, which is produced due to the broad-based flat tumour with central ulcer and elevated margins in the lesser curvature, producing a convex inner border directed towards the lumen and concave outer border. Niche is common in the lesser curvature and is due to barium accumulating in ulcer projecting beyond the wall. This produces a corresponding spasm in the greater curvature, called notch.

46. **A-T, B-F, C-F, D-T, E-F**

47. **A-T, B-T, C-F, D-T, E-T**

48. **A-F, B-T, C-F, D-T, E-F**
Presents with severe retching, but no vomiting. Nasogastric tube cannot be passed into the stomach. The combination of pain, retching and inability to pass tube is Borchardt's triad. Volvulus is due to long suspensory gastrohepatic and gastrocolic mesenteries, large hiatal/diaphragmatic hernias/phrenic N palsy/eventration. Organoaxial volvulus is seen around a line from cardia to pylorus. Barium does not enter stomach completely.

49. **A-T, B-T, C-T, D-T, E-T**

50. **A-T, B-T, C-F, D-T, E-T**
A crude estimation of widening of retrogastric space is when the space is more than 3/4th of the corresponding vertebral AP diameter. Pancreatic and mesenteric tumours are other causes of widening of retrogastric space.

51. **A-T, B-F, C-F, D-T, E-F**
Almost 1-5% of stomach malignancies are lymphomas. Stomach is the most common site of extranodal lymphoma, accounting for 25% of such cases. Majority of stomach lymphomas are non-Hodgkin's. There is no specific predilection for any portion of the stomach. The gastric wall is flexible and this is the salient feature of lymphoma unlike carcinoma.

52. **A-F, B-T, C-T, D-T, E-F**
The wall thickening is on an average about 4-5 cm, which is more than carcinoma. Lymphoma is more diffuse than carcinoma. Lymph nodes are larger and usually extend below the renal pedicle level. Homogeneous contrast enhancement is a feature of lymphoma.

53. **A-T, B-T, C-T, D-T, E-T**

54. **A-F, B-F, C-F, D-T, E-F**
    Polyp is the most common benign tumour of stomach followed by leiomyoma.
    Majority are submucosal, 35% are subserosal. Submucosal type forms right angle with the mucosa. Haemorrhage, obstruction, perforation, infection and malignancy are common complications. Surface is usually smooth. May show ulcer.

55. **A-F, B-T, C-T, D-T, E-F**
    It is sometimes difficult to differentiate leiomyoma and leiomyosarcoma even in pathology. More than 25 mitotis per high power field is suggestive of malignancy.
    Associated with hamartomas and extra-adrenal paragangliomas in Carney's triad (Epitheloid leiomyosarcomas).
    The tumour is very large, extends outside stomach, has central necrosis and heterogeneous enhancement. The ulcer can communicate with the stomach lumen, giving leak of contrast. Does not involve lymph nodes. Hematogeneous spread is more common.

56. **A-F, B-T, C-T, D-F, E-T**
    GIST is gastrointestinal stromal tumour, which arises from interstitial cells of Cajal.
    These tumours were previously classified as leiomyoma and leiomyosarcoma and thought to arise from smooth muscle cells, but they are considered a distinct entity now arising from stroma. Arise from mutation of CD117, tyrosine kinase gene, which regulates the stromal cell growth. Imaging appearances are similar to that of leiomyosarcoma. The stomach capacity is increased.

57. **A-F, B-T, C-T, D-T, E-T**
    Gastric atony is seen in 10% of truncal and selective vagotomy and only 3% of highly selective vagotomy. In truncal vagotomy, the vagal trunk is removed, denervating stomach, biliary tract, pancreas, small intestine and proximal large bowel. In selective vagotomy, the motor and acid secretory apparatus of the entire stomach is denervated, with preservation of hepatobiliary innervation. In highly selective vagotomy, denervation of motor and acid secretory apparatus of fundus and body with preservation of antrum. The gastric stasis after gastric surgery is a predisposing factor for bezoar formation.

58. **A-T, B-T, C-T, D-T, E-T**
    Diarrhoea is due to alklanisation of upper GIT content with colonisation with intestinal bacteria and altered gastric empyting times. Leak from duodenal stump is due to devascularisation or

postoperative pancreatitis or afferent loop obstruction. Afferent loop obstruction results in accumulation of pancreatic and biliary secretion and produces high pressure in the loop resulting in duodenal leak and pancreatitis. Pancreatitis is seen in 5% of instances and also can be seen secondary to trauma during surgery. Since the hepatic branch of the anterior vagal trunk is involved with control of gallbladder motility, denervation results in stasis and stone formation.

59. **A-T, B-T, C-F, D-T, E-F**
    Layer 1—echogenic mucosa, 2—hypodeep mucosa, muscularis mucosa, 3—echogenic—submucosa, 4—hypomuscularis propria, 5—echogenic—serosa, adventitia.
    Air has to be evacuated before scanning.

60. **A-T, B-T, D-T, E-T, E-T**
    In linear array and radial array scanners (7.5 MHz), five layers are seen. In miniprobes, up to nine layers are seen.

61. **A-F, B-T, C-F, D-T, E-T**
    T1—layers 1-3, T2—layer 4, T3—layer 5, T4—beyond wall. Accuracy is highest for esophageal cancers. In linitis, submucosa and muscularis propria are involved. Mucosa is preserved and the architecture of different layers are not affected.

62. **A-F, B-F, C-T, D-T, E-F**
    > 10 mm, round contour are other features which suggest malignancy. Peripheral halo is not a very useful sign.

63. **A-F, B-T, C-F, D-T, E-F**
    Recurrence is more common in duodenal than gastric ulcer. Incomplete vagotomy, hypercalcemia, hyperparathyroidism, Zollinger-Ellison syndrome, G cell hyperplasia, drugs and smoking are causes of recurrent ulcers. If pain is relieved and there is no bile and food in vomit, it is afferent loop obstruction; but if pain is unrelieved and the vomit has food and bile, it indicates chronic alkaline reflux esophagitis. Billroth II is gastrectomy with gastrojejunostomy, Billroth I is gastrectomy with gastroduodeno-stomy. Gastrocolic fisulta is best diagnosed by barium enema than a meal, since the pressure difference is greater with barium enema.

64. **A-T, B-T, C-F, D-F, E-F**
    Anticholinergics, morphine, levo dopa, acute gastroenteritis, hypokalemia and hyperglycemia are other causes.

65. **A-F, B-F, C-T, D-T, E-F**
    Duodenal ulcer, gastric surgery and other causes of malabsorption are other causes of abnormally rapid emptying of stomach.

66. A-T, B-T, C-T, D-T, E-T

67. A-T, B-T, C-F, D-T, E-T
The most common polyp in stomach is hyperplastic, which constitutes 75-90% of all polyps. It is usually less than 1 cm, usually multiple, common in fundus and there is no lobulation. Adenomatous polyps are more than 1 cm, constitute 10%, common in antrum, lobulated, solitary and are premalignant.
In duodenum, adenomatous polyps are more common than hyperplastic polyps.

68. A-T, B-T, C-T, D-F, E-F
Villous adenomas are common anywhere in stomach and in the second part of duodenum. They are premalignant. They have characteristic soap bubble appearance. About 50% of villous adenomas less than 4 cm are malignant. Leiomyoma is a submucosal lesion, with intact mucosa, hence there is no distortion of areae gastricae. Bulls eye lesion is due to central ulceration of submucosal lesion and is seen in leiomyoma itself and does not indicate malignant transformation.

69. A-T, B-T, C-F, D-T, E-T
Pancreatic lesions, stomach tumours, tumours in adjacent organs, obesity, aneurysm, ascites, enlarged caudate lobe, aortic aneurysm, omental hernia.

70. A-F, B-F, C-F, D-F, E-T
Villous adenomas are very soft and do not cause obstruction. Lipomas are also very soft and they have characteristic change in appearance and size in fluoroscopy. About 80% of leiomyomas are endogastric growing towards the lumen and only 15% are exogastric. Ectopic pancreatic rests are present only in this typical location. Size is not a criterion for differentiating leiomyomas and sarcomas, since malignancy can be found in small tumours.

71. A-F, B-F, C-T, D-T, E-T
Stomach is the most common organ affected (80%), with fragments of pancreatic anlage implanted into the bowel wall during development. In heterotopic or ectopic pancreatic rest there is good differentiation, hence acini, ducts and islet cells are present, but arranged haphazardly. Poorly differentiated lesions are called adenomyosis. The central umbilication measures 1-5 mm and is 5-10 mm deep. Reflux of barium into the duct will terminate in a tiny club-shaped pouch which is pathognomonic.

72. **A-F, B-T, C-T, D-F, E-T**

73. **A-T, B-F, C-T, D-T, E-F**
Benign ulcer—Hampton's line, crescent sign, deeper, projects beyond the walls, convergence of folds towards the edge of the crater, smooth radiating folds, ulcer—round, oval or linear, mound central, smooth symmetrical ulcer collar and margin. Normal peristalsis present, healing in weeks, uncommon in fundus or proximal greater curvature.
Malignant ulcer—Carman-Kirklin meniscus sign, folds stop short of the crater edge, thick irregular radiating folds, eccentric ulcer mound, irregular ulcer, shallow, nodular ulcer margin and eccentric ulcer collar, no peristalsis, no ulcer healing, can occur anywhere.

74. **A-T, B-T, C-T, D-F, E-F**
Erosive gastritis can be: a. Complete—collections of barium surrounded by halo due to elevated mucosa or b. incomplete—collections of barium with no halo, without mucosal elevation. Hypertrophic gastritis is common in the fundus and body and is due to hyperplasia of gastric glands. The folds are thickened. Acid production is increased, but there is no protein losing enteropathy, like Ménètrier's disease.

75. **A-T, B-T, C-T, D-T, E-T**

3

Small Intestine

1. **Duodenum:**
   A. The duodenum is completely retroperitoneal
   B. The duodenal cap has a rugal pattern similar to that of pylorus
   C. The first part of the duodenum is called the duodenal cap
   D. The epiploic foramen lies posteriorly to the first part of the duodenum
   E. The gastroduodenal artery runs inferiorly behind the first part of the duodenum

2. **Duodenum:**
   A. The accessory pancreatic duct opens caudal to the ampulla of Vater
   B. The transverse mesocolon crosses the midpoint of second part of duodenum
   C. The right ureter is situated posterior to the third part of the duodenum
   D. The superior mesenteric artery runs anterior to the third part of the duodenum
   E. The duodenojejunal flexure is situated at the level of L1

3. **Duodenum:**
   A. The appearance of the duodenal cap varies with the body habitus of patient
   B. Aortic impression is seen in the third part of the duodenum
   C. The first part of the duodenum shows small plicae circularis
   D. The ligament of Trietz at the duodenojejunal flexure extends to the right crus of the diaphragm
   E. The duodenum drains into the prepyloric veins

4. **Small bowel:**
   A. The jejunum comprises 3/5ths of the small bowel length
   B. The small bowel mesenteric root measures approximately 6.5 m
   C. The mesenteric root extends from the right of L2 to the right sacroiliac joint

    D. Plica circulares encircle the inner two-thirds of inner surface of jejunum

    E. The plicae are more prominent in the distal ileum

5. **Small bowel studies:**
    A. Gastrograffin slows the gastrointestinal transit
    B. Lying on the left side accelerates the small bowel transit
    C. Glucagon is preferred if barium meal and follow through are combined
    D. In peroral pneumocolon, air is insufflated through the enteroclysis catheter
    E. Images are acquired preferably in the supine position

6. **The following are true about arteries of gastrointestinal tract:**
    A. Arcus of Hyrtl formed by right and left epiploic arteries
    B. Arcus of Barkow formed by right and left gastroepiploic arteries
    C. Wilkies artery—gastroduodenal artery
    D. Arc of Riolan—superior and inferior mesenteric artery anastomosis through middle colic artery branch
    E. Drummond's artery—main branch of superior mesenteric artery
    F. Dwights artery—arc parallel to the small bowel wall

7. **GIT vessels:**
    A. Superior terminal branches of splenic artery are longer than the inferior terminal branches
    B. Inferior polar artery is seen in spleen in 82%
    C. Short gastric branches of splenic artery are best seen if there is hiatal hernia
    D. The left gastroepiploic artery is larger than the left epiploic artery
    E. Short gastric arteries supply the antrum of stomach

8. **Jejunum and ileum:**
    A. The jejunal mesenteric vessels form one or two arcades
    B. Numerous short vessels supply the jejunal wall from the mesenteric vessels
    C. The plicae are deeper set in the jejunum
    D. The ileum is wider than jejunum
    E. The distal ileum drains into the inferior mesenteric vein

9. **Small bowel and large bowel:**
    A. Mesenteric angiography will detect small intestinal hemorrhage only if there is active bleed at the rate of 1 ml/minute
    B. The ileocaecal valve is seen as filling defect in the barium studies

C. The ileocaecal valve prevents the reflux from caecum into terminal ileum

D. The caecum is completely enclosed by peritoneum

E. Appendix is commonly retrocaecal in position

10. **Appendix:**
   A. The appendicular artery is a branch of the posterior caecal artery
   B. Failure of appendix to fill in barium enema indicates disease
   C. The appendix is attached to the anteromedial surface of the caecum
   D. The appendix arises from caecum 2.5 cm below the ileocaecal junction
   E. Appendiculoliths are seen in 15% of normal population

11. **Duodenal leisons:**
   A. 95% of duodenal ulcers are seen in the bulbar region
   B. Thickened folds converging towards the ulcer is seen, similar to gastric ulcer
   C. Gastroduodenal fistula is more common due to duodenal ulcer than gastric ulcer
   D. Common site of gastroduodenal fistula is between greater curvature of antrum and bulbar region
   E. Duodenojejunal intussusceptions are always associated with benign duodenal tumours

12. **Differential diagnosis of polypoid lesions in duodenum:**
   A. Brunner's gland hamartoma
   B. Prolapsed gastric mucosa
   C. Pseudolesion
   D. Leiomyoma
   E. Crohn's disease

13. **Zollinger-Ellison syndrome clinical features:**
   A. Gastrin > 1000 ng/L
   B. Basal acid output > 15 mEq/L
   C. Diarrheoa
   D. Gastric hypersecretion
   E. Fall in serum gastrin secretion after administration of secretin

14. **Duodenal ulcers:**
   A. 50% of ulcers are bulbar and 50% are postbulbar
   B. Any ulcer below the level of ampulla of Vater should alert to possibility of Zollinger-Ellison syndrome
   C. 50% affect anterior wall
   D. Postbulbar ulcers are commonly situated just below the ampulla of Vater
   E. Healing produces scarring in the longitudinal direction of the duodenal bulb

15. **Impressions of adjacent organs on duodenum:**
    A. Normal right adrenal causes anterior displacement of duodenum
    B. Hepatomegaly causes inferior and lateral displacement of the bulb
    C. Hepatic flexure does not produce any impression
    D. Transverse colon impresses the posterior wall of duodenum
    E. Right kidney indents the posterolateral aspect of duodenal sweep

16. **Common causes of diminished duodenal peristalsis:**
    A. Chagas' disease
    B. Thiamine deficiency
    C. Schistosomiasis
    D. Ascariasis
    E. SLE

17. **Common causes of multiple duodenal ulcers:**
    A. Tuberculosis
    B. Sarcoidosis
    C. Lymphoma
    D. Crohn's disease
    E. Syphilis

18. **Ulcer:**
    A. A fistula between the stomach and duodenum improves the patient's symptoms
    B. Perforation through the posterior wall of the stomach produces a gas collection in the left upper quadrant
    C. Mottled collection of gas indicates extension into retroperitoneum
    D. Ulcer in greater curvature is known to form a confined perforation into the liver
    E. In confined perforation extraluminal gas collection is seen only in 50% of times

19. **Peptic ulcer:**
    A. In gasroduodenal fistula, the fistulous tract is the one situated along the lesser curvature
    B. Gastrocolic fistulas are better demonstrated by barium meal than enema
    C. NSAIDs are common causes of gastrocolic fistula
    D. Majority of choledochoduodenal fistulas are caused by bulbar ulcers
    E. Duodenocolic fistula is the most common into the transverse colon

20. **Differential diagnosis of multiple nodular lesions in duodenum:**
    A. Brunner's gland hyperplasia
    B. Duodenitis
    C. Heterotopic gastric mucosa
    D. Lymphoma
    E. Lymphoid hyperplasia

21. **Duodenum:**
    A. Brunner's gland hyperplasia is actually a hamartoma
    B. High acid output is an etiology of Brunner's gland hamartoma
    C. Cobblestone appearance is typical in Brunner's gland hyperplasia
    D. Leiomyoblastomas are very aggressive tumors
    E. Brunner's gland hyperplasia is highly premalignant

22. **Duplication cysts:**
    A. No smooth muscle lining in duplication cysts
    B. Seen in antimesenteric side of bowel
    C. Duodenum is the most common site involved in gastrointestinal tract
    D. Pancreatitis is a complication
    E. Majority communicate with the bowel lumen

23. **Arteries of GIT:**
    A. The anatomical end point of superior mesenteric artery is the anastomosis between most distal ileal artery and ileal branch of ileocolic artery
    B. The persistent vitellointestinal artery arises at level of anatomical end point
    C. The right colic artery commonly arises together with the middle colic artery
    D. There are more ileal branches than jejunal branches, from SMA
    E. Terminal ileum is relatively avascular in angiography

24. **Inferior phrenic artery supplies the following structures:**
    A. IVC
    B. Renal capsule
    C. Liver
    D. Spleen
    E. Stomach

25. **The anatomical level of origin of the arteries in abdomen:**
    A. Inferior phrenic artery—D11
    B. Celiac artery—D12-L1
    C. SMA—L1
    D. Renal—L1-2
    E. Inferior mesenteric artery—L3

26. **Zollinger-Ellison syndrome:**
    A. The diarrhoea characteristically occurs in night
    B. The most common location of ulcer is in the duodenal bulb
    C. The ulcers are multiple in 30%
    D. Postgastrectomy the ulcers are seen in the antimesenteric side of efferent loop
    E. Gastric peristalsis is fast

27. **Ulcer:**
    A. Bulbar ulcer rarely causes obstruction
    B. In gastric outlet obstruction, stomach should always be decompressed before barium
    C. Perforation in posterior wall is usually a free perforation into the peritoneal cavity
    D. Anterior wall perforation is more common in gastric than duodenal ulcer
    E. Water-soluble contrast should be performed for diagnosing perforation if there is no pneumoperitoneum and there is clinical suspicion

28. **Malrotation of bowel is associated with:**
    A. Femoral hernia   B. Congenital heart disease
    C. Omphalocele   D. Gastroschisis
    E. Caroli's disease

29. **Widened duodenal sweep is seen in:**
    A. Aortic aneurysm
    B. Chronic pancreatitis
    C. Pancreatic carcinoma
    D. Mesenteric lymphangioma
    E. Choledochal cyst

30. **Duodenum:**
    A. Has both endodermal and mesodermal components
    B. The first part is the most common site of diverticula
    C. Diverticulum perforates into the retroperitoneum
    D. Intraluminal diverticulum produces windsock deformity
    E. ERCP is difficult with duodenal diverticulum

31. **Duodenal duplication:**
    A. Common in the lateral aspect of second part of duodenum
    B. Typically communicate with the duodenal lumen
    C. Carcinoma can rise inside the duplication cyst
    D. Presence of mural nodule inside duplication cyst is not uncommon
    E. Usually calcified

32. Plain film signs of small bowel obstruction:
A. Dilated bowel in loops in the periphery of abdomen
B. > 2 dilated small bowel loops
C. String of beads indicates peristaltic hyperactivity
D. More the number of dilated bowel loops, more distal the obstruction
E. Gasless abdomen

33. Annular pancreas:
A. Presents in adults in 50% of cases
B. Formed due to persistence of the two ventral buds
C. Adherence of ventral bud to duodenum
D. Increased incidence of pancreatic carcinoma
E. Colon is seen in the right side of abdomen

34. Duodenal trauma:
A. Commonly crushed against the vertebra
B. Intramural haematoma warrants urgent surgery
C. Clinical diagnosis is difficult in duodenal injuries
D. Endoscopic perforation is usually managed surgically
E. In endoscopic perforation, fluid is seen around duodenum

35. Signs of duodenal injury:
A. Air in retroperitoneum
B. Duodenal wall edema
C. Peripancreatic stranding
D. Biliary ductal dilatation
E. Pancreatic transection

36. Duodenal tumours:
A. Villous adenomas have malignant potential
B. Lymphoma is the most common malignant neoplasm of duodenum
C. Lipoma is the most common benign lesion of duodenum
D. Ovarian carcinoma produces metastases to duodenum
E. Lymphoma of duodenum is associated with parasite infestation

37. Duodenal ulcers:
A. Giant ulcer always seen in the bulb
B. Trifoil deformity is due to multiple pseudodiverticula
C. Pyloric channel ulcers are common along the lesser curvature and are treated as duodenal ulcers
D. Barium has only 50% sensitivity in finding the bleeding site in ulcer
E. Barium does not give good coating when ulcer is bleeding

38. Carcinoid tumour of the ileum:
   A. Desmoplastic reaction is seen
   B. Selective mesenteric angiogram is normal
   C. Tumour less than 1 cm is nonmalignant
   D. Patients are usually asymptomatic
   E. Mimics Crohn's disease in barium study

39. Primary carcinoid tumour occurs in the following organs:
   A. Liver   B. Pancreas
   C. Stomach   D. Esophagus
   E. Ileum

40. Tethered small bowel folds are seen in:
   A. Lymphoma
   B. Carcinoid
   C. Retractive mesenteritis
   D. Adhesions
   E. Endometriosis

41. Small bowel cancers:
   A. There is 100-fold increased risk in Crohn's disease
   B. Ulcerative colitis does not increase the risk of small bowel cancer
   C. Increased risk in Meckel's diverticulum
   D. Extension of Crohn's disease into new portions of small bowel indicates development of carcinoma
   E. Sprue increases the risk of adenocarcinoma, not lymphoma

42. Meckel's diverticulum:
   A. Bleeding is more common in children rather than adults
   B. Presents with chronic bleeding in adults
   C. Occurs in 20% of population
   D. Increased incidence in colonic carcinoma
   E. Active bleeding is likely to be picked up by pertechnate scans

43. Features of Zollinger-Ellison syndrome:
   A. Malignant islet cell tumour is seen in 60%
   B. In a gastrinoma with liver metastasis, the resection of tumour will stop the acid production
   C. Gastroesophageal reflux is seen
   D. Rapid small bowel transit
   E. Large areae gastricae

44. The following are complications of Meckel's diverticulum:
   A. Intestinal obstruction   B. Volvulus
   C. Intussusception   D. Carcinoid
   E. Sarcoma

45. **Tc 99m pertechnate scan for Meckel's diverticulum:**
   A. Excretion is dependent on the presence of parietal cells
   B. Uptake is seen twenty minutes following the uptake in stomach mucosa
   C. Serial images are taken every half hour for two hours
   D. Enema should be administered 24 hours before procedure
   E. Fasting should be avoided before the procedure, since it degrades image quality

46. **The following drugs increase the uptake in technetium Meckel's scan:**
   A. Glucagon
   B. Atropine
   C. Cimetidine
   D. Pentagastrin
   E. Somatostatin

47. **Ribbon-like bowel is seen in:**
   A. Allergy
   B. Graft-versus-host disease
   C. Metastasis
   D. Amyloidosis
   E. Crohn's disease

48. **Common causes of widening of the aortomesenteric angle:**
   A. Pancreatitis
   B. Peptic ulcer
   C. Strongyloidosis
   D. Crohn's disease
   E. Tuberculosis

49. **Anatomical variations:**
   A. As many as 20% of normal individuals have the right hepatic artery arising from the superior mesenteric artery
   B. 0.5% have a common celiac and superior mesenteric artery
   C. Common origin of splenic, hepatic and superior mesenteric artery is seen in 2%
   D. Arc of Buhler (the anastomosis between the right and left gastroepiploic arteries), seen 75% of population.
   E. Only 65% of normal individuals have the typical left gastric, splenic common hepatic arterial branching from celiac trunk

50. **Crohn's disease:**
   A. Very high incidence in jews
   B. Males and females are equally affected
   C. Familial association seen
   D. Peak occurrence 15-35 years
   E. Two-thirds need at least one surgery

51. Crohn's Disease:
A. Mortality is 5-10%
B. The main cause for mortality is infection
C. The inflammation is confined to mucosa and submucosa
D. Granulomas are seen in pathological sections
E. Coarse granular pattern in the earliest stage

52. Yersinia enterocolitica infection:
A. Erythema nodosum is a recognized feature
B. Diagnosis made by stool culture
C. Is a recognized cause of acute ileitis
D. Recognised complication of antibiotic treatment
E. Polyarthritis is a feature

53. Abdominal veins:
A. Inferior mesenteric vein drains into superior mesenteric vein in 30%
B. Superior mesenteric vein drains into inferior mesenteric vein in 20%
C. Left gastric vein drains into splenic vein
D. Right gastric vein drains into the left branch of portal vein
E. The anterior and posterior inferior pancreaticoduodenal veins drain into the inferior mesenteric veins

54. The following structures form the posterior relation of the root of the mesentery:
A. Right gonadal vessels
B. Fourth part of duodenum
C. IVC
D. Aorta
E. Right ureter

55. Yersinia enterocolitica infection:
A. Mimics appendicitis
B. Gram positive rods are the causative agents
C. Mimics tuberculosis in barium
D. Causes aphthoid ulceration
E. Causes deep ulceration

56. Bowel obstruction is precipitated by:
A. Radiotherapy
B. Talc
C. Heparin
D. Barium

57. **Small bowel pseudodiverticula is seen in:**
    A. Lymphoma   B. Mesenteric ischemia
    C. Giant ulcer   D. Crohn's
    E. Ileal duplication

58. **Diseases producing huge ulcers in small bowel:**
    A. Tuberculosis
    B. Meckel's
    C. Crohn's
    D. Actinomycosis
    E. Salmonella

59. **Multiple small bowel ulcers are seen in:**
    A. Steroids
    B. Celiac disease
    C. Bacillary dysentery
    D. Lymphoma
    E. Leukemia

60. **Cavitary small bowel lesions are seen in:**
    A. Leiomyosarcoma
    B. Lymphoma
    C. Adenocarcinoma
    D. Crohn's disease
    E. Metastasis

61. **Aortoenteric fistula:**
    A. Esophagus can be involved
    B. Third part of duodenum is the most common site in GIT
    C. Secondary type is more common than primary type
    D. CT is more sensitive than endoscopy
    E. Gas in aorta with focal duodenal thickening is highly
       suggestive

62. **Duodenal tumours:**
    A. Majority involve the first portion
    B. 40% of small bowel tumours occur in the duodenum
    C. Duodenal lymphoma produces more intestinal obstruction than
       carcinoma
    D. Aneursymal dilatation is suggestive of carcinoma
    E. Concentric ring sign in MRI is suggestive of leiomyosarcoma

63. **Separation of small bowel loops is seen in:**
    A. Cirrhosis   B. Carcinoid
    C. Whipple's   D. Amyloidosis
    E. Radiation injury

64. **Sand-like lucencies in small bowel:**
    A. Cystic fibrosis
    B. Waldenström's macroglobulinemia
    C. Mastocytosis
    D. Lymphoma
    E. Yersinia

65. **Causes of megaduodenum:**
    A. Wilkinson syndrome
    B. Annular pancreas
    C. Ladds bands
    D. Pancreatitis
    E. SLE

66. **Thickened duodenal folds are seen in:**
    A. Strongyloides
    B. Eosinophilia
    C. Mastocytosis
    D. Melanoma
    E. Sarcoma

67. **Protein losing enteropathy occurs in:**
    A. Cardiac failure   B. Actinomycosis
    C. Brucellosis   D. Gastric carcinoma
    E. Regional ileitis

68. **Pseudo-obstruction of the gut:**
    A. Normally affects the left side
    B. Causes recurrent dilatation
    C. Peristalsis is absent in all subtypes
    D. Scleroderma is the most common cause
    E. Bowel sounds are not altered in pseudo-obstruction

69. **Carinoid syndrome:**
    A. Causes flushing exacerbated by sunlight
    B. 90% of primary carcinoids occur in the ileocaecal region
    C. Tumour embolisation releases pressor substances into the circulation
    D. A recognized cause of aortic stenosis
    E. Not caused by lung tumours

70. **Thickened irregular valvulae conniventes are seen in:**
    A. Carcinoid
    B. Zollinger-Ellison syndrome
    C. Giardiasis
    D. Radiotherapy
    E. Celiac disease

71. **Following are features of small bowel haemorrhage rather than mesenteric occlusion:**
    A. Complete resolution
    B. Presence of mesenteric mass
    C. Small bowel obstruction
    D. Prominent spasm and irritability
    E. Stacked coin appearance of mucosal folds

72. **Causes of small bowel haemorrhage:**
    A. Henoch-Schönlein purpura
    B. Abdominal aortic aneurysm
    C. Ischemia
    D. Multiple myeloma
    E. Lymphoma

73. **Radiation injury to bowel:**
    A. The critical dose is 3000 rad
    B. Increased risk after pelvic surgery
    C. Separation of bowel loops is seen
    D. Obstruction is uncommon
    E. Mesentery shows decreased attenuation in CT scans

74. **Common causes of small bowel obstruction in adults:**
    A. Gallstone
    B. Appendicitis
    C. Volvulus
    D. Tumour
    E. Hernia

75. **Small bowel strictures are seen in:**
    A. Radiation
    B. Enteric coated tablets
    C. Ischemia
    D. Whipple's
    E. Amyloidosis

76. **Celiac disease:**
    A. Increased incidence of lymphoma
    B. Transient intussusception commonly seen
    C. Mucosal folds show a picket fence appearance
    D. Small bowel transit time is decreased
    E. Dilatation of small bowel is common

77. **Celiac disease:**
    A. There is a strong association with HLA DR 3 histocompatibility gene
    B. The amino acid tryptophan is believed to be the etiological factor
    C. A specific peptidase is absent in the small bowel mucosa
    D. Improvement of the disease after a gluten-free diet is the most specific diagnostic indicator
    E. Although clinical improvement occurs after using gluten-free diet, the histological changes are persistent

78. **Indications for enteroclysis:**
    A. Upper gastrointestinal bleeding
    B. Intestinal obstruction
    C. Gastric ulcer
    D. Post op assessment for ileus
    E. Malabsorption

79. **Enteroclysis:**
    A. Double contrast technique uses 100% of weight/volume
    B. 1-2 liters of methylcellulose are used in double contrast technique
    C. 200 ml of barium should be given in single contrast enteroclysis
    D. Infusion rate is 20 ml/min
    E. The radiation dose is less than of CT of abdomen

80. **In enteroclysis:**
    A. The upper limit of ileal lumen diameter is 3 cm
    B. The No of jejunal folds is 2-3 folds/inch
    C. Normal ileal fold thickness is less than 2 mm
    D. Normal jejunal fold thickness is less than 4 mm
    E. The normal jejunal loop measures less than 4 cm

81. **Scleroderma:**
    A. Dermatomyositis can be differentiated from scleroderma by its normal motility
    B. It is not possible to differentiate scleroderma and sprue radiologically
    C. Colonic diverticula seen in the mesenteric side through areas of smooth muscle atrophy
    D. Barium impaction is a life-threatening complication
    E. Loss of haustration indicates inflammatory bowel disease than scleroderma

82. **Small bowel:**
    A. Barium enema is better for assessing terminal ileal Crohn's disease than barium follow through
    B. Enteroclysis can accurately diagnose celiac disease
    C. Barium follow through is better than enteroclysis for small bowel tumours
    D. Barium will cause impaction in small bowel obstruction patients
    E. No bowel preparation is required for enteroclysis

83. **Delayed small bowel transit is seen in:**
    A. Tuberculosis   B. Anxiety
    C. Diabetes   D. Hyperthyroidism
    E. Hyperkalemia

84. The following are common causes of neonatal distal bowel obstruction:
  A. Hirschsprung's disease
  B. Meconium ileus
  C. Jejunal atresia
  D. Ileal atresia
  E. Malrotation

85. Multiple stenotic lesions in small bowel are seen in:
  A. Metastasis
  B. Endometriosis
  C. Tuberculosis
  D. NSAIDs
  E. Radiation

86. Causes of aortoduodenal fistula:
  A. Whipple's
  B. Atherosclerosis
  C. Radiation
  D. Peptic ulcer
  E. Lymphoma

87. Small bowel tumours:
  A. Malignant melanoma deposits rarely ulcerate
  B. Bowel wall metastasis may calcify
  C. Carcinoid is associated with celiac disease
  D. Obstruction is rare in leiomyosarcoma
  E. Symptoms of Crohn's disease paradoxically resolve after development of carcinoma

88. Features of GIT scleroderma:
  A. Pneumatosis cystoides intestinalis
  B. Hide bound sign is seen in 60% of cases
  C. Folds are widely separated
  D. Thickened folds
  E. Intussusception is uncommon in scleroderma due to absence of lead point

89. Small bowel nodules are seen in:
  A. Typhoid
  B. Waldenström's macroglobulinemia
  C. Leukemia
  D. Zollinger-Ellison syndrome
  E. Whipple's disease

90. Peutz-Jeghers syndrome:
A. Increased incidence of gastric carcinoma
B. Increased incidence of breast carcinoma
C. Autosomal dominant
D. GI haemorrhage is a life-threatening complication
E. Increased incidence of adenomatous polyps in the stomach

91. Small bowel:
A. Polyps of the stomach and duodenum may be associated with hyperchlorhydria
B. In AIDS lymphoma, multiple nodules are seen in small bowel
C. Duodenal ulcers are most commonly seen on the anterior aspect of the duodenal bulb
D. Polyps are associated with hyperkalemia
E. Filling defects are caused by duodenal varices

92. Crohn's disease:
A. Even in late stages the haustral pattern is preserved unlike ulcerative colitis
B. Increased density of mesenteric fat
C. Anorectal disease is seen in 65% of Crohn's with colonic disease
D. Sinus tracts are produced due to raised intraluminal pressure and not due to mucosal disease
E. In cobblestoning, the intervening mucosa is normal

93. GIT manifestations of HIV:
A. Kaposi's sarcoma is usually associated with skin lesions
B. Diamond ulcers are seen in candida infections of esophagus
C. Lymphoma is rarest in esophagus
D. Cryptosporidium can cause cholangitis
E. MAI causes small bowel polyps
F. Duodenum most common site of Kaposi's

94. Celiac disease:
A. Transit time is markedly reduced
B. Sacroilitis is a recognized feature
C. Jejunal ulceration occurs
D. Carcinoma esophagus is associated
E. Increased incidence of carcinoma pharynx

95. Thickened small bowel folds without obstruction:
A. Amyloidosis
B. Whipple's
C. Eosinophilic enteritis
D. Crohn's disease
E. Hodgkin's lymphoma

96. Thickened duodenal folds are seen in:
A. Amyloidosis
B. Tapeworm
C. Haemotoma
D. Peptic ulcer
E. Pancreatitis

97. Tuberculosis of small bowel:
A. Most common in the terminal ileum
B. <2% of patients have active lung disease
C. Noncaseating granulomas are seen in the active phase of the disease
D. Associated with increased incidence of sclerosing cholangitis
E. Most common in young adults

98. Gastrointestinal haemorrhage:
A. Angiography is more useful for lower GI haemorrhage than upper GI haemorrhage
B. Tc sulphur colloid is more useful for upper GI haemorrhage
C. Tc labelled RBCs are the best for lower GI haemorrhage
D. In technetium pertechnate scans, the tracer uptake is seen in mucus secreting cells
E. Delayed images in gallium scans can be used for detecting gastrointestinal haemorrhage

99. Atrophy of small bowel folds is seen in:
A. Amyloidosis
B. Celiac disease
C. Radiation
D. Tuberculosis
E. Whipple's

100. Tc sulfur colloid for GI haemorrhage:
A. Bleeding must be active at the time of examination
B. Present in blood for 30 min
C. Very useful for upper gastrointestinal haemorrhage
D. Study terminated if no abnormality is seen in 2 hours
E. Flow study is performed for one minute

101. Crohn's disease:
A. Large and small bowel are involved in 30%
B. Skip areas are characteristic
C. Linear ulcers are seen in the antimesenteric border
D. Aphthous ulcers indicate late, chronic stage
E. Polyps are seen in late stages

102. Tc labelled RBCs:
A. Has prolonged stay in the blood pool
B. Correlation of 83% with angiography
C. Best isotope for localisation of bleeding site
D. Images acquired every two seconds
E. High target to background ratio

103. False positive for Tc RBC:
A. Hemangioma
B. Renal pelvis uptake
C. Physiological uptake in intestine
D. Intussusception
E. Enteric duplication

104. Meckel's diverticulum:
A. Located wihin 2 feet of the duodenojejunal flexure
B. Seen in 5% of population
C. Asymptomatic in 40%
D. Seen in the mesenteric border of the ileum
E. Inverted Meckel's diverticulum is seen as elongated mass perpendicular to the axis of ileum

105. False positive Meckel's scan (Tc pertechnate):
A. Malrotation of ileum
B. Zollinger-Ellison syndrome
C. Irritable bowel syndrome
D. Tuberculosis
E. Pancreatitis

106. Appendicitis:
A. Normal plain film excludes appendicitis
B. Appendicolith is the most reliable plain film sign of appendicitis
C. Non-filling of appendix in barium enema indicates appendicitis
D. Air in the appendix in plain film is a reliable sign of appendicitis
E. Pneumoperitoneum often follows ruptured gangrenous appendicitis

107. Small bowel carcinoid:
A. All carcinoids are considered malignant unless proved otherwise
B. 95% of tumours more than 2 cm, metastasise
C. Extensive desmoplastic reaction is a characteristic feature of carcinoid and is due to serotonin
D. Bowel resection is indicated for all tumours more than 1 cm and bowel symptoms
E. 30% of carcinoids are multiple

108. Appendicitis:
A. Fluid around appendix is highly suggestive of appendicitis
B. 10% have appendicolith
C. 45-50% of normal appendices are visualized in CT
D. Ultrasound-guided compression is 75-90% sensitive
E. Normal appendix is visualized in 90% of ultrasound examinations

109. Small bowel nodules are seen in:
A. Typhoid
B. Waldenström's macroglobulinemia
C. Leukemia
D. Zollinger-Ellison syndrome
E. Whipple's disease

110. Ileal lymphoid hyperplasia is seen in:
A. Crohn's disease
B. Hypogammoglobulinemia
C. Children
D. Yersinia
E. Carcinoid

111. Small bowel obstruction:
A. Adhesions are seen after 90% of laparatomies
B. 30% of obstruction is caused by adhesion
C. Adhesion is clearly seen in CT scan with reconstructed images
D. 95% of hernias causing obstruction are external hernias
E. Most of the internal hernias are acquired and not congenital

112. Small bowel tumours:
A. The most common tumour in the small bowel is adenocarcinoma
B. The most common primary tumour in small bowel is carcinoid
C. Obstruction in carcinoid is due to desmoplastic response
D. Carcinoma lung is the most common cause of submucosal metastasis
E. 25% of intestinal obstructions end in strangulation

113. Common causes of subserosal small bowel metastasis:
A. Stomach
B. Lung
C. Breast
D. Pancreas
E. Uterus

114. Appendiceal tumours:
A. 90% present with acute appendicitis
B. Carcinoids are the most common tumours
C. Mucoceles are always malignant
D. Retention cysts are less than 2 cm
E. Appendicitis is less common in mucinous tumours than non-mucinous tumours

115. Thickened irregular volvulae conniventes are seen in:
   A. Whipple's disease   B. Crohn's disease
   C. Tuberculosis   D. Mastocytosis
   E. Scleroderma

116. Appendicial lesions:
   A. Presence of mucin inside the lesion is highly specific for malignancy
   B. Dense opacities inside mucoceles indicate infection
   C. All appendiceal neoplasms are seen above 50 years
   D. Colonic type adenocarcinomas only half as common as mucinous neoplasms
   E. Mucoceles are formed even in colonic type adenocarcinomas

117. Celiac disease:
   A. Presence of four folds/per inch of jejunum is diagnostic
   B. In ileum, there are more than 5 folds per inch
   C. Lymphomas in celiac disease are B cell type
   D. Weight loss in a patient who responded well with gluten-free diet indicates lymphoma
   E. Development of obstruction in a patient with celiac disease indicates lymphoma

118. Appendiceal lesions:
   A. 20% of Crohn's disease patients have involvement of appendix
   B. 90% of carcinoids are seen in appendix
   C. Appendix measuring more than 6 mm in compression sonography is abnormal
   D. Appendiculolith indicates appendicitis complicated by perforation or abscess
   E. The nidus of appendiculolith is vegetable matter

119. Recognised causes of appendiceal mucocele:
   A. Caecal bascule
   B. Appendicular volvulus
   C. Endometrioma
   D. Fecolith
   E. Polyp

120. Complications of celiac disease:
   A. Osteoporosis
   B. Macrocytic anemia
   C. Malignancy
   D. Hypoglycemia
   E. Dermatitis herpeteformis
   F. Splenomegaly

121. **Scleroderma:**
    A. Marked dilatation of duodenum is a feature
    B. Bacterial overgrowth in the small bowel results in malabsorption
    C. Colonic pseudodiverticula are narrow necked
    D. Esophageal involvement leads to esophageal stricture
    E. Small bowel transit time is decreased

122. **False-positive uptake in Meckel's scan is seen in:**
    A. Hydronephrosis
    B. Meninomyelocele
    C. Hemangioma
    D. Intussusception
    E. Ulcerative colitis

123. **Celiac disease:**
    A. Increased association with primary sclerosing cholangitis
    B. In those patients who respond well to gluten-free diet, the number of ileal folds decrease since the jejunal function is restored
    C. In nonresponders, the ileal folds increase
    D. Moulage sign is due to flocculated suspension
    E. Mosaic pattern is a specific pattern seen in endoscopy and not in barium

124. **Meckel's diverticulum:**
    A. Is a remnant of omphalomesenteric duct
    B. Tc 99m uptake is seen in 60%
    C. Causes rectal bleeding
    D. Normal isotope scan excludes Meckel's
    E. May have colonic tissue

125. **Common sites for lodgement of gallstone:**
    A. Proximal ileum
    B. Distal ileum
    C. Proximal jejunum
    D. Rectum
    E. Stomach

126. **Bouveret's syndrome:**
    A. Gastric outlet obstruction is seen
    B. Pneumobilia is seen
    C. Causes intrahepatic ductal dilatation
    D. Premalignant
    E. Produces osteoporosis

127. **Bowel obstruction:**
    A. 40% of surgical admissions for acute abdomen are due to intestinal obstruction
    B. 80% of bowel obstructions are at the level of the small bowel
    C. 70% of small bowel obstructions are due to tumours
    D. CT is superior to plain film in detection of small bowel obstruction
    E. Thin sections should be taken at the level of the transition point

128. **Protein losing enteropathy occurs in:**
    A. Vagotomy
    B. Constrictive pericarditis
    C. Crohn's disease
    D. Jejunal diverticulosis
    E. Intestinal lymphangiectasia

129. **Small bowel lymphoma:**
    A. Aneurysmal dilatation is seen in the mesenteric border
    B. Cavitation is more common in the antimesenteric border
    C. Sandwich configuration is suggestive of lymphoma
    D. Cobblestone pattern is seen
    E. The volvulae conniventes are thick

130. **Tuberculosis:**
    A. Sterling's sign indicates rapid emptying of the distal ileum
    B. Fleischner's sign is associated with narrowed ileocaecal valve
    C. Nodes are common in the retroperitoneum than the mesentery
    D. Lymph nodes are of high density in the acute phase
    E. Ascites is of high density

131. **False positive sulfur colloid scans for gastrointestinal haemorrhage:**
    A. Transplanted kidney   B. Arterial graft
    C. Aortic aneurysm   D. Male genitalia
    E. Accessory spleen

132. **Failure of air reduction or intussusception occurs in the following circumstances:**
    A. Ileo ileo colic type   B. Presence of lead point
    C. Early recurrence   D. Palpable mass in abdomen
    E. Viral illness

133. **Hernias:**
    A. Richter's hernia contains the Meckel's diverticulum
    B. Spigelian hernia happens through the rectus abdominis
    C. Littre's hernia—entrapment of antimesenteric border of bowel loop
    D. Femoral hernia is the most common hernia in females
    E. Anterior perineal hernia is through a defect in the levator ani

134. Appendiceal mucoceles:
   A. A broad-based smooth filling defect in the medial aspect of caecum is highly likely to be an appendiceal neoplasm
   B. Curvilinear calcification is seen in majority of appendiceal mucoceles
   C. The most common differential diagnosis is ovarian lesion
   D. Irregularity of the wall of mucocele indicates malignancy
   E. Gas bubbles inside lesion exclude the diagnosis

135. Internal hernia:
   A. Accounts for 5% of mechanical small bowel obstruction
   B. The most common location is in lesser sac
   C. Majority of paraduodenal hernias occur on the right side
   D. The fossa of Waldeyer is caudal to the superior mesenteric artery and inferior to the third portion of duodenum
   E. The jejunal loops are commonly involved rather than the ileal loops, in the lesser sac hernia

136. Features of advanced Crohn's disease:
   A. Enteroclysis can differentiate stricture from spasm secondary to inflammation
   B. Pseudopolyps are produced due to elevated normal mucosa in between ulcers
   C. Ileosigmoid fistula causes improvement of symptoms
   D. The most common enterocolic fistula is between ileum and caecum
   E. Perforation is very common in advanced Crohn's

137. Whipple's disease:
   A. Caused by a gram-negative bacteria
   B. Foamy macrophages in submucosa with PAS positive material is characteristic appearance
   C. More common in females
   D. Arthritis precedes intestinal disease in 25%
   E. Generalised lymphadenopathy is seen in 50%

138. Features of Whipple's disease:
   A. Dilatation of small bowel
   B. Rigid folds
   C. Rapid transit
   D. Thick folds
   E. Small nodules

139. Intussusception:
   A. Most common cause of bowel obstruction in children
   B. More common in summer
   C. There is no sex predominance

D. 75% occur under two years

E. Bleeding per rectum indicates bad success rate for air reduction

140. **Gastrointestinal haemorrhage:**
    A. Tc sulphur colloid requires bleeding of 0.5 ml/min
    B. Tc labelled RBCs require bleeding of 0.35 ml/min
    C. Angiography requires bleeding of 0.1 ml/min
    D. Tc 99m pertechnate 0.5 ml/min
    E. Nuclear medicine scans are more sensitive than angiography

141. **Tropical sprue:**
    A. Caused by infection
    B. Cured by antibiotics and folic acid
    C. Affects proximal small bowel more than distal small bowel
    D. Flocculation of barium is not seen, unlike celiac disease
    E. Megaloblastic anemia is seen at presentation

142. **Metabolic conditions producing malabsorption:**
    A. Hyperthyroidism
    B. Hypothyroidism
    C. Hyperparathyroidism
    D. Diabetes mellitus
    E. Zollinger-Ellison syndrome

143. **Causes of lead point in intussusception in children:**
    A. Duplication cyst
    B. Appendicitis
    C. Henoch-Schönlein purpura
    D. Teratoma
    E. Scleroderma

144. **Crohn's disease:**
    A. Only the perianal region is invovled in 2-3% of Crohn's disease
    B. Lymphoid hyperplasia is the earliest finding in Crohn's
    C. Rose thorn ulcers are very specific of Crohn's disease
    D. Mesentery is sclerosed adjacent to the involved bowel wall
    E. Sacculations are seen in the mesenteric border

145. **Causes of malabsorption and typical biopsy features:**
    A. Diltated lacteals—abetalipoproteinemia
    B. Noncaseating granuloma—tuberculosis
    C. Proteins—sarcoidosis
    D. High lymphocytes, absent plasma cells—Whipple's
    E. PAS positive lymphocytes—agammaglobulinemia

146. **Bacterial overgrowth syndromes:**
     A. More than 10^6 bacteria are seen per ml
     B. Majority of bacteria are aerobic
     C. B_6 deficiency caused by bacterial consumption
     D. Fistulas are predisposing factors for overgrowth
     E. Normal peristalsis is an important factor preventing the development of bacterial overgrowth

147. **Malabsorption:**
     A. Gastrointestinal tract is involved in 70% of primary amyloidosis
     B. Malabsorption is seen in 75% of cases of scleroderma
     C. In intestinal lymphangiectasia, the folds are thickened and there are large nodules
     D. In eosinophilia, small nodules are seen in proximal ileum than terminal ileum with thickened folds
     E. In primary idiopathic pseudo-obstruction, there is prolonged transit time due to damage to myenteric plexus

148. **Jejunal diverticulosis:**
     A. Progressively increase in size when moving from proximal to distal jejunum
     B. Diffuse involvement of jejunum rather than a focal segmental involvement
     C. Involves the antimesenteric border
     D. Fabry's disease is jejunal diverticulosis with anemia and bacterial overgrowth
     E. Warrants surgery if inflamed

149. **Recognised causes of lymphangiectasia:**
     A. Retroperitoneal fibrosis
     B. Tuberculosis
     C. Metastasis
     D. Whipple's dissese
     E. Constrictive pericarditis

150. **Short bowel syndrome:**
     A. With intact colon, at least 200 cm of small bowel should be present to sustain oral autonomy
     B. Ileum can take the functions of jejunum when it is lost
     C. In complete loss of ileum, jejunum takes over the metabolic function of ileum
     D. Increased renal stone formation in short bowel syndrome
     E. In total parenteral nutrition the adaptation of the ileal mucosa to jejunal loss is lost

151. Chronic intestinal pseudo-obstruction is caused by:
- A. SLE
- B. Hypothyroidism
- C. Diverticulosis
- D. Blind loop syndrome
- E. Scleroderma

152. Superior mesenteric artery syndrome:
- A. Compresses the second part of the duodenum
- B. The angle between aorta and superior mesenteric artery is decreased to 45 degrees in this disease
- C. The compression is relieved by turning the patient in the left anterior oblique position
- D. A transverse linear compression defect can be seen over the duodenum
- E. The duodenum is dilated proximal and distal to the site of compression

153. Causes for superior mesenteric artery syndrome:
- A. Malrotation
- B. Volvulus
- C. Pregnancy
- D. Weight gain
- E. Burns

154. Small bowel cancers:
- A. Accounts for 10% of bowel cancers
- B. Rapid transit in the small bowel is a factor which decreases the incidence of small bowel cancers
- C. Alkalinity of small bowel contents increases the risk of small bowel cancer
- D. Adenocarcinomas are highest in the ileum
- E. The highest incidence of carcinoids is in the jejunum

155. The following are risk factors of development of small bowel tumours:
- A. Neurofibromatosis
- B. Ileocystoplasty
- C. Familial adenomatosis polyposis
- D. Peutz-Jeghers syndrome
- E. Crohn's disease

156. Whipple's disease:
- A. Pseudo-Whipple's disease is seen in AIDS
- B. Pseudo-Whipple's is caused by *Mycobacterium avium intracellulare*
- C. Hepatosplenomegaly is common
- D. Segmentation and fragmentation are common in barium studies
- E. It is differentiated from sprue absence of dilatation and fold thickening

157. Tuberculosis:
A. String sign indicates presence of stenosis
B. Presence of interloop ascites is highly suggestive of tuberculosis
C. Enteroliths are seen invariably proximal to a stricture
D. The bowel wall thickening in tuberculosis is variegated
E. Heterogeneous echogenicity in a single lymph node group indicates lymphoma

158. Small bowel lymphoma:
A. Majority of lymphomas are primary lymphomas
B. Bowel is involved in 30% of bowel lymphomas
C. Bowel is involved in up to 20% of all NHL
D. Diffusely infiltrative type is the most common type
E. Small bowel is the most common site in the gastrointestinal tract

159. Small bowel carcinoid:
A. The incidence of carcinoid is higher in small bowel than appendix
B. Flushing is the most common symptom in small bowel carcinoid
C. Serotonin is the agent responsible for diarrhoea in carcinoid syndrome
D. Vasoactive intestinal peptide is the major agent producing telangiectasia
E. Increased excretion of 5 Vanillyl mandelic acid in urine

160. The following are associations of small bowel lymphoma:
A. Celiac disease
B. Crohn's
C. SLE
D. Chemotherapy
E. Radiation

161. Small bowel carcinoid:
A. The incidence of carcinoid syndrome is more when the tumour drains directly into the systemic circulation
B. It is uncommon for carcinoid tumour metastasising to liver to produce carcinoid syndrome, since liver Monoamine oxidase deactivates the serotonin produced by the tumour
C. Defecation increases the risk of development of carcinoid syndrome
D. Carcinoid tumours arise from the crypts of Leiberkuhn
E. The incidence of liver metastasis is highest in colonic carcinoids than small intestine tumours

162. **Radiological features of small bowel carcinoid:**
    A. Intussusception
    B. Hernias
    C. Crowding of folds
    D. Calcified mesenteric mass
    E. Mucosal elevation

163. **Small bowel carcinomas:**
    A. Most common cause of apple core deformity in small bowel
    B. Ulcerative type is more common than polypoidal type in duodenum
    C. Annular constrictive type is the most common type in ileum and jejunum
    D. The strictures of carcinomas are longer than in metastatic lesions
    E. Overhanging edges are highly suggestive of a benign pathology rather than carcinoma

164. **The following are recognized clinical findings in malabsorption:**
    A. Night blindness   B. Osteoarthropathy
    C. Haemorrhage   D. Nocturia
    E. Peripheral neuropathy

165. **Adenocarcinoma small bowel:**
    A. There is no relationship between the size of small bowel cancer and invasiveness of tumour
    B. The lymph nodes are very bulky in adenocarcinoma
    C. A soap bubble pattern in duodenum indicates adenocarcinoma
    D. Familial adenomatous polyposis produces adenomas in periampullary region
    E. Villous adenomas more than 5 mm should be considered invasive

166. **Intussusception:**
    A. The segment of bowel which invaginates is called intussuscipiens
    B. 90% of intussusceptions are ileocolic
    C. 90% of intussusceptions are without a lead point
    D. Meckel's diverticulum is the most common lead point
    E. The most common site of filling defect in barium enema is the transverse colon

167. **Causes of intussusception in adults:**
    A. Scleroderma   B. Whipple's
    C. Anxiety   D. Starvation
    E. Celiac disease

168. **Air reduction of intussusception:**
    A. Each attempt lasts at least 10 min
    B. Only three attempts at maximum
    C. Reduction should be obtained within 10 minutes
    D. In hydrostatic reduction, the bag is kept at height of 1 m
    E. Maximum pressure allowed is 150 mm Hg

169. **Air reduction of intussusception:**
    A. Lesser intracolonic pressure than for barium
    B. Slower than barium, due to low pressure
    C. Radiation dose is more than barium, since air is less dense than barium
    D. Perforation is sterile
    E. Larger tears than in barium

170. **Contraindications for air reduction of intussusception:**
    A. 12 hours since onset
    B. Pneumoperitoneum
    C. Obstruction
    D. Hirschsprung's disease
    E. Ascites

171. **Appendiceal carcinoids:**
    A. Majority are seen within 1 cm of the base
    B. Carcinoid syndrome is very unlikely
    C. Even tumours 5 cm are considered benign and managed by local resection
    D. Irregular soft tissue mass at the base of mesentery is a characteristic finding
    E. Malignant mucinous neoplasms of appendix require right hemicolectomy

172. **Small bowel lymphoma:**
    A. Most common malignant small bowel tumour
    B. The most common cause of intussusception in children less than six years
    C. Multicentric in 40%
    D. Most common site is the ileum
    E. Infiltrative type is the most common

173. **Tuberculosis:**
    A. Sterling sign is highly specific for tuberculosis
    B. Hypertrophic form is the most common form
    C. Ulcers are parallel to the long axis of the intestine
    D. Tuberculin skin test is negative
    E. Tuberculosis of the ileocaecal areas is the most common presentation in the abdomen

174. Intussusception:

A. Fluid seen within the intussusception is a contraindication for air reduction
B. No blood flow in intussusception indicates bowel wall necrosis
C. Contrast flow into the ileum during barium enema excludes intussusception
D. Coiled spring pattern is seen in antegrade barium examination but not in retrograde study
E. Plain film shows soft tissue mass in 50% of cases

175. Adynamic ileus is seen in:

A. Hypokalemia
B. Diabetes
C. Lymphoma
D. Glucagon
E. Vagotomy

176. Pseudosacculation is seen in:

A. Scleroderma
B. Ulcerative colitis
C. Ischemic bowel disease
D. Diverticular disease
E. Crohn's disease

177. Scleroderma:

A. Small intestine is the most common involved region in the gut
B. Involvement of small intestine indicates rapid progression
C. Dilated small bowel loops indicate obstruction
D. Abrupt cut off at IMA level
E. Sacculations are seen in the mesenteric side

ANSWERS

1. **A-F, B-T, C-F, D-F, E-T**
   The first 2.5 cm of duodenum is intraperitoneal and situated in between the folds of the greater and the lesser omentum. The rest of duodenum is retroperitoneal. The duodenal cap is the first 2 cm of duodenum. The epiploic foramen lies superior to the first part of the duodenum.

2. **A-F, B-T, C-T, D-T, E-F**
   The accessory pancreatic duct opens cranial to the ampulla of Vater. The duodenojejunal flexure situated at level of L2.

3. **A-T, B-T, C-F, D-T, E-T**
   The duodenum drains into the prepyloric vein and from there to the portal vein. Plicae begin from 2nd part of duodenum.
   The hepatic and gastroduodenal arteries send small branches to the duodenum. Proximal duodenum drains into celiac and distal duodenum into superior mesenteric nodes.

4. **A-F, B-F, C-F, D-T, E-F**
   The small intestine measures approximately 6.5 m and jejunum constitutes 2/5ths of it.
   The small bowel mesenteric root, measures 15 cm from the left of L2 to Rt Sacroiliac joint. Plicae are more prominent in the jejunum, less in the proximal ileum and absent in the distal ileum.

5. **A-F, B-F, C-T, D-F, E-F**
   Gastrograffin 10 ml or metoclopramide 20 mg accelerates the transit time. Lying on the right side is another maneuver. Glucagon does not affect small bowel transit and hence it is preferred over buscopan. Images are acquired every 20 min for one hour, and 30 min after that, in the prone position, to separate the bowel loops. In peroral pneumocolon, a barium follow through is performed, and air is insufflated through the rectum once the barium enters the ileocaecal region.

6. **A-F, B-F, C-F, D-T, E-F, F-T**
   Arcus of Hyrtl—anastomosis between right and left gastroepiploic arteries
   Arcus of Barkow—anastomosis between right and left epiploic arteries
   Wilkies artery is the supraduodenal artery, a branch of right gastric artery.
   Arc or Riolan—a branch of middle colic artery, runs parallel to it and links the SMA and IMA, thus forming an important collateral channel.

Drummond's artery—marginal artery. This is the arc which parallels the bowel wall and gives the vasa recta, formed by anastomosis between ileocolic A, right, middle and left colic A.

7. **A-T, B-T, C-T, D-F, E-F**

Splenic artery divides into superior, inferior and middle terminal branches, which further divide intrasplenic branches. Superior polar artery is seen in 65% and inferior polar artery is seen in 82%. Short gastric arteries supply the cardia and fundus.

The left epiploic artery, a branch of left gastroepiploic artery, is larger and is seen easily in angiogram.

8. **A-T, B-F, C-T, D-F, E-F**

The jejunal mesenteric vessels form one or two arcades and the branches are long and less numerous. The ileal mesenteric vessels form three or four arcades and the branches are small and more numerous. The jejunum is wider and has more and deeper plicae. The distal ileum drains into the superior mesenteric vein, just like the rest of the small bowel.

9. **A-F, B-T, C-F, D-F, E-T**

Mesenteric angiography will detect active bleed of 0.5 ml/min. The ileocaecal valve has two folds the superior and inferior, but it does not prevent reflux. The terminal ileal wall is thickened and acts as sphincter to prevent reflux. The caecum has peritoneum in anterior aspect and on the sides.

10. **A-T, B-F, C-F, D-T, E-T**

Appendix drains into the posterior caecal vein, into the superior mesenteric vein.

The lymph nodes drain into the epicolic nodes and thence into the superior mesenteric nodes. The appendix is attached to the posteromedial surface of the caecum.

Appendiculoliths when seen in symptomatic patients have a 90% predictability for acute appendicitis. Failure of appendix to fill during barium does not indicate disease.

11. **A-T, B-F, C-F, D-F, E-T**

Duodenal ulcers do not show the converging folds which are typically seen in gastric ulcers. Gastroduodenal fistula is more common due to gastric than duodenal ulcer and is seen between lesser curvature of antrum and base of duodenal bulb. Gastro-duodenal intussusceptions are associated with benign gastric or duodenal tumours.

12. A-T, B-T, C-T, D-T, E-F
Prolapsed antral polyp is another cause. Pseudolesion is caused by redundant mucosa in the duodenal flexure at the junction of the first and second part.

13. A-T, B-T, C-T, D-T, E-F
Serum gastrin rises by >200 ng/l after administration of secretin.

14. A-F, B-T, C-T, D-F, E-F
About 95% ulcers are situated in the bulb and only 5% are situated in the postbulbar region. The high incidence in the bulb is believed to be due to jets of acid striking the bulb through the sphincter, presence of mucosal transitional zone and poor vascularity. In postbulbar region, the most common location is seen just proximal to the ampulla of Vater. Healing produces scarring in the transverse direction of duodenal bulb.

15. A-T, B-F, C-F, D-F-, E-T
Hepatomegaly causes displacement of the duodenal bulb to the left side. Hepatic flexure indents the right side of the descending duodenum. Transverse colon indents the anterior wall of the descending duodenum. CBD produces a linear or a small round impression on the bulb. Enlarged GB causes impression on the superior aspect. Dilated vessels will be seen as single or multiple impressions on the outer wall of the duodenal bulb and sweep.

16. A-T, B-T, C-F, D-F, E-T
Diabetes, scleroderma, dermatomyositis, porphyria and anticholinergic drugs are other reasons.

17. A-T, B-T, C-T, D-T, E-T
Peptic ulcer, Zollinger-Ellison syndrome, caustics and cytomegalovirus are other causes.

18. A-T, B-T, C-T, D-F, E-T
A fistula between the stomach and duodenum produces the typical double pyloric channel and this opens an alternate pathway for gastric emptying thus improving the symptoms of gastric outlet obstruction. Perforation through posterior wall can produce a confined perforation, which involves the pancreas in 75% of cases. The lesser omentum, transverse mesocolon, colon can be involved. The spleen is involved in greater curvature ulcers and left lobe of liver is involved in lesser curvature ulcers. Gastrograffin studies are performed when plain X-ray is noncontributory, but even this is positive in only 50% of cases.

19. **A-T, B-F, C-T, D-F, E-F**

    Gastrocolic fistulas are produced by ulcers in the greater curvature which perforate into the transverse colon. It is common with greater curvature ulcers produced by NSAIDs. The characteristic clinical triad is diarrhoea, fecal vomiting and foul-smelling eructation. Barium meal will show the ulcer and can show early filling of transverse colon. But barium enema is better for demonstration of the fistula, due to higher pressure in the colon. About 95% of choledochoduodenal fistulas are caused by gall-stones and only 5% are caused by duodenal ulcers. Duodenocolic fistula is common into the hepatic flexure. Other rarer fistulas include gastropericardial fistula from an ulcer in hiatal hernia or gastric pull through and a duodenorenal fistula into the right kidney.

20. **A-T, B-T, C-T, D-T, E-T**

21. **A-T, B-T, C-T, D-F, E-F**

    Brunner's gland hyperplasia is also called hamartoma. It is also believed to be formed secondary to high acid output from stomach. It can be a diffuse hyperplasia or a focal hamartoma. Diffuse lesion is seen as cobblestone appearance with central flecks of barium. Hamartoma is seen as a submucosal tumour. They do not have atypical cells or mitosis and are not called adenomas. Leiomyo-blastoms are benign tumours composed of epithelioid cells. They are a component of Carney's triad, which also includes pulmonary hamartomas and extradrenal pheochromocytoma.

22. **A-F, B-F, C-F, D-T, E-F**

    Duplication cysts are lined by epithelium and smooth muscle. They can arise anywhere in the GIT and the epithelium is identical to the parent organ. They usually do not communicate with the bowel, but occasionally communicate. They are seen in the mesenteric border of the bowel. They are most common in ileum. In stomach they are seen in the greater curvature and in the duodenum, the medial part is involved. It can ulcerate or bleed or obstruct or produce jaundice by CBD compression or pancreatitis by MPD compression. The shape and size change with fluoroscopy.

23. **A-T, B-F, C-T, D-T, E-T**

    The embryological end point is 5 cm proximal to the anatomical end point. The persistent vitellointestinal artery which supplies the Meckel's diverticulum, arises from this point.
    There are 9-13 ileal arteries and 4-6 jejunal arteries.

24. **A-T, B-T, C-T, D-T, E-T**

    Also supplies the esophagus and suprarenal glands.

25. **A-F, B-T, C-T, D-T, E-T**
Inferior phrenic artery—D12, celiac artery—D12-L1, SMA-L1, Renal L1-L2, IMA-L3.

26. **A-T, B-T, C-F, D-F, E-F**
Diarrhoea occurs characteristically in the night, since the increased acid neutralizes the pancreatic enzymes. The ulcers are solitary in 90%. But multiple ulcers are quite frequent. The most common location is in duodenal bulb (65%). Atypical ulcers are common, such as near the ligament of Trietz, C loop of duodenum and distal esophagus. In postgastrectomy patients, it is seen on the gastric side of the anastomosis and mesenteric border of the efferent loop. The peristalsis is sluggish.

27. **A-T, B-T, C-F, D-F, E-T**
Obstruction is usually caused by edema or scarring in a postbulbar ulcer. Obstruction is very rare in bulbar ulcer. Perforation in posterior wall is usually confined. Perforation in anterior wall is free, into the peritoneal cavity. Perforation of anterior wall is more common in duodenal ulcer than gastric ulcer. The development of pneumoperitoneum depends on the rate of sealing of perforation. If the ulcer is sealed quickly, there may not be any pneumoperitoneum. Water-soluble contrast can be instilled to confirm perforation. Even this may be false negative in 50% if it has been sealed fast.

28. **A-F, B-T, C-T, D-F, E-F**

29. **A-T, B-T, C-T, D-T, E-T**

30. **A-T, B-F, C-T, D-T, E-T**
Duodenum develops from midgut. At 8 weeks, the mucosa proliferates and there is no lumen. Recanalisation occurs at 10 weeks. The second and third part, especially within 2 cm from ampulla, is the most common site. Diverticulum can be inflamed and can perforate into the retroperitoneum. Occasionally, intra-luminal diverticulum is seen in the second or third part. If the ampulla drains into the diverticulum, cannulation of CBD is difficult.

31. **A-F, B-F, C-T, D-F, E-F**
It is common in the medial aspect of second part of duodenum. It does not usually communicate with the duodenal lumen. Calcification is uncommon.
Presence of mural nodules and vegetation inside duplication is suspicious for carcinoma.

32. **A-F, B-F, C-T, D-T, E-T**
> 3 small bowel loops. > 3 cm is suggestive of small bowel obstruction.
Step ladder sign—dilated bowel loops, string of beads sign, candy cane appearance, stretch sign (completely encircling of bowel lumen by volvulae conniventes). In small bowel obstruction, the dilated small bowel loops are placed in the center of the abdomen, unlike large bowel loops which are peripheral.

33. **A-T, B-T, C-T, D-F, E-F**
Annular pancreas is due to persistence of two ventral buds or adherence of the remnant ventral bud to duodenum.

34. **A-T, B-F, C-T, D-F, E-T**
Common cause is a blunt injury crushing duodenum against vertebra or deceleration force. Intramural haematoma usually managed conseratively, perforation managed surgically. Because of retroperitoneal location, clinical diagnosis is difficult.
Endoscopic perforation is due to rupture from the scope or sphincterotomy. If small, it managed conservatively. Fluid and air are seen around the duodenum in CT scan.

35. **A-T, B-T, C-T, D-F, E-T**
Extravasation of oral contrast can be seen in retroperitoneum.

36. **A-T, B-F, C-F, D-T, E-T**
Villous adenomoas are more malignant than tubular adenomas. Adenocarcinoma is the most common primary malignant tumour in duodenum. Leiomyoma is the most common benign tumour. Lipoma and paraganglioma are less common benign tumours. Lymphoma is associated with HIV, celiac disease and parasitic infestation.
Colon, ovary and melanoma produce metastasis to duodenum.

37. **A-T, B-T, C-F, D-F, E-T**
Giant duodenal ulcer is more than 2 cm and is exclusively seen in the bulb, sometimes replacing the entire bulb. Retraction and scarring of bulb during healing occurs asymmetrically and the uninvolved portions will balloon out producing pseudodiverticula. This gives the characteristic trifoil or cloverleaf or jockey cap deformity of head. Barium has 80-90% sensitivity in detecting bleeding site. Endoscopy has higher sensitivity. Pyloric channel ulcers are treated as gastric ulcers and management is similar to gastric ulcer.

38. **A-T, B-F, C-T, D-T, E-T**
Tumour < 2 cm is likely to be benign. 65% of tumours are asymptomatic. Desmoplastic reaction produces extensive fibrosy can be vascular in angiography.

39. A-F, B-T, C-T, D-F, E-T

40. A-T, B-T, C-T, D-T, E-T
Peritoneal implants, tuberculosis and mesothelioma are other causes.

41. A-T, B-F, C-T, D-T, E-F
Crohn's disease-relapse of symptoms after prolonged quiesence and late development of stricture, mass and obstruction are suggestive of obstruction. It is more common in males and seen in terminal ileum, the tumours occurring ten years earlier than in non Crohn's patients. Duodenal diverticulum, Meckel's diverticulum, duplication, heterotopias all show increased incidence of small bowel cancer.

42. A-T, B-F, C-F, D-F, E-F
GI bleeding is due to ulceration of the ectopic gastric mucosa. Occurs in 2% of population. Pertechnate will pick up only the gastric mucosa, not bleeding. It is usually symptomatic in children, especially less than 2 years, but it is asymptomatic in adults.

43. A-T, B-F, C-T, D-T, E-T
Liver metastasis will continue to secrete gastrin and increases gastric secretion.

44. A-T, B-T, C-T, D-T, E-T
Bleeding is a common complication.

45. A-F, B-F, C-F, D-F, E-F
Excretion depends on the presence of ectopic gastric mucosa in the Meckel's diverticulum and not on the presence of parietal cells. Uptake is seen at the same time as that in stomach, in the right lower quadrant. No irritative procedures such as enema, endoscopy, cathartics, contrast studies and drugs, should be carried out within 48 hours of the procedure. Fasting increases the quality of image, due to decreased gastric secretion and peristalsis. Images are obtained every 5-10 minutes for one hour.

46. A-T, B-F, C-T, D-T, E-F
Glucagon decreases peristalsis. Cimetidine inhibitis secretion. Pentagastrin stimulates uptake. Atropine decreases uptake.

47. A-T, B-T, C-F, D-T, E-T
Ribbon bowel is featureless small bowel with effacement of folds. It is also seen in celiac disease, radiation, ischemia and lymphoma are other causes.

48. A-T, B-T, C-T, D-T, E-T
All the above disease produce thickening of bowel wall or mesenteric mass, which occupy the aortomesenteric angle. Metastasis and lymphadenopathy are other common causes.

49. A-T, B-T, C-F, D-F, E-T

0.25% have common splenic, hepatic and superior mesenteric artery. Two percent have the arc of Bühler which is an anastomosis between celiac, common hepatic or splenic artery and superior mesenteric artery, representing persistent ventral longitudinal anastomosis.

50. A-T, B-T, C-T, D-T, E-T

Crohn's etiology is still uncertain, infection, inflammation and immune-related etiologies proposed. It is common in Caucasians, with Jews having three times normal incidence.
Familial association seen in 2-5%.

51. A-T, B-T, C-F, D-T, E-T

Inflammation is transmural. Affects all the layers.

52. A-T, B-F, C-T, D-F, E-T

Stool culture is negative in Yersinia, but serum agglutination tests are very helpful to make the diagnosis. Reactive arthritis is a recognised feature. Antibiotics produce pseudomembranous colitis and is commonly due to *Clostridium difficile*.

53. A-T, B-F, C-T, D-T, E-F

Inferior mesenteric vein commonly drains into the splenic vein, but 30% each drain into the SMV and the SMV-splenic vein confluence. Left gastric vein usually (65%) drains into the confluence, but can drain into splenic V (15%), portal V (25%). Right gastric V drains into main or left portal vein intrahepatic portal venous branch, which causes a perfusion defect in CT arterioportography or triple phase helical CT.
The anterior and posteroinferior pancreaticoduodenal veins drain into the superior mesenteric vein.

54. A-T, B-T, C-T, D-T, E-T

The right psoas muscle is another structure that lies posterior to mesentery.

55. A-T, B-F, C-T, D-T, E-F

Yersinia is a gram negative bacillus. Ulceration is superficial, differential diagnosis is TB, Crohn's, radiation and lymphoma.

56. A-T, B-T, C-T, D-T, E-F

Talc causes adhesive peritonitis and heparin causes haemorrhage.

57. A-T, B-T, C-T, D-T, E-T

Scleroderma is the most common cause. Communicating ileal duplication can cause pseudodiverticula.

58. A-T, B-T, C-T, D-F, E-T
Yersinia, Shigella are other causes.

59. A-T, B-T, C-T, D-T, E-F
NSAIDs and carcinomas are other causes.

60. A-T, B-T, C-T, D-F, E-T

61. A-T, B-T, C-T, D-T, E-T
Aortoenteric fistula can affect any part of bowel. Third part of the duodenum is the most common site due to the proximity with the abdominal aorta. Secondary type, due to surgical repair is more common than primary types. Endoscopy is limited by pooling of blood in the lumen. CT is very sensitive and demonstrates aneurysm, perianeurysmal haematoma, extravastation of contrast, air in aorta and focal duodenal thickening.

62. A-F, B-T, C-F, D-F, E-F
Majority of duodenal tumours involve the second or third part. Almost 25-40% of small bowel tumours occur in the duodenum. Duodenal lymphoma is more extensive than carcinoma, but intestinal obstruction is less common. Aneurysmal dilatation is seen either due to lymphoma or leiomyosarcoma. Concentric ring sign in MRI in duodenum is specific for haematoma.

63. A-T, B-T, C-T, D-T, E-T
Cirrhosis causes ascites, which separates the bowel loops. Inflammation, infection, tumours, deposits, ascites and extrinsic masses are causes for separation of bowel loops.

64. A-T, B-T, C-T, D-T, E-T
Nodular lymphoid hyperplasia, lymphangiectasia and Whipple's are other causes.

65. A-T, B-T, C-T, D-T, E-F
Bands, atresia, stenosis, annular pancreas, superior mesenteric artery syndrome (Wilkinson, nutcracker syndrome), paralytic ileus due to pancreatitis, scleroderma.

66. A-T, B-T, C-T, D-T, E-F
Thickened folds are: Inflammatory—duodenitis, pancreatitis, Zollinger-Ellison syndrome; Crohn's disease; Infection—tapeworm, hookworm, strongyloides, giardiasis; Infiltrative—amyloidosis, eosinophilic enteritis, mastocytosis, Whipple's Vascular— haematoma, ischemia; Edema—lymphatic obstruction, venous obstruction, hypoproteinemia, Tumours—lymphoma, metastasis.

67. **A-T, B-F, C-F, D-T, E-T**
   Causes of protein losing enteropathy are CA stomach/colon, leukemia/lymphoma, celiac disease, tropical sprue, Whipple's disease, Crohn's disease, ulcerative colitis, radiotherapy, retroperitoneal fibrosis, cirrhosis, IVC thrombosis, villous adenoma.

68. **A-F, B-T, C-F, D-F, E-F**
   In visceral neuropathy there is no peristalsis. But in visceral myopathy, nonpropulsive contractions are seen.

69. **A-F, B-T, C-T, D-F, E-F**
   Carcinoid causes right heart lesions such as tricuspid regurgitation and pulmonary stenosis. The flushing is exacerbated by food and alcohol.

70. **A-T, B-T, C-T, D-F, E-F**
   Thickened, irregular folds in small bowel are seen in
   A. Inflammatory—Crohn's disease, Zollinger-Ellison syndrome
   B. Infections—Tuberculosis, Giardiasis, Strongyloidosis
   C. Inflitrative—Amyloidosis, eosinophilic enteritis, Whipple's disease, mastocytosis.

71. **A-T, B-T, C-T, D-F, E-T**
   Complete resolution occurs in 2-6 weeks and mechanical small bowel obstruction occurs. There is no prominent spasm and irritability. Picket fencing and thumbprinting are seen in ischemic colitis.

72. **A-T, B-F, C-T, D-T, E-T**
   Henoch-Schönlein purpura, idiopathic thrombocytopenic purpura, DIC, haemophilia, trauma, ischemia, leukemia, lymphoma and multiple myeloma.

73. **A-F, B-T, C-T, D-F, E-F**
   Critical dose is 4500 rad and it takes 1-2 years for the changes to take place. The incidence is 5% and it increases with pelvic surgery, especially in cervical, ovarian, endometrial and bladder cancers. Obstruction is common due to strictures. Mesentery shows increased density in CT scans. The bowel loops are separated, fixed, with thickened walls and serrated margin.

74. **A-T, B-F, C-T, D-T, E-T**
   Appendicitis is not a common cause of obstruction in adults.

75. **A-T, B-T, C-T, D-F, E-F**
   Causes of small bowel strictures are adhesions, Crohn's, tuberculosis, radiation, ischemia,tumours (carcinoma, lymphoma, sarcoma, carcinoid, metastasis) and enteric coated potassium tablets.

76. **A-T, B-T, C-F, D-F, E-T**
    The small bowel is dilated and measures more than 3 cm. Painless, transient intussusception is seen in fluoroscopy. Mucosal folds are thickened, if there is associated edema.

77. **A-T, B-F, C-T, D-T, E-F**
    There are many theories of formation of celiac disease. It is believed to be autosomal dominant disease with incomplete penetrance. The common mechanism is consumption of rice, which has gluten, rich in glutamine and gliadin polypeptides associated with the absence of a specific peptidase in mucosa which fails to hydrolyse the gluten peptides into simpler peptides. Gluten can also cause immunological reactions in the mucosa. After using a gluten-free diet, there will be clinical, histological and biochemical improvement.

78. **A-T, B-T, C-F, D-T, E-T**
    It is used in the early postoperative period to differentiate ileus from mechanical obstruction.

79. **A-T, B-T, C-F, D-F, E-T**
    Single contrast—18% w/v—800-1200 ml—75 ml/min. Double contrast—85-100%—200 ml with 1-2 l of 0.5% methylcellulose. Radiation dose is less than 1.5-2 mSv which is less than 8 mSv for CT abdomen.

80. **A-T, B-F, C-T, D-F, E-T**
    Normal luminal diameters—Upper jejunum < 4 cm, Lower jejunum < 3.5 cm, Ileum < 3 cm; Normal fold thickness—Jejunum <2.5 mm, ileum < 2 mm; Normal number of folds in jejunum 4-6 folds/inch, Ileum 2-3 folds/inch.

81. **A-F, B-F, C-F, D-T, E-F**
    Dermatomyositis is indistinguishable radiologically from sclero-derma. Sprue-normal motility, dilation more in midjejunum, increased secretions and segmentation. Colonic diverticula are seen in the antimesenteric side. Loss of haustration can be seen in scleroderma.

82. **A-T, B-F, C-F, D-F, E-F**
    Barium enema with reflux of contrast into the ileum is better in assessing terminal ileum than barium follow through. Celiac disease can be diagnosed only by biopsying the jejunal mucosa and imaging findings are nonspecific. Barium follow through can show tumours in the jejunum, but majority are found in the terminal ileum, a situation in which enteroclysis is better than follow through. Bowel prepration is required for enteroclysis.

83. **A-F, B-T, C-T, D-F, E-F**
    The normal transit time is 6 hours. Scleroderma, sprue, hypothyroidism, hypokalemia, atropine, opiates and phenothiazines are other causes. Tuberculosis and hyperthyroidism cause rapid transit.

84. **A-T, B-T, C-F, D-T, E-F**
    Meconium plug syndrome and colonic atresia are other causes.

85. **A-T, B-T, C-T, D-T, E-T**

86. **A-F, B-T, C-T, D-T, E-F**

87. **A-F, B-T, C-F, D-F, E-F**
    Malignant melanoma is characteristically known to ulcerate centrally producing the characteristic bulls eye appearance along with other submucosal lesions.

88. **A-T, B-T, C-F, D-F, E-F**
    Hide bound sign, indicates closely spaced, normal thickness folds in small bowel, within a dilated segment. Intussusception without lead point is common in scleroderma.

89. **A-T, B-T, C-F, D-F, E-T**

90. **A-T, B-T, C-T, D->, E-F**
    Almost 2-3% incidence of gastric carcinoma 13% incidence of breast carcinoma.
    GI bleed is seen in 30% and 25% incidence of adenomatous polyps in stomach.

91. **A-T, B-T, C-T, D-F, E-T**
    Villous polyps secrete potassium producing hypokalemia.

92. **A-F, B-T, C-F, D-T, E-F**
    The haustral pattern is lost in Crohn's disease in later stages. Increased density in mesenteric fat is due to inflammation. Anorectal region is involved in 35% of Crohn's disease, 67% of those with colonic disease and 25% of those with small intestinal disease. Rose thorn ulcer is a deep ulcer. Sinus tracts, tissues, fistulas, pseudopolyps, abscesses, strictures, sacculation and haustration loss are late features. Cobblestoning is produced due to coalescence of ulcers to form a network of longitudinal linear ulcers with intervening normal mucosa.

93. **A-T, B-T, C-T, D-T, E-T**
    Skin is the most common site of Kaposi's sarcoma and occurs before visceral involvement. MAI causes proximal small bowel thickening, resembling Whipple's disease.

94. **A-F, B-T, C-T, D-T, E-T**
There is increased incidence of carcinoma esophagus, pharynx, duodenum, rectum and jejunum.

95. **A-T, B-T, C-T, D-T, E-F**
NHL causes thick folds, Hodgkin's dose not.

96. **A-T, B-T, C-T, D-F, E-T**
NHL causes thickened folds but Hodgkin's does not.

97. **A-T, B-F, C-F, D-F, E-T**
The common locations of tuberculosis in the appropriate order are, ileocaecal region, ileum, caecum, ascending colon, jejunum, colon, rectum duodenum, stomach, esophagus. It is usually seen in 15-30 year group. 25% of cases with active advanced pulmonary disease have GIT tuberculosis. Caseating granulomas are seen.

98. **A-F, B-F, C-F, D-T, E-F**
Angiography has higher sensitivity for detecting upper GI haemorrhage. Tc sulphur colloid is not useful in upper GI haemorrhage due to background uptake in liver and spleen. Tc labelled RBCs are very useful for detecting upper GI haemorrhage. Gallium scans are not useful in GI bleeding.

99. **A-F, B-T, C-T, D-F, E-F**

100. **A-T, B-F, C-F, D-F, E-T**
Bleeding must be active at the time of tracer administration. The tracer has a half-life in the blood for 3.5 min, because of clearance by reticuloendothelial cells. It is not useful in upper GI bleed because of uptake in liver and spleen. Images are acquired every 5 sec for one minute, 60 sec images at 2, 5, 10, 15, 20, 30, 40, 60 min. Usually, study is terminated if no abnormality is seen at 30 minutes. Delayed images can be taken at 2, 4, 6, 12 hours.

101. **A-F, B-T, C-F, D-F, E-F**
Coarse granular pattern, linear ulcers along the mesenteric border, apthrous ulcers, fold thickening and inflammatory polyps are seen in early stages. The distribution is in a skip pattern with intervening normal areas. Cobblestone pattern is produced due to alternating inflamed and normal mucosa. Strictures, abscesses and fistula are seen in later stages.
Small bowel alone involved in 20%, large bowel alone in 20% and both in 60%. Upper GIT involved in 5-10%.

102. **A-T, B-T, C-F, D-T, E-F**
It stays for a longer time in the blood pool than the sulphur colloid. It is not very useful in localising the bleeding site, because of the rapid transit time of the isotope. Images are acquired every

2 seconds for 60 seconds, static images at 2, 5 minutes and then every five minutes till 30 minutes and every 10 min till 90 min. Delayed images at 2, 4, 6, 12, 24, 36 hours. Target to background ratio is low due to uptake in a lot of structures such as liver, spleen, kidneys, stomach and colon.

103. **A-T, B-T, C-T, D-F, E-F**

104. **A-F, B-F, C-T, D-F, E-F**
Located within 2 feet of the ileocaecal junction, in the antimesenteric border of the ileum. It is seen in 2% of the population and is asymptomatic in 20-40%. Inverted Meckel's is seen in 20%, and is seen as elongated mass parallel to the long axis of ileum.

105. **A-F, B-F, C-F, D-F, E-F**
Also seen in other conditions producing increased bood pool such as hemangioma, AVM, aneurysm and vascular tumours. Ectopic gastric mucosa are seen in a variety of other conditions such as duplication cyst, Barrett's esophagus and normal small bowel. Volvulus, intussusception, duodenal ulcer, Crohn's disease and appendicitis.

106. **A-F, B-T, C-F, D-F, E-F**
Rupture is usually localized, not generalized. Appendiculolith is the only reliable sign of acute appendicitis. Mass indenting the caecum, scoliosis with concavity to the right side, blurring of the psoas outline and widening of properitoneal line are other recognised plain X-ray features of acute appendicitis. Air in appendix is not reliable and is also seen in normal population, large bowel obstruction and paralytic ileus.

107. **A-T, B-T, C-T, D-T, E-T**
About 50% of tumours more than 1 cm and 95% of tumours more than 2 cm, metastasise, hence all carcinoids are considered malignant until proved otherwise. Tumours more than 1 cm are usually managed by bowel resection and less than 1 cm, require only local excision. 75% of carcinoids in appendix are benign. Desmoplastic reaction is extensive fibrotic reaction in the soft tissue and results in bowel kinking, adhesions and obstruction.

108. **A-F, B-T, C-T, D-T, E-F**
Normal appendix visualised in 4-64% of patients. Appendix diameter > 6 mm, noncompressibility, round shape in cross section, fluid inside lumen, absence of gas, fat inflammation, nodes, cecal wall thickening, hyperemia in Doppler are other findings.

109. **A-T, B-T, C-F, D-F, E-T**
Nodules are seen in lymphoid hyperplasia, lymphoma, metastasis (melanoma, breast, ovary), mastocytosis, polyposis, pseudopoly-

posis, Whipple's, Waldenström's macroglobulinemia, infection (typhoid and yersinia) and inflammatory (Crohn's).

110. **A-T, B-T, C-T, D-T, E-F**
Nodular lymphoid hyperplasia is characterized by small 2-4 mm nodules without fold thickening in the terminal ileal region. This is usually associated with hypogammaglobulinemia. This is normally seen in children and in adults it may be an earlier sign of Crohn's disease. This is also associated with malabsorption and infections such as giardiasis, strongyloides and moniliasis.

111. **A-T, B-F, C-F, D-T, E-F**
Adhesions contribute to 60% of small bowel obstruction. Adhesion is a diagnosis of exclusion, and is not visualized in CT scan images. It can be seen as an abrupt tapering of the bowel caliber. Internal hernias are usually congenital, not acquired.

112. **A-F, B-T, C-T, D-T, E-T**
The most common tumour in small bowel is metastasis and the most common primary tumour is carcinoid (varies with the series, adenocarcinoma is the most common in some series). Lung tumour and malignant melanoma are common causes of submucosal metastasis to small bowel.

113. **A-T, B-F, C-T, D-T, E-F**
Colon and ovary are other common causes.

114. **A-F, B-F, C-F, D-T, E-T**
Up to 50% of appendiceal neoplasms present as appendicitis. The most common neoplasm is mucin-producing tumour. Mucocele is a descriptive term for a lesion with abundant mucin and this can be produced by benign or malignant or non-neoplastic disease. Other presentations include obstruction, intussusception and abdominal mass.

115. **A-T, B-T, C-T, D-T, E-F**

116. **A-F, B-F, C-F, D-T, E-F**
Mucin can be found even in benign adenomas. Histologically, there should be neoplastic infiltration to diagnose malignancy. Carcinoids are found before 50 years. Colonic type adenocarcinomas are uncommon. Mucoceles are not formed in these lesions. Dense opacities inside the mucocele is not due to infection, but due to myxoglobosis, which has calcified spherules.

117. **A-F, B-T, C-F, D-T, E-T**
Normally, there are more than 5 folds per inch of jejunum and 2-4 folds per inch of ileum.

In celiac disease, the number of jejunal folds are decreased. Four-folds are nondiagnostic. Three and less are indicative. Ileal folds are increased to 4-6 folds per inch. The folds are thickened and measure more than 1 mm. There is increased fluid inside the lumen. Development of abdominal pain, weight loss, malabsorption, bleeding, obstruction, perforation haemorrhage in a patient with good response to gluten-free diet, indicates lymphomatous development. It is usually T cell type. The lymphoma can appear after or with the development of celiac disease.

118. **A-T, B-T, C-T, D-T, E-T**
Up to 20% of those with appendiceal Crohn's have Crohn's disease elsewhere in the bowel. Appendicolith is 1-4 cm and is made up of inspissated feces and calcium salts around vegetable matter. Graded compression sonography is used for diagnosing appendicitis. In appendicitis, the appendix is inflamed and measures more than 6 mm and is not compressible.

119. **A-T, B-T, C-T, D-T, E-T**
Appendiceal carcinoma, carcinoid, endometrioma, polyp, volvulus and caecal carcinoma are other recognized causes of volvulus.

120. **A-F, B-T, C-T, D-F, E-T,F-F**
Splenic atrophy and not splenomegaly. There is diabetes mellitus, not hypoglycemia.

121. **A-T, B-T,C-F, D-T, E-F**
Scleroderma is a common cause of megaduodenum. Bacterial overgrowth in scleroderma is called pseudobacterial overgrowth. Pseudodiverticula have characteristic wide necks.
Stricture is often the end result of esophageal involvement in scleroderma. Small bowel transit time can be increased up to 24 hours due to slow peristalsis.

122. **A-T, B-T, C-T, D-T, E-T**

123. **A-T, B-F, C-T, D-T, E-F**
There is increased association with primary sclerosing cholangitis and primary bilary cirrhosis. In celiac disease, the number of jejunal folds is decreased and ileal folds are increased. After treatment, if there is good response, the number of jejunal folds is increased, but the ileal folds will not decrease. If there is no response, the jejunal folds will not increase, but the ileal folds increase for compensating. Moulage sign is smooth elongated clumps of flocculated barium. Mosaic pattern is barium seen in grooves 1-3 mm apart. It is seen in barium and in endoscopy.

124. A-F, B-T, C-T, D-F, E-T
Sensitivity of isotope scan is 85% and specificity is 95%. Gastric, pancreatic and colonic tissue may be seen.

125. A-T, B-T, C-T, D-F, E-T
Lodgement in stomach is called Bouveret syndrome.

126. A-T, B –T, C-F, D-F, E-F
Bouveret's syndrome is migration of gallstone into stomach and duodenum, with resultant gastric outlet obstruction.

127. A-F, B-T, C-F, D-F,E-T
Bowel obstruction makes up for 20% of those who are admitted for acute abdomen in a surgical unit. Eighty percent of the obstruction occurs at the level of small bowel and a majority of them (70%) are due to surgical adhesions as sequelae of previous laparotomies. CT scan and plain X-ray have almost equal sensitivities for the diagnosis of small bowel obstruction. However, CT is more useful in finding out the cause and severity of the obstruction.

128. A-F, B-T, C-T, D-F, E-T

129. A-F, B-F, C-T, D-T, E-T
Aneurysmal dilatation is due to destruction of the autonomic nerves in the infiltrative type and is common in the antimesenteric border, whereas the cavitation is more common in the endo-exenteric type of lymphoma. Sandwich sign is due to engulfment of mesenteric vessels by enlarged lymphomatous lesions. Cobble-stone pattern is due to multiple lymphomatous nodules.

130. A-T, B-F, C-F, D-F, E-T
Fleischner's sign—also called inverted umbrella sign, is due to thickening of ileocaecal valve, producing a broad-based triangular shape with base towards the caecum.
Sterling's sign—due to extreme irritability of the ulcerated portion of the terminal ileum, there is nonretention of barium in the inflamed segment, with normal column of barium on either side. Nodes are common in the mesentery, but are also seen in the retroperitoneum. It also affects the nodes in the mesenteric root, porta hepatis, celiac and peripancreatic region depending on the segment of bowel affected.
Lymph nodes are of low density due to central ceasation necrosis. Ascites is very dense.

131. A-T, B-T, C-T, D-T, E-T

132. A-T, B-T, C-T, D-F, E-F
Ileo ileo colic type has more edema and usually has a lead point. Presence of lead point indicates poor success rate and early

recurrence indicates the presence of a lead point as the etiology. Palpable mass, vomiting, pain and viral illness are not bad predictors.

133. **A-F, B-F, C-F, D-F, E-F**
Littre's hernia contain Meckel's diverticulum. Richter's hernia is entrapment and ischemia of antimesenteric border of bowel. Spigelian hernia occurs through semicircular line, which is lateral to the rectus abdominis muscle. Femoral hernia is more common in females, but inguinal hernia is still the most common hernia in females. Anterior perineal hernia is through a defect in the urogenital membrane and the posterior hernia occurs through a defect in levator ani.

134. **A-T, B-T, C-T, D-T, E-F**
Ovarian lesions such as abscess and cystic neoplasm, duplication cyst and abscess are common differential diagnosis. Infiltration of fat is another indicator of malignancy. Gas bubbles can be seen inside when there is superinfection and this will produce clinical symptoms of acute appendicitis.

135. **A-F, B-F, C-F, D-T, E-F**
Internal hernias account for 1% of mechanical small bowel obstruction. The most common location is paraduodenal region. It is more common in the right side, where it occurs lateral to the 4th portion of duodenum and behind transverse and descending mescolon (Landzert fossa). In the left side (fossa of Waldeyer), it happens caudal to superior mesenteric artery and inferior to third portion of duodenum. The lesser sac hernia (foramen of Winslow) and ileal loops are common than the jejunal loops.

136. **A-T, B-T, C-T, D-F, E-T**
Features of advanced Crohn's are fissures, pseudopolyps, cobblestoning, ulcernodular pattern, large flat ulcers, bowel wall thickening and progression of disease. Strictures produce the string sign of Kantor, and this has to be differentiated from simple spasm in an inflamed area. Fistulas can be enterocolic, the most common between transverse colon and duodenum, enterocutaneous and enterovesical. Perforations are very rare in Crohn's because fissures deepen slowly and adhesions form.

137. **A-F, B-T, C-F, D-F, E-T**
Whipple's disease is caused by *Tropheryma whippeli*, a gram-positive organism. It is characterized by presence of PAS positive, material in the foamy macrophages in the submucosa os small bowel. It is eight times common in males. Arthritis precedes intestinal disease in 10%. Generalised lymphadenopathy is seen in 50%.

138. A-F, B-F, C-F, D-T, E-T
Radiological features are—no dilation of small bowel, moderately thickened but not rigid folds, nodules, hypersecretion, fragmentation, segmentation, normal transit time, hepatosplenomegaly.

139. A-T, B-T, C-F, D-T, E-T
More common in males by a ratio of 2:1.

140. A-F, B-T, C-F, D-F, E-T
Angiography—0.5 ml/min
Tc labelled RBC—0.35 ml/min
Tc sulfur colloid—0.05-0.1 ml/min
Tc pertechnate—does not depend on the rate of bleeding
Angio has a sensitivity of 65% for upper GI and 40% for lower GI bleed.

141. A-T, B-T, C-F, D-F, E-T
As the name implies, tropical sprue occurs in the tropics, has epidemic and endemic forms. Believed to be caused by infection (*E. coli*) or toxin or nutritional deficiency. Tetracycline or sulpha drugs and folate for one month cure the disease. There is a uniform distribution in small bowel unlike celiac disease which is more common in the proximal bowel. The small bowel is dilated with thick folds and flocculation of barium.

142. A-T, B-F, C-F, D-T, E-T
Hyperparathyroidism, adrenal insufficiency and carcinoid are other metabolic/endocrine disorders producing malabsorption.

143. A-T, B-T, C-T, D-F, E-F
Other causes are enterogenous cyst and meconium impaction.

144. A-T, B-T, C-T, D-T, E-F
In early stages there is lymphoid hyperplasia, villi thickening and aphthous ulcers, which will be seen as thick, regular folds, coarse villous pattern and 1-3 mm bulls eye ulcers surrounded by halo respectively. In intermediate stage, there is submucosal edema—thumb printing, stellate or rose thorn ulcers, thickening/sclerosis/retraction of mesentery and long linear ulcers along mesenteric border. The mesenteric side is more commonly involved in the disease and hence the unaffected antimesenteric side bulges when there is increase in intraluminal pressure.

145. A-F, B-F, C-F, D-F, E-F
Whipple's—PAS positive macrophages: Abetalipoproteinemia-Normal villi, vacuolation.
Lymphangiectasia—dilated lacteals, villi clubbing. Agammaglobulinemia—absent plasma cells, high lymphocytes, flat or absent villi;

amyloidosis—proteins; Regional enteritis—noncaseating granulomas. Eosinophilic enteritis—eosinophilic infiltrate; Mastocytosis—mast cells, lymphoma—malignant cells. Other diseases have nonspecific appearance with short villi or atrophied villi. Scleroderma—fibrosis around Brunner's gland. Collagen sprue—marked collagen deposition.

146. A-T, B-F, C-F, D-T, E-T

In normal small intestine, less than 10^4 bacteria are seen/ml of aspirin. Most of these are aerobic bacteria. The protective factors that prevent bacterial overgrowth are acidic stomach contents, peristalsis, mucous layer, rapid turnover of enterocytes (2-4 days), immunoglobulins and intact ileocaecal wall. Any factor that causes stasis, increased bacterial entry due to impaired gastric acid output or abnormal sources of bacteria or immunodeficiency are risk factors for development of bacterial overgrowh. Sugar malabsorption is also seen since bacteria destroy disaccharidase and decreased absorption of amino acids are seen. B_{12} deficiency is caused by bacterial consumption. $> 10^5$/ml is diagnostic, anaerobes are common.

147. A-T, B-F, C-F, D-F, E-T

GIT is involved in 70% of primary and 55% of secondary amyloidosis. Micronodules, polyps, large nodules, fold thickening, narrowed lumen and separated loops are other features. Malabsorption is seen in one-third of scleroderma. Other findings are hide bound sign, sacculations, pneumoperitoneum; in lymphangiectasia, there are thickened folds but the nodules are micronodular. In eosinophilia, stomach antrum is more commonly affected than small intestine. In small intestine, terminal ileum is commonly involved than proximal ileum. The disease can affect mucosa, muscular layer or serosa. In mucosal disease, there are nodules and thickened folds, especially in the terminal ileum. In muscular disease, there is thickened wall. In serosal disease, serosa is thickened with intact mucosa. Primary idiopathic pseudo-obstruction is diagnosed after excluding mechanical obstruction, ileus and secondary pseudo-obstruction. In visceral neuropathy, myenteric plexus is damaged by drugs, chemicals and viruses. There are nonpropulsive contractions. But in visceral myopathy, there are aperistaltic loops.

148. A-F, B-F, C-F, D-T, E-T

Jejunal diverticulosis have mucosa and submucosa. It is seen in the mesenteric side where the vasa recti penetrate the wall. It usually involves a confined segment of the jejunum and the size progressively decreases when moving from the proximal to the distal small bowel. X-ray will show multiple fluid levels which may be mistaken for obstruction. Surgery is indicated if there is haemorrhage, obstruction, perforation, abscess and malabsorption. Also associated with pseudo-obstruction and vacuolation of jejunal musculature.

149. **A-T, B-T, C-T, D-T, E-T**
In lymphangiectasia, there is lymphatic obstruction from bowel to body resulting in decreased uptake of chylomicrons and fat-soluble vitamin. The high pressure in peripheral lymphatics results in leakage of lymph from gut surface to lumen and escape of chylomicrons, lymphocytes and proteins, producing hypoalbuminemia and lymphocytopenia. This can be a primary congenital obstruction or acquired. Other causes of acquired obstruction include Crohn's disease, congestive cardiatic failure, chronic pancreatitis and carcinoma.

150. **A-F, B-T, C-F, D-T, E-T**
With intact colon, only 50-70 cm of small bowel is required to sustain oral autonomy. With loss of colon, 150 cm of small bowel is required. When jejunum is lost, ileum can take over its function, unless TPN affects the adaptation. But the loss of ileum is metabolically irreplaceable, since the enterohepatic circulation is cut off. Vit B_{12} deficiency, hyperoaxaluria and calculi are the sequelae.

151. **A-T, B-T, C-T, D-T, E-T**
Chronic intestinal pseudo-obstruction can be primary or secondary. Other causes of secondary pseudo-obstruction include side-to-side anastomosis bypassed bowel, pouches, dermatomyositis, polymyositis, amyloidosis, Chagas' disease, diabetes, tricyclic antidepressants and NSAIDs.

152. **A-F, B-F, C-F, D-F, E-F**
Compresses the third, transverse portion of the duodenum.
The normal angle between SMA and aorta is 45-65 degrees and it is reduced to 10-20 in this condition.
The compression is worse when the patient is in the supine position and is relieved in the prone position.
A vertical linear compression defect is seen in the third part of the duodenum.
There is gross dilatation of the duodenum proximal to the level of compression and the distal portion is collapsed.

153. A-F, B-F, C-T, D-F, E-T
Weight loss, prolonged bedrest and exaggerated lumbar lordosis are recognised causes of superior mesenteric artery syndrome.

154. A-F, B-T, C-F, D-F, E-F
Small bowel cancers account for only 1% of all bowel cancers. The incidence of cancer is very low in small bowel due to a number of reasons, including, the high alakalinity, rapid transit, decreased mechanical trauma due to liquid content, low IgA level, low bacterial content, high benzopyrene hydroxylase activity in bowel wall and high small bowel epithelial cell turnover. Adenocarcinomas are most common in the duodenum (40%), followed by jejunum (38%) and ileum (22%). Malignant carcinoids are most common in the ileum (84%), jejunum (10%) and duodenum (6%). Leiomyosarcomas are most common in the ileum (53%), followed by jejunum (37%) and duodenum (10%). Lymphomas are most common in jejunum (48%), followed by ileum (36%), duodenum (16%).

155. A-T, B-T, C-T, D-T, E-T
Neurofibromatosis, celiac sprue, Crohn's, FAP, ileostomy and ileal conduit are all risk factors for adenocarcinoma. Nodular lymphoid hyperplasia, AIDS and celiac sprue are risk factors for lymphoma.

156. A-T, B-T, C-T, D-T, E-T
The differential diagnosis is sprue, in which there is marked dilatation of the small bowel, no fold thickening and marked segmentation and fragmentation.

157. A-T, B-T, C-T, D-F, E-F
String sign is a persistence of a narrow column of barium in the small bowel and indicates stricture. Enterolith is calcification in the bowel lumen, seen in 2-4% of cases, and is invariably proximal to stricture. The bowel wall thickening is circumferential and homogeneous in both ultrasound and CT. In malignancy, the thickening is variegated, along the mesenteric border in Crohn's disease. Heterogeneous opacity in a single lymph node group indicates tuberculosis. Lymphoma is more homogeneous.

158. A-F, B-F, C-T, D-F, E-F
Majority of bowel lymphomas are secondary. Bowel is involved in 10-20% of abdominal lymphomas. The four types are polypoidal, nodular, ulcerative and infiltrative of which polypoidal is the most common. Stomach is the most common site in the GIT followed by the small bowel and colon.

159. **A-F, B-F, C-T, D-T, E-F**
Carcinoid tumours are more common in appendix than in small bowel. Up to 95% of GIT carcinoids occur in the appendix, small intestine and rectum. Diarrhoea is the most common symptom, followed by flushing, asthma and pellagra. There are many chemical mediators producing carcinoid syndrome—flushing by bradykinin, diarrhoea by serotonin, telangiectasia by VIP, bronchospasm by bradykinin, endocardial fibrosis, hypotension and arthropathy by serotonin. There is increased excretion of 5 hydroxy indole acetic acid in urine, more than 50 mg/day (normal is 2-9 mg/day).

160. **A-T, B-T, C-T, D-T, E-F**

161. **A-T, B-F, C-T, D-T, E-T**
All carcinoid tumours do not produce carcinoid syndrome. The chemical mediators produced by carcinoid tumours will produce carcinoid syndrome, when the tumour drains directly into the systemic circulation such as from ovaries or from bronchi. The liver has monoamine oxidase, which can deactivate the serotonin and other mediators. In liver metastasis, the capacity of liver to deactivate these enzymes is often overcome and carcinoid syndrome is produced. Liver massage, Valsalva's maneuver, meals and sex are other factors which increase the occurrence of carcinoid syndrome. The tumours arise from enterochromatin cells situated at the base of crypts of Leiberkuhn. About 50% of colonic tumours metastasise, while one-third of small intestinal carcinoids metastasise.

162. **A-T, B-F, C-T, D-T, E-T**
Kinking of bowel loops, narrowing of bowel loops, annular mass, ridigity, fixation and stranges in soft tissue are other radiological features.

163. **A-F, B-F, C-T, D-F, E-F**
The most common cause of apple core deformity in small bowel is metastasis, especially from carcinoma colon, followed by adenocarcinomas. About 70% of duodenal tumours are polypoidal and 20% are ulcerative, 10% infiltrative. In jejunum and ileum, 75% of tumours are annular stenosing, usually involving a small segment, with overhanging edges, with mucosal ulcerations and proximal dilatation. The differential diagnosis will include Crohn's, radiation, benign stricture and benign ulcer, but none of these have overhanging edges. The strictures in metastasis are longer, with more pronounced narrowing and obstruction.

164. **A-T, B-F, C-F, D-T, E-T**
Nocturia—hypokalemia, delayed absorption of water, azotemia—fluid depletion, hypotension—electrolyte depletion, amenorrhea—protein depletion, secondary hypopituitarism, anemia—iron, folate, pyridoxine, B_{12}, Haemorrhage—vitamin K, Bone pain—vit D, tetany—calcium, magnesium, weakness—anemia, hypokalemia, osteoarthropathy, night blindness, xerophthalmia—A, peripheral neuropathy—B_6, purpura—K, hyperkeratosis—A.

165. **A-T, B-F, C-F, D-T, E-T**
In large bowel cancers, there is a direct relationship between the size of the tumour and the invasiveness; but in small bowel cancers, there is no direct relationship. Hence, a small tumour can be very invasive and a large tumour can be noninvasive. Lymph nodes are very bulky in lymphoma, but not in adenocarcinoma. Adenomas are most common in the periampullary region. A pain brush or lazy pattern is typical of villous adenoma, but seen only in one-third of cases. Villous adenomas are very prone for malignancy and 30% have associated cancers.

166. **A-F, B-T, C-T, D-T, E-T**
The segment which invaginates is called intussusceptum and the one into which it invaginates is called intussuscipiens. Other causes of lead points are lymphoid hyperplasia, lymphoma, polyps and other tumours.

167. **A-T, B-T, C-T, D-T, E-T**
Tumours are the most common cause.

168. **A-F, B-T, C-T, D-T, E-F**
Each attempt lasts 3 minutes, with a gap of three minutes in between the three attempts.
Maximum pressure is 120 mm Hg.

169. **A-F, B-F, C-F, D-T, E-F**
Higher intracolonic pressure is required for satisfactory reduction and the pressure is higher in air reduction than barium reduction. This is a faster technique with lesser radiation dose. The tears are small.

170. **A-F, B-T, C-F, D-F, E-F**
Onset more than 48 hours is contraindication. Perforation and gangrene are absolute contraindications. Obstruction is not a contraindication but success rate is low.

171. **A-F, B-T, C-F, D-T, E-T**
Majority are seen in the distal tip of the appendix and hence do not obstruct and appendicitis is very uncommon. Tumours larger

than 2 cm are considered malignant and require right hemico-
lectomy. They do not metastasise and hence carcinoid syndrome
is not seen.

172. **A-F, B-T, C-F, D-T, E-T**
Metastasis is the most common malignant tumour in the small
intestine. Adenocarcinomas constitute 25-50% of primary tumours,
lymphomas 10-25%, malignant carcinoid 15-40% and leiomyosarcoma 10-20%. In another series, malignant carcinoid accounted
for 41% of cases, adenocarcinoma 24%, lymphoma 22% and
sarcoma 11%.
It is multicentric in 20%. Infiltrative type is the most most common
type in small bowel. The other types are polypoidal, nodular,
endoexoenteric and mesenteric types.

173. **A-T, B-F, C-F, D-T, E-F**
It is very rare to find evidence of associated pulmonary tuberculosis. There are two types of lesions in the GIT. The ulcerative
form is more common than the hypertrophic type. Sterling's sign
is also seen in Crohn's disease. The ulcers are usually perpendicular to the axis of the intestine. They are parallel in typhoid.
Tuberculin skin test is often negative.
Although ileocaecal region is the most common site in the
gastrointestinal tract, tuberculous peritonitis is the most common
presentation in abdomen. Sterling sign—direct emptying of
terminal ileum into stenotic ascending colon without visualization
of fibrosed contractecd caecum.

174. **A-T, B-T, C-T, D-F, E-T**
Occasionally, peritoneal fluid can be seen within the wall of the
intussusception and indicates necrosis. Coiled spring pattern can
be seen in both barium follow through and enema procedure.

175. **A-T, B-T, C-F, D-T, E-T**

176. **A-T, B-F, C-T, D-F, E-T**
Scleroderma, Crohn's and ischemia are the three causes of
pseudosacculation.

177. **A-F, B-T, C-F, D-F, E-T**
Esophagus is more commonly involved than small intestine.
Involvement of small intestine and esophagus indicate rapid
progression of the disease. Dilated small bowel, especially duo-
denum and jejunum are common and do not indicate obstruction.
Abrupt cut off is seen at the superior mesenteric artery level.
Diverticula are seen due to smooth muscle atrophy.

4 *Large Bowel*

1. **Colon:**
   A. The proximal transverse colon is supplied by the right colic artery and the distal thirds by the left colic artery
   B. Both the superior and inferior mesenteric vessels supply the transverse colon
   C. The left limb of the sigmoid mesocolon lies lateral to the iliac vessels
   D. The right limb of sigmoid mesocolon extends up to S3
   E. Sigmoid colon drains into the inferior mesenteric nodes

2. **Best positions in the barium enema for the following structures:**
   A. Caecum—left anterior oblique
   B. Hepatic flexure—left anterior oblique erect
   C. Splenic flexure—right anterior oblique erect
   D. Sigmoid—prone
   E. Rectum—lateral

3. **Colon:**
   A. There are three bands of taenia
   B. Taenia are condensations of the longitudinal muscle layer of colon
   C. Appendices epiploicae are prominently seen in the caecum
   D. Haustrations are not complete
   E. Haustrae are caused by the taenia

4. **Arterial supply to the rectum:**
   A. Median sacral artery from aorta
   B. Superior rectal artery from superior mesenteric artery
   C. Middle rectal artery from inferior mesenteric artery
   D. Inferior rectal artery from internal pudendal artery
   E. Lateral sacral artery

5. **Colon:**
   A. The iliohypogastric nerve lies posterior to the ascending colon
   B. The ascending colon is intraperitoneal
   C. Transverse colon measures 25 cm
   D. Transverse colon is attached to the stomach by the gastrocolic ligament
   E. The hepatic flexure is attached to the diaphragm by the phrenicocolic ligament

6. **Rectum:**
   A. Rectum has no haustrations
   B. The middle third of the rectum is covered by peritoneum in the front and the sides
   C. The rectal ampulla lies on the pelvic diaphragm
   D. The rectal ampulla is convex to the right side
   E. The rectum has three Houston valves, two the left and one on the right side

7. **Relations of rectum:**
   A. The rectum is related directly to the uterus anteriorly in the females
   B. The pelvic fascia encloses the anteriorly placed seminal vesicles and ductus deferens in males
   C. Sigmoid colon is seen anteriorly in the upper two-thirds
   D. Lower third of rectum is related to vagina in females
   E. Sacral plexus is seen in the posterior aspect of rectum in both males only

8. **Normal constrictions seen in the colon:**
   A. Rossi—just before splenic flexure
   B. Peyerstrauss—rectosigmoid junction
   C. Busci—midtransverse colon
   D. Moulgi—sigmoid descending colon
   E. Balli—proximal descending clolon

9. **Anal canal:**
   A. The puborectal sling angles the anal canal forwards
   B. Anus has up to 10 horizontal anal columns
   C. The valves of ball join the lower end of anal folds
   D. Hilton's line is a demarcation between the arterial and venous supply between the upper and lower parts of rectum
   E. The part of rectum above Hilton's line drains into systemic venous system

10. **Defecation proctography:**
    A. At rest, the anorectal junctions, is at the level of ischial tuberosities
    B. During evacuation the pelvic floor descends at least 50 mm
    C. Anorectal angle decreases from 120-90 degrees on defaecation
    D. Hirschsprung's disease is an indication
    E. Not useful when patient has fecal incontinence

11. **Anal sphincters:**
    A. The internal and external sphincters overlap in the middle third of the rectum
    B. Internal sphincter is thicker posteriorly
    C. Musculus submucosus ani is condensation of the longitudinal muscle layer of anus
    D. The superficial external sphincter is attached to the perineal body
    E. The deep external sphincter merges with the puborectalis

12. **Anterior relations of anal canal in a male:**
    A. Anococcygeal body
    B. Perineal body
    C. Urogenital diaphragm
    D. Penis
    E. Urethra

13. **Barium enema:**
    A. Use of balloon retention catheter increases risk of perforation
    B. Perforation by a balloon is more apparent when the balloon is fully inflated
    C. Endotoxic shock results from barium perforation
    D. Barium perforation requires resection of perforated segment
    E. Ureteric obstruction is a sequelae of barium perforation

14. **The following structures posterior to the descending colon:**
    A. Left kidney
    B. Left adrenal
    C. Lateral cutaneous nerve of the thigh
    D. Transverses abdominus
    E. Quadratus lumborum

15. **Barium enema:**
    A. Antibiotic prophylaxis is indicated for high risk patients
    B. Cefuroxime is the routinely used antibiotic
    C. Transient bacteremia occurs only in those with colonic disease
    D. Glucagon is contraindicated in cardiac conditions
    E. Air in portal vein during procedure indicates bad prognosis

16. **Barium enema:**
    A. According to present guidelines, antibiotic prophylaxis is not indicated
    B. If antibiotics are used, it is not required after procedure
    C. Plain X-ray should be obtained if inadequate poor bowel preparation is suspected
    D. If buscopan is required, it should be given before the start of the procedure only
    E. If caecum is not visualized properly, postevacuation film should be performed

17. **Barium enema:**
    A. Cardiac arrhythmia is the most common cause of death
    B. Pre-existing heart disease increases risk of arrhythmia
    C. ECG changes of arrhythmia occurs most commonly in the post-evacuation phase
    D. After biopsy, a gap of at least five days should be given for barium enema
    E. Barium column should not be elevated to more than 1 m from table top

18. **The following views are best for the corresponding views of large bowel:**
    A. LAO—hepatic flexure
    B. Supine 45 degree caudal angulation—sigmoid colon
    C. Head up—caecum
    D. Lateral wall of descending colon—left lateral decubitus
    E. Transverse colon—erect views

19. **Common causes of lead point in intussusception in adults:**
    A. Lipoma
    B. Typhoid
    C. Gastroenteritis
    D. Prolapsed gastric mucosa
    E. Ectopic pancreas

20. **Large bowel obstruction:**
    A. The critical diameter of caecum is 6 cm
    B. Transverse colon is the most dilated portion
    C. Gas fluid levels distal to the caecum is/are abnormal
    D. If both the colon and small bowel are dilated, it indicates incompetent ileocaecal valve
    E. Transverse colon is the most common portion involved in diaphragmatic hernia

21. **Barium enema—venous intravasation:**
    A. Patient is placed in head down position to treat intravasation
    B. Mortality with venous intravasation has a direct correlation with the amount of barium intravasated
    C. Once recognised, patient should be placed in the left lateral position
    D. The complication rate is higher when the barium extravasates into the portal sytem than systemic circulation
    E. High rectal tears will cause portal and low rectal tears cause systemic extravasation

22. **Gas fluid levels in colon are seen in:**
    A. Diarrhoea   B. Obstruction
    C. Cathartics   D. Enema
    E. Diverticulosis

23. **Contraindications for emergency barium enema:**
    A. Toxic megacolon
    B. Obstruction
    C. Portal venous gas
    D. Pneumatosis intestinalis
    E. Extraluminal gas

24. **X-ray abdomen:**
    A. Fluid levels after enema are small and multiple
    B. There is no significant bowel distension in high small bowel obstruction
    C. If there is gas seen beyond the obstruction, it indicates incomplete obstruction
    D. Majority of obstructing gallstones are calcified
    E. Air is seen in gallbladder and cystic duct in all cases of gallstone ileus

25. **X-ray abdomen:**
    A. Gas is seen in plain X-ray abdomen for 30 days after normal laparatomy
    B. Fluid levels are not seen in obstruction before 12 hours
    C. Large bowel fluid levels are shorter than those of small bowel
    D. Fluid levels are seen in uremia and hypokalemia
    E. In incompetent ileocaecal valve, fluid levels take longer time to develop

26. **Causes of toxic megacolon:**
    A. Ischemia   B. Tuberculosis
    C. Yersinia   D. Typhoid
    E. Pseudomembranous colitis

27. **Features of toxic megacolon:**
    A. Barium enema is diagnostic
    B. Pseudopolyps seen
    C. Pneumatosis coli
    D. Multiple air fluid levels
    E. Haustral loss

28. **Common causes of large bowel obstruction:**
    A. Mesenteric ischemia
    B. Acute pancreatitis
    C. Schistosomiasis
    D. LGV
    E. Diverticulitis

29. **Tc labelled RBCs:**
    A. Bleeding site confirms to bowel anatomy
    B. Progressively increased tracer accumulation with time
    C. The appearance progressively changes
    D. Not useful if the bleeding is less than 500 ml in 24 hours
    E. Glucagon is contraindicated during the procedure

30. **Extrinsic causes of large bowel obstruction:**
    A. Endometriosis
    B. Distended bladder
    C. Mesenteritis
    D. Bad colostomy
    E. Pelvic abscess

31. **Gastrointestinal tract:**
    A. In mesenteric angiography, the superior mesenteric artery should be examined first
    B. 500 ml of barium paste is used for evacuation proctography
    C. Anorectal incontinence is a contraindication of evacuation proctography
    D. A control film should always be obtained before performing sinogram
    E. Barium can be used for suspected large intestinal obstruction, if surgery is indicated

32. **Recognized associations:**
    A. Celiac disease and CA esophagus
    B. Crohn's disease and lymphoma
    C. Laxative abuse and melanosis coli
    D. Ulcerative colitis and renal calculi
    E. Lymphoid hyperplasia and lymphoma

33. Colon cut off sign is seen in:
    A. Mesenteric thrombosis
    B. Ischemic colitis
    C. Chronic pancreatitis
    D. Yersinia
    E. Obstruction

34. Common causes of rectal narrowing:
    A. Rectal ulcer
    B. Radiation
    C. Pelvic lipomatosis
    D. Ulcerative colitis
    E. Amoebiasis

35. Lesions in the pouch of Douglas:
    A. Chronic pelvic sepsis
    B. Endometriosis
    C. Internal iliac artery aneurysm
    D. Uterine tumour
    E. Chordoma

36. Large bowel strictures are seen in:
    A. Hirschsprung's disease
    B. Pericolic abscess
    C. Lymphoma
    D. Amoebiasis
    E. Distended bladder

37. Pseudopolyposis coli occurs in:
    A. Ulcerative colitis
    B. Crohn's disease
    C. Pneumatosis coli
    D. Hirschsprung's disease
    E. Celiac disease

38. Carpet lesions of colon:
    A. Rectal varices   B. Familial polyposis
    C. Colonic urticaria   D. Endometriosis
    E. Villous adenoma

39. Increased risk of malignancy in ulcerative colitis occurs:
    A. Females
    B. After 10 years
    C. Beginning in childhood
    D. Pancolitis
    E. Filiform pseudopolyps
    F. Sclerosing cholangitis

40. Ulcerative colitis and peripheral arthritis:
   A. Associated with HLA B27
   B. Improves with colectomy
   C. Nonerosive
   D. Severity parallels disease
   E. There is slight increase in incidence of rheumatoid arthritis

41. Familial polyposis coli associated with:
   A. Duodenal carcinoma
   B. Gastric hamartomas
   C. Always involves the rectum
   D. Autosomal recessive
   E. Associated with berry aneurysm

42. Colonic duplication:
   A. Associated with genitourinary anomalies
   B. Heterotropic mucosal lining is seen in majority
   C. Associated with Meckel's diverticulum
   D. Postevacuation film is required for demonstrating communication point
   E. Transverse colon is the most common part affected

43. Causes of colonic narrowing:
   A. Diverticulosis
   B. LGV
   C. Actinomycosis
   D. Colitis
   E. Amoebiasis

44. Submucosal tumours in colon:
   A. Leiomyoma
   B. Lymphoma
   C. Hemangioma
   D. Carcinoid
   E. Lipoma

45. Well-known causes of ileocaecal disease:
   A. Appendicitis
   B. Amebiasis
   C. Graft-versus-host disease
   D. Lymphoma
   E. Diverticulitis

46. Common causes of proctosigmoiditis:
   A. Herpes
   B. Crohn's
   C. Gonorrhoea
   D. Chlamydia
   E. Lymphoma

47. **Thumbprinting is seen in:**
    A. Lymphoma
    B. Amoebic colitis
    C. Schistosomiasis
    D. Ischaemic colitis
    E. Pneumatosis coli

48. **Villous polyps:**
    A. Villous adenoma presents with low potassium
    B. Benign and malignant villous tumours can be easily differentiated at barium
    C. Villous polyps have less malignant potential than tubular adenomas
    D. Villous polyps are generally pedunculated
    E. Barium coating is generally poor in villous adenoma

49. **Skip lesions are seen in:**
    A. Tuberculosis
    B. Ulcerative colitis
    C. Amoebiasis
    D. Crohn's disease
    E. LGV

50. **Recognised causes of deep ulcers in the colon:**
    A. Ischemia
    B. Amoebiasis
    C. Strongyloidosis
    D. LGV
    E. Yersinia

51. **Recognised extraintestinal manifestations of inflammatory bowel disease:**
    A. Pancreatitis
    B. Perinephric abscess
    C. Fatty liver
    D. Amyloidosis
    E. Rheumatoid arthritis

52. **Ulcerative colitis:**
    A. The annual incidence is 10-15/100000
    B. Peak incidence 15-25 and 55-65 years
    C. In transverse colon there is a radiolucent stripe parallel to the transverse colon
    D. Mucosal islands are pathologically due to thick colonic wall
    E. 75% have one attack and no subsequent symptoms

53. Extraintestinal manifestations:
A. Pyoderma gangrenosum is not seen in Crohn's disease
B. Peirpheral joint disease is episodic in Crohn's and nonepisodic in ulcerative colitis
C. Ocular lesions are more common in ulcerative colitis
D. Sclerosing cholangitis is seen only in Crohn's disease
E. Amyloidosis is seen only in Crohn's disease

54. The following are in favour of ulcerative colitis than Crohn's:
A. Rectal involvement
B. Perianal abscess
C. Ulcers on background of normal mucosa
D. Cobblestone mucosa
E. Asymmetrical thickening

55. Plain X-ray findings of ulcerative colitis:
A. Extent of formed fecal residue is a reliable indicator of extent of bowel involvement
B. Fecal residue method underestimates the level of colitis
C. Irregular edge of the mucosa indicates normal variant
D. Haustral loss should be diagnosed only if the colon is fully distended
E. Thinned colonic wall

56. Villous adenomas:
A. May cause massive bleeding
B. Transverse colon is the most common site
C. Rarely malignant
D. Lacy reticular pattern seen in double contrast enema
E. Causes hypocalcemia

57. Villous adenoma:
A. May completely encircle the colon
B. Large amount of mucus produced
C. If villous elements constitute more than 75% of the tumour, diagnosis can be made by barium enema
D. 30% of the polyps in familial adenomatous polyps are the villous types
E. The tumour decreases in size in the postevacuation film

58. Differential diagnosis of colitis:
A. Salmonella
B. Cytomegalovirus
C. Amebiasis
D. Graft-versus-host disease
E. Diverticulitis

59. **Giant sigmoid diverticulum:**
    A. Lined by granulation tissue
    B. Formed due to a ball valve mechanism
    C. A communication between the giant diverticulum and lumen is seen only in 10%
    D. Air fluid levels seen
    E. Subserosal perforation is seen

60. **The following are differential diagnosis of a giant sigmoid diverticulum:**
    A. Meckel's diverticulum B. Carcinoma colon
    C. Carcinoma bladder D. Vesicoenteric fistula
    E. Tubo-ovarian abscess

61. **Antibiotic enterocolitis:**
    A. *Clostridium perfringens* is the cause
    B. Short segments of bowel are involved
    C. Oral clindamycin is the treatment of choice
    D. Barium enema shows mucosal edema
    E. Nodular haustral thickening is highly specific

62. **Coning of caecum is seen in:**
    A. Amebiasis B. Ulcerative colitis
    C. Tuberculosis D. Appendicitis
    E. Carcinoma

63. **Extraintestinal manifestations of inflammatory bowel disease:**
    A. Ankylosing spondylitis
    B. Uveitis
    C. Pyoderma gangrenosum
    D. Renal calculi
    E. Pleuropericarditis

64. **Caecal filling defect indicates:**
    A. Appendicitis
    B. Caecal volvulus
    C. Appendiceal intussusception
    D. Ileocolic intussusception
    E. Endometriosis

65. **Colonic tuberculosis:**
    A. A long segment tuberculosis of colon always involves the ileocaecal region
    B. The most common location of a short segment stricture is the proximal caecum
    C. Ulceration is seen in the mesenteric border
    D. Fistulae is more more common than in Crohn's
    E. Perforation is more common in Crohn's than in tuberculosis

66. **Caecal volvulus:**
   A. Occurs only if there is long caecal mesentery
   B. Caecum is fixed
   C. Small bowel is dilated
   D. Distal large bowel is dilated
   E. Obstruction at level of ascending colon

67. **Sigmoid volvulus:**
   A. Majority have a 540 degree rotation
   B. Common in elderly
   C. Fluid-fluid level seen within the sigmoid
   D. Lies under the left dome of diaphragm
   E. Midline crease is due to mesentery

68. **Signs of sigmoid volvulus:**
   A. Rigler's sign
   B. Overlapping the left iliac bone
   C. Left flank overlap is due to overlapping the properitoneal fat stripe in the left flank
   D. Air fluid ratio is more than 2:1
   E. Barium enema is contraindicated

69. **Double tracking of colon seen in:**
   A. Ulcerative colitis
   B. Crohn's disease
   C. Diverticulitis
   D. Lymphoma
   E. Adenocarcinoma

70. **Caecal volvulus:**
   A. CT shows swirlling of caecum and mesentery in the left upper quadrant
   B. Mortality is 40%
   C. X-ray shows the caecum in the left upper quadrant
   D. The smooth surface of coffee bean faces the left lower quadrant
   E. The caecum is seen posterior to the stomach

71. **Volvulus:**
   A. In transverse colon volvulus, the splenic and hepatic flexure are close to each other
   B. In caecal bascule, there is folding without twisting
   C. Caecal bascule does not perforate
   D. In ileosigmoid knot, dilatation of sigmoid colon is seen in the right side
   E. The radiology of transverse colon volvulus is the same as sigmoid volvulus

72. **Associations of ulcerative colitis:**
    A. Cirrhosis
    B. Erythema multiforme
    C. Clubbing
    D. Mouth ulcers
    E. Bile duct carcinoma

73. **Causes of colonic cancer:**
    A. Left-sided ulcerative colitis
    B. Diverticular disease
    C. Gardner's syndrome
    D. Lynch syndrome
    E. Ischaemic colitis

74. **Risk factors for colonic cancer:**
    A. Ureterosigmoidostomy
    B. History of endometrial cancer
    C. Radiation
    D. Cholecystectomy
    E. Prominent lymphoid follicles

75. **Colonic cancer:**
    A. It takes 10 years for a colonic adenoma of 1 cm to develop into cancer
    B. The number of right-sided lesions increases with age
    C. Rectosigmoid is the most common region involved in colon
    D. Anemia is the presenting feature in left-sided colonic lesions
    E. FOBT has a positive predictive value of 35%

76. **Complications of colonic carcinoma:**
    A. Intussusception
    B. Pneumatosis cystoides intestinalis
    C. Pseudymyxoma peritonei
    D. Perforation
    E. Volvulus

77. **Colonic cancer:**
    A. Barium enema has a sensitivity of 83% for detecting polyps less than 1 cm
    B. Calcification is characteristic of mucinous adenocarcinoma
    C. Scirrhous carcinoma is often seen in ulcerative colitis
    D. Annular carcinoma is due to infiltration of lymphatics in the circle muscle layer
    E. Screening for first degree relatives of patients with colon cancer should start at 30 years

78. **Staging of colonic cancer:**
    A. Dukes A is limited to mucosa
    B. Dukes B2 is involvement of the serosa
    C. Dukes C2 has lymph nodal involvement
    D. More than 2 pericoloic nodes is N2
    E. Metastasis occurs early due to lymphatics in the lamina propria

79. **Staging of colorectal tumour:**
    A. In MRI, bowel wall is better seen in the lower part of rectum
    B. The layers of rectum are better seen in T1W images
    C. MRI with body coil has high accuracy than CT in staing
    D. Infiltration of fat is better seen in T2W images
    E. CT is good for assessing depth of extension within the rectal wall

80. **FDG PET for colonic cancer:**
    A. Very useful for necrotic tumours
    B. Not useful for submucosal tumours
    C. Within six months of radiation, it is not possible to differentiate radiation-induced change and recurrence
    D. Pulmonary metastasis does not occur without liver metastasis in colonic cancer
    E. False positive rate is 4%

81. **Postoperative imaging in colonic cancer:**
    A. Recurrence peaks between 9 and 18 months
    B. Seeding of neoplastic cells at surgery is the most important factor
    C. MRI gives high signal within fibrous tissue after radiotherapy
    D. Clinical presentation is early in recurrence due to invasion of local structures
    E. MRI can differentiate fibrosis from recurrence with high specificity in the first year after surgery

82. **Presacral space widening is seen in:**
    A. Diverticulitis
    B. Radiotherapy
    C. Duplication cysts
    D. Normal
    E. Prostatic metastasis

83. **Familial adenomatous polyposis:**
    A. X-linked dominant inheritance
    B. Called Turcot's syndrome when extracolonic findings are present
    C. 95% develop polyps by 35 years
    D. The number of adenomas is less than 20
    E. Prophylactic colectomy indicated for preventing colorectal cancer

84. **Sigmoid volvulus:**
    A. The apex lies on the right side
    B. Apex lies above level of T10
    C. Overlaps the liver in the right upper quadrant
    D. Inferior convergence is seen to right of midline, below lumbosacral junction
    E. Summation line is due to convergence of medial walls of the sigmoid loops

85. **Cancer polyposis syndromes:**
    A. Pigmented penis is seen in Turcot's syndrome
    B. High incidence of carcinoma breast in Peutz-Jeghers syndrome
    C. Medulloblastoma is seen in Ruvalcaba-Muire-Smith syndrome
    D. Juvenile polyps are seen except esophagus in Cronkhite Canada syndrome
    E. Thyroid carcinoma is seen in Cowden's syndrome

86. **Fistula:**
    A. A pelvirectal type of fistula is classifed as a high type of fistula
    B. Colostomy is required for high fistulas
    C. In fistulography, presence of contrast in rectum indicates rectal opening
    D. Hydrogen peroxide is injected into the tract for better images in endoscopic ultrasound
    E. Internal opening can be visualised directly in anal ultrasound

87. **Carcinoma colon:**
    A. In Lynch syndrome I, TCC is associated
    B. Lynch syndrome affects proximal colon
    C. Increased risk in hyperparathyroidism and acromegaly
    D. High association with streptococcal infection
    E. Up to 8% have synchronous or metachronous cancers

88. **Polyps with high risk of malignancy:**
    A. Size > 2 cm, 10% risk
    B. Tubular rather than villous architecture
    C. Less dysplasia
    D. Pedunculated than sessile
    E. Location in proximal large bowel

89. **Inflammatory bowel disease and cancer:**
    A. There is direct correlation between extent of bowel involvement and carcinoma
    B. Higher incidence in proctitis than left-sided colitis
    C. 2% risk in first ten years of ulcerative colitis and 20 times risk in Crohn's disease
    D. Small bowel cancers are more common than large bowel cancers in Crohn's disease
    E. High risk of carcinoma in fistulous tracts

90. Diverticular disease of the colon:
- A. The second most common disease of colon in western countries
- B. 50% of people over 50 years have diverticular disease
- C. 12% have isolated caecal involvement
- D. 95% have sigmoid involvement
- E. 17% have diffuse colonic involvement

91. Diverticulitis:
- A. 35% of diverticular disease patients develop diverticulitis
- B. 5% of general population develop diverticulitis
- C. It is usually self-limiting and surgery is not required
- D. Double tracking of contrast is pathognomonic of peridiverticulitis
- E. Pneumoperitoneum is an earlier sign
- F. Colovaginal fistula is the most common fistula that is formed

92. The following features indicate diverticula rather than polyps:
- A. Meniscus sign, with the contrast fading outwards
- B. Boweler's hat sign with the contrast pointing away from the center of the long axis of colon
- C. Fluid level
- D. Filling defect in barium
- E. Any part seen outside the bowel wall

93. Diverticulosis:
- A. Concertina effect indicates development of cancer
- B. In diverticular disease, the haustra indent alternately from one border to another border
- C. There is strong correlation between the number and size of phleboliths and degree of diverticular disease
- D. 50% of those after 80 years are affected
- E. Both the haustra and interhaustral segments contract alternately in diverticulosis

94. Fistula in ano:
- A. The site of crossing of sphincters best seen in axial MRI
- B. Horse shoe extension better seen in coronal MRI images
- C. CT with thin slices can show relation of fistula to the levator ani
- D. Contrast fistulography is better than MRI in assessing the internal openings
- E. The internal opening is usually at the level of crypts

95. Diverticular disease:
A. Sigmoid is most common segment involved because the stool is most dehydrated here
B. The most common location of diverticula is between taenia omentalis and taenia libera
C. Diverticula produce bubbly appearance of sigmoid in plain films
D. A diverticulum obstructed by feces mimicks polyp
E. The appearance of diverticulum should be the same regardless of the view and position of patient

96. Colonic cancer:
A. 95% of cancers arise from polyps
B. A patient with adenoma has 30% risk of developing carcinoma in the next fifteen years
C. 10 mm is the critical mass of intraepithelial neoplasia
D. 15% of adenomas, 5 mm in size, develop into cancer
E. Malignancy is seen in 40% of tubular adenomas

97. The following indications for FDG PET scanning in colonic cancer:
A. Rising CEA without radiological abnormality
B. Hepatic metastasis in known colonic cancer
C. Extrahepatic metastasis in known colonic cancer
D. Preoperative staging in recurrent disease
E. Differentiating cancer and scar in postoperative patients

98. Colonic cancer:
A. 5% incidence of synchronous cancer
B. 80% survival with Dukes A
C. The lymph nodes are of higher density in mucinous adenocarcinoma
D. 4% incidence of extracolonic malignancy
E. Colonoscopy misses 5% of colonic polyps

99. Diverticulitis:
A. Haemorrhage occurs in 30% of diverticular disease
B. Haemorrhage is more common in right-sided diverticulitis
C. Diverticular neck is larger on the left colon
D. Increased density of pericolic fat in CT is indicator of diverticulitis
E. Abscess more than 5 cm is stage 2 of diverticulitis and is the most severe form

100. Colorectal lymphomas:
A. Account for 10% of colonic tumours
B. Transverse colon is the most common segment involved in colonic lymphoma
C. The mucosa of large bowel is intact in nodular disease
D. Polypoidal mass with terminal ileal involvement is highly indicative of carcinoma rather than lymphoma
E. The strictures are shorter in lymphoma than carcinoma

101. Colon:
A. An irregular base in a polyp is seen only in malignancy
B. Polyps between 0.5 and 1 cm need not be biopsied
C. In polyp, there is 20% risk of additional polyp
D. Saddle tumour involves only a wall of the bowel
E. Single contrast enema is preferred in elderly patients

102. Colon:
A. PEG used for bowel preparation causes excretion of potassium and chloride
B. Balloon inflation in colostomy is avoided
C. There is no need for waiting for two weeks for barium enema if polypectomy is endoscopic
D. PEG leaves a lot of fluid residue and hampers coating before barium enema
E. If cleansing enemas are used for bowel preparation, they should be given at least 12 hours before

103. Polyps and carcinoma:
A. There is high risk of developing metachronous cancer if there are more than one polyp
B. There is 25% risk of developing cancer in polyp in 20 years time
C. Two-thirds of resected cancers have adenomatous polyps within them
D. There is high incidence of synchronous cancer if there are more than one polyp
E. Tumours with Lynch syndrome have better prognosis

104. Contrast agents used in MR colonography:
A. Air
B. Water
C. Gadopentetate dimeglumine
D. Iron glycerophosphate enema
E. Manganese chloride

105. MR colonography using half fourier RARE sequences:
- A. Susceptibility artefacts are common
- B. Heat deposition in tisuses is increased
- C. Acquisition time is subsecond
- D. Lesions less than 5 mm are not detected
- E. Three-dimensional volumetric breath hold MR technique is superior to RARE (rapid acquisition relaxation enhancement)

106. Imaging for detection of colonic lesions:
- A. Barium enema has a sensitivity of 70-90%
- B. CT has a specificity of 60-70%
- C. Barium enema has false positivity of 5-10%
- D. CT colonography has sensitivity up to 100%
- E. MR colonography has sensitivity of over 90%

107. GI manifestations of chronic renal failure:
- A. Pancreatitis
- B. Pseudo-obstruction
- C. Lymphoma
- D. Diverticulitis
- E. Colonic perforation

108. Angiodysplasia of colon:
- A. Diagnosed by pertechnate
- B. Common in the left colon
- C. Early filling of ileocaecal veins
- D. Multiple in majority
- E. Associated with aortic stenosis
- F. Diagnosis is made on barium enema

109. Solitary rectal ulcer syndrome:
- A. Polypoid lesions can be seen
- B. Caused by prolapse of posterior rectal wall
- C. Bleeding requires transfusion
- D. Stricture seen
- E. Failure of anorectal angle to open while straining

110. Diverticulitis in ascending colon:
- A. Colonic carcinoma and diverticulitis can be coexistent in 30% of cases
- B. Thick-walled diverticula are very specific for diverticulitis
- C. Preservation of normal layers of the wall indicates malignancy
- D. Thick wall with normal enhancement indicates diverticular disease
- E. Diverticulitis produces more concentric thickening in right colon

111. **Diverticulitis and carcinoma colon:**
    A. There is more bowel wall thickening than pericolonic infiltration in diverticulitis than carcinoma
    B. Vascular engorgement if present is very reliable for diverticulitis
    C. Saw tooth type of muscular hypertrophy is the earliest appearance of diverticulosis in the right-sided colon
    D. Arrow head sign, (arrow-shaped stasis of contrast in the ileocaecal region) is highly specific for right-sided diverticulitis
    E. Pericolic abscess is uncommon in the right side

112. **The following are features of carcinoma sigmoid than diverticular disease:**
    A. Progressive obstruction
    B. Long segment
    C. Preservation of mucosa
    D. Shouldering
    E. Spastic bowel

113. **Common causes of multiple external openings in a perianal fistula:**
    A. Lymphogranuloma venereum
    B. Colloid carcinoma
    C. Crohn's disease
    D. Schistosomiasis
    E. Ulcerative colitis

114. **Fistulae in ano:**
    A. External types are more common
    B. Intersphincteric involves the external sphincter
    C. Sagittal images show fistula best
    D. Transphincteric is more common
    E. Crohn's disease is the most common cause

115. **Fistulae in ano:**
    A. Suprasphincteric fistula goes through the ischiorectal fossa
    B. Secondary tracks can occur in any direction
    C. Horseshoe-shaped fistula extends into intersphincteric, ischiorectal and supralevator spaces
    D. Horseshoe extensions are always located posteriorly
    E. Horseshoe extensions are most common in the intersphincteric plane

116. **Fistula in ano:**
     A. Supralevator sepsis can arise only with suprasphincteric fistula
     B. Intersphincteric space is best assessed in the coronal images
     C. Internal opening of fistula is best seen in coronal images
     D. The fistula is dark in MRI STIR images
     E. Levator ani is best assessed in the axial images

117. **Fistula in ano:**
     A. Endoscopic ultrasound is contraindicated
     B. Best seen in T1W MR sequences
     C. Intersphincteric is the most common form
     D. If the external opening lies further from anal margin, it is likely to be trans-sphincteric
     E. On endorectal ultrasound, they appear hyperechoic

118. **Diverticular disease:**
     A. Causes small bowel obstruction
     B. Volvulus of a giant diverticulum is a cause of large bowel obstruction
     C. Abscesses can compress the bowel lumen to produce large bowel obstruction
     D. A common cause of pseudo-obstruction
     E. A significant risk factor of sigmoid volvulus

119. **Fistula in ano:**
     A. Supralevator fistula is usually secondary to drainage of a high abscess
     B. External opening in relation to the anterior half of anus is likely to be horseshoe type
     C. Adenocarcinoma and squamous cell carcinoma can arise from the sinus tract
     D. MRI is mainly done for diagnosing the fistulous tract
     E. Infection of anal glands is the primary event in formation of fistula in ano

120. **Excessive pelvic floor descent:**
     A. Resting anorectal junction is more than 3 cm below level of ischial spine
     B. Descent of more than 5 cm on defecation
     C. Descent of the posterior part of pelvic floor during defecation with sparing of anterior portion
     D. Associated with chronically elevated intrarectal pressure
     E. The lesion is in the pudendal nerves

121. **Functional causes of constipation:**
  A. Anismus is due to paradoxical contraction of puborectalis
  B. Associated with sexual abuse
  C. Proctography shows excessive opening of anorectal junction
  D. Proctography shows prominent puborectalis impression
  E. Associated with pelvic incoordination

122. **Large bowel obstruction:**
  A. Onset is more acute than in small bowel obstruction
  B. Abdominal distension is more than small bowel
  C. Abdominal mass indicates presence of strangulation
  D. Vomiting is not as frequent as in small bowel obstruction
  E. There is hemoconcentration rather than anemia

123. **Large bowel obstruction:**
  A. Adhesion is the most common cause of large bowel obstruction
  B. Caecal distension is more prominent if the ileocaecal valve is incompetent
  C. Dilatation of bowel loops is mainly due to swallowed air
  D. In a large bowel tumour causing obstruction, the perforation is more common at the caecum which distends maximally than at the level of the tumour
  E. Caecum perforates when the pressure is more than 55 mmHg

124. **The following portions of gastrointestinal tract can show normal gas in plain film:**
  A. Transverse colon inferior to level of stomach
  B. Sigmoid
  C. Rectal gas
  D. Ascending colon
  E. Descending colon

125. **Large bowel obstruction:**
  A. Appendagitis epiploicae can cause obstruction of rectosigmoid
  B. Inflammation of greater omentum causes obstruction of transverse colon
  C. Gallstone ileus is more common in sigmoid diverticular disease
  D. The most common site of faecal impaction is the sigmoid colon
  E. Obstruction after acute pancreatitis is seen after 21 days

126. **Large bowel obstruction:**
  A. The most common site to be obstructed in carcinoma colon is the splenic flexure
  B. A higher percentage of tumours in splenic flexure cause obstruction than those in rectosigmoid
  C. Obstruction is more common with a right-sided colonic tumour than a left-sided one

    D. Diverticulitis contributes to 12% of large bowel obstruction

    E. Caecal caliber is best assessed in the supine film

127. Ogilvies syndrome (colonic pseudo-obstruction):
    A. This is due to unopposed sympathetic stimulation
    B. Sigmoid colon is not commonly distended in pseudo-obstruction
    C. Barium enema is indicated to rule out obstruction
    D. Presence of intramural gas is a sign of impending perforation
    E. 100% of caecum more than 15 cm will perforate

128. Causes of colonic pseudo-obstruction:
    A. Alcoholism
    B. Retroperitoneal disease
    C. Pregnancy
    D. Colonic cancer
    E. Ischemia

ANSWERS

1. A-F, B-T, C-F, D-F, E-T
The proximal transverse colon is supplied by middle colic branch of superior mesenteric A and the distal third is supplied by left colic branch of inferior mesenteric A.
The left limb of sigmoid mesocolon is medial to the iliac vessels.

2. A-T, B-F, C-F, D-T, E-T
Best Positions
Caecum—left anterior oblique; Hep flexure—right anterior oblique; Spl flexure—left anterior oblique. Sigmoid and rectum—prone, lateral, right anterior oblique and left posterior oblique.

3. A-T, B-T, C-F, D-T, E-T
Taenia are produced due to the longitudinal muscle layer and there are three bands, anteriorly, posteromedially and posterolaterally extending from caecum to the rectum.
Since the taenia are shorter than the colon, they produce colonic haustrations due to their contraction. The haustrations are not complete, unlike the volvulae conniventes.
Appendices epiploiecae are collections of fat and are prominent in the sigmoid colon.

4. A-T, B-F, C-F, D-T, E-F
The upper third is supplied by superior rectal A, a branch of IMA.
Mid third by middle rectal A, branch of Internal iliac artery.
Distal third by inferior rectal artery, branch of internal pudendal artery.
Lymphaticcs from upper two-thirds drain into inferior mesenteric nodes and from lower third drains into internal iliac nodes.

5. A-T, B-F, C-F, D-T, E-F
Iliohypogastric and ilioinguinal nerves are seen posterior the ascending colon running over the quadratus lumborum. The ascending colon is retroperitoneal
Transverse colon measures 45 cm. Transverse colon is attached to the greater curvature of stomach by the gastrocolic ligament. The splenic flexure is attached to the diaphragm by the phrenicocolic ligament.

6. A-T, B-F, C-T, D-F, E-T
The upper third of rectum has peritoneum on front and the sides. The middle third has only on the front. There is no peritoneal covering for the lower third of the rectum.
The dilated lower part of the rectum, the ampulla, is convex to the left lies over the pelvic diaphragm. This produces three lateral curves in the rectum.

7. **A-F, B-T, C-T, D-T, E-F**

   Posteriorly, the rectum is related to levator ani, coccygeus, piriformis, sacrum, coccyx and sacral sympathetic nerves. Anteriorly: Males—upper two-thirds—sigmoid, ileal loops; lower third—bladder, prostate, vas deferens, seminal vesicles, in visceral pelvic fascia; Females—upper two-thirds—pouch of Douglas with sigmoid, ileal loops, ovaries, separating from the uterus; Lower one-third—vagina.

8. **A-F, B-F, C-T, D-T, E-T**

   Rossi—rectosigmoid junction
   Grish—proximal sigmoid colon
   Moulgi—sigmoid descending colon junction
   Balli—proximal descending colon
   Peyerstrauss—descending colon before splenic flexure
   Campis—transverse colon just beyond splenic flexure
   Buscis—midtransverse colon

9. **A-T, B-F, C-T, D-T, E-F**

   Puborectal sling marks the anorectal junction, where the anus angles forwards, after which it angles posteriorly at right angles. Anus has 6-10 vertical folds, called anal columns, which join at the lower aspect forming the valves of ball. Hilton's line demarcates the arterial, venous, lymphatic supply. Above this line—hindgut, lined by mucosa, sup Rect A (IMA branch), sup rect V (portal vein), inferior mesenteric nodes
   Below this line—epithelium—lined by skin, Inf Rect A (int pud A), inf rect V (iliac V), superficial inguinal nodes.

10. **A-F, B-F, C-F, D-T, E-F**

    At rest, the anorectal junction is above the level of ischial tuberosities
    During evacuation, the pelvic floor descends by 30 mm. Ano rectal angle increases from 90 degrees to 115 degrees during defecation. Conspitation, fecal incontinence, levator ani syndrome, proctalgia fugax and Hirschsprung's disease are the indications.

11. **A-T, B-F, C-T, D-T, E-T**

    Internal sphincter lines the upper two-thirds and external sphincter lines the lower two-thirds; hence, there is a overlap in the middle. Internal sphincter—thickened circular muscle layer of upper two-thirds, which surrounds the submucosa, involuntary. Musculus submucous ani—fascial condensation of longitudinal muscle layer, identified in MRI.
    External sphincter—subcutaneous part- thick muscle below the skin

Superficial part—attached to coccyx posteriorly and perineal body anteriorly.
Deep part—annular, blends with puborectalis and lower part of internal sphincter.

12. **A-F, B-T, C-T, D-T, E-T**
Anococcygeal body is posterior. Ischiorectal fossa is posterior. Membranous urethra, bulb of penis, urogenital diaphragm and perineal body are anterior. In females, lower part of vagina, membranous urethra and perineal body are seen.

13. **A-T, B-F, C-T, D-T, E-T**
Balloon inflation can cause rectal tear and perforation. However, it may be sealed with inflated balloon and becomes more apparent only when it is deflated. If perforation is recognized, surgical management with resection of affected segment and peritoneal lavage is indicated. Barium in peritoneum can cause peritonitis and fibrosis which will cause bowel and ureteric obstruction.

14. **A-T, B-F, C-T, D-T, E-T**
Psoas, iliacus, iliac crest, ilioinguinal nerve and iliohypogastric nerve and are the other structures.

15. **A-T, B-F, C-F, D-F, E-F**
The Royal College guidelines support the use of antibiotic prophylaxis for high risk cardiac patients. It is usually amoxicillin 1 g IM or IV with Gentamicin 120 mg 15 minutes before procedure and Amoxicillin 500 mg oral six hours after procedure. Transient bacteremia can occur regardless of presence or absence of colonic disease. Glucagons is preferred in cardiac disease instead of buscopan. Air in portal vein is benign, barium in portal vein is not.

16. **A-F, B-F, C-T, D-F, E-T**
Antibiotic prophylaxis is indicated for high risk patients. Usually, Amoxicillin 1 g and Gentamicin 120 mg IV are administered before the procedure. Amoxicillin 500 mg is given orally six hours after procedure. Buscopan can be given in the middle of procedure.

17. **A-T, B-T, C-T, D-T, E-T**
It is common in elderly patients, who have to be monitored for at least one hour after procedure, because arrhythmia can manifest at this time.

18. **A-F, B-F, C-F, D-F, E- T**
LAO—splenic flexure, RAO—hepatic flexure, head down with right tilt—caecum, prone with 45 degree caudad angulation—sigmoid

colon, lateral wall of descending colon and medial wall of ascending colon—right lateral decubitus, medial wall of descending colon and lateral wall of ascending colon—left lateral decubitus film.

19. **A-T, B-T, C-T, D-T, E-T**
Tumours are the most common cause.

20. **A-F, B-F, C-F, D-F, E-T**
The critical diameter of caecum is 10 cm. The caecum is the most dilated portion in obstruction. Gas fluid levels in caecum and ascending colon can be normal.
If both colon and small bowel are dilated, it indicates ileocaecal valve obstruction secondary to caecal overdistension. If only small bowel is dilated, it indicates incompetent ileocaecal valve.

21. **A-F, B-T, C-F, D-F, E-F**
Venous intravasation is the most feared complication of barium enema. It can go into systemic circulation if there is tear in the lower rectum or vagina and goes into portal circulation in upper rectal tears. Complication rate is approximately 15% for portal (mainly liver abscess) and 75% for systemic circulation. The patient should be placed in the right side with head tilted up to prevent entry of barium into lungs.

22. **A-T, B-T, C-T, D-T, E-F**

23. **A-T, B-F, C-T, D-T, E-T**

24. **A-T, B-T, C-T, D-F, E-F**
Fluid levels after an enema can be confused with obstruction, but the fluid levels are small and multiple. The higher the obstruction, lesser the dilatation. Majority of obstructing gallstones are cholesterol and may not be seen in plain X-rays. Air is seen in gallbladder and cystic duct only if the cystic duct is patent. It may be occluded after acute cholecystitis and there may be no gas in it.

25. **A-F, B-F, C-F, D-T, E-T**
Gas is normal till 5-10 days after laparatomy. Fluid levels are seen in 6 hours. Fluid levels in small bowel is/are shorter than large bowel. Fluid levels can be seen in metabolic conditions also and do not necessarily indicate mechanical obstruction.

26. **A-T, B-F, C-F, D-T, E-T**
Megacolon is diagnosed when transverse colon is more than 5.5 cm. Ulcerative colitis is the most common cause. Crohn's and amebiasis are other recognised causes.

27. **A-F, B-T, C-T, D-F, E-T**
Barium enema is contraindicated and will lead to perforation. Few air fluid levels. Mucosal islands are seen.

28. A-T, B-T, C-T, D-T, E-T
Other causes are tumours, volvulus, inflammation and hernias.

29. A-T, B-T, C-T, D-T, E-F
The appearance progressively changes due to bowel peristalsis. The sensitivity decreases if the bleeding is little. Glucagon can be administered during the procedure to decrease the gastric peristalsis. It has 90% sensitivity for bleeding more than 500 ml/24 hours and only 50% if the bleeding is less than 500 ml/24 hours.

30. A-T, B-T, C-T, D-T, E-T

31. A-F, B-F, C-F, D-T, E-F
Inferior mesenteric arteriogram should be used first, otherwise the distal branches of inferior mesenteric arteries will be obscured by contrast filled bladder. 120 ml of barium paste is introduced using Foley's catheter, in evacuation proctography. Anorectal incontinence is an indication for defecation proctography. Barium is contraindicated for obstruction, since it will preclude surgery.

32. A-T, B-T, C-T, D-T, E-F
Nodular lymphoid hyperplasia is a benign finding. Low magnesium/citrate in relation to calcium causes stones in UC. High oxalic acid causes stones in Crohn's disease.

33. A-T, B-T, C-F, D-F, E-T
Colon cut off sign is abrupt termination of air column in large bowel. Acute pancreatitis causes cut off at transverse colon.

34. A-F, B-T, C-T, D-T, E-F
LGV is another cause. Schistosomiasis, pericolic abscess, endometriosis, carcinoma and lymphoma and other causes. Amoebiasis affects descending colon.

35. A-T, B-T, C-T, D-T, E-F
Ascites, peritoneal metastases are other lesions.

36. A-T, B-T, C-T, D-T, E-T
Physiological causes, infections, inflammation, tumours and extrinsic diseases are common causes of large bowel strictures.

37. A-T, B-T, C-T, D-F, E-F
Ulcerative colitis, Crohn's disease, Pneumatosis coli, Lymphoma, Lymphoid hyperplasia.

38. A-T, B-T, C-T, D-T, E-T
Carpet lesions are very often villous tumours, predominantly in caecum, ascending colon, rectum. They can have malignant degeneration.

39. **A-F, B-T, C-T, D-T, E-F, F-T**

    Filiform polyps indicate burnt out disease. 20 years of left colitis increases risk. No risk in proctitis. Sclerosing cholangitis, sialosyl-In antigen, p53 mutations increase.

40. **A-F, B-T, C-T, D-T, E-F**

    Fifteen percent incidence of arthritis—Peripheral (Elbow, wrist, hip, ankle), spondylitis, ankylosing spondylitis. Peripheral—Monoarticular, asymmetrical, nosynovial destruction, controlling inflammation relieves symptoms spondylitis—Starts before symptoms of UC—No relief/correlation with control of inflammation/colectomy. Ankylosing spondylitis is rare, associated with B-27, young males. Once spine is fused, there is no response to treatment of IBD.

41. **A-T, B-T, C-T, D-F, E-F**

    FAP-Autosomal dominant-APC gene. Thousands of polyps. Males=females; mean age of onset—16 years. Mean age of cancer—39 years. Desmoids, carcinoma duodenum/periampullary, medulloblastomas, hepatoblastoma, thyroid cancer, adrenal hyperplasia, cancer. Gastric-Fundal (hamartoma)/Adenomatous.

42. **A-T, B-F, C-T, D-T, E-F**

    Colonic duplication is very rare congenital anomaly. Heterotropic mucosal lining is not common. Can be associated with a lot of GI conditions such as ileal duplication, diverticulosis, etc. Sigmoid colon is the most common portion of large bowel affected. There are two broad types, Type I—duplication confined to alimentary tract, Type II—associated with duplication of lower genitourinary tract.

43. **A-F, B-T, C-T, D-T, E-T**

    Diverticulitis causes narrowing, but not diverticulosis. Schistosomiasis, radiation, endometriosis carcinoma, lymphoma, tuberculosis and ischemia are other causes.

44. **A-T, B-F, C-T, D-T, E-T**

    Melanoma mets is another recognised cause.

45. **A-T, B-T, C-T, D-F, E-F**

    Tuberculosis, Crohn's, yersinia, typhlitis and carcinoma are other causes.

46. **A-T, B-F, C-T, D-T, E-F**

    Ulcerative colitis is the common cause. Herpes simplex virus is another known cause.

47. **A-T, B-T, C-T, D-T, E-F**

    Ischaemic colitis, ulcerative colitis, Crohn's disease are other causes.

48. **A-T, B-F, C-F, D-F, E-T**
Villous adenomas secrete potassium. It is difficult to differentiate benign and malignant villous adenomas
Villous polyps have more malignant potential than simple tubular adenomas. Villous adenomas are usually sessile.
Barium coating is poor giving a lacy appearance.

49. **A-T, B-F, C-T, D-T, E-T**
Normal mucosa seen in between affected areas.

50. **A-T, B-T, C-T, D-F, E-F**

51. **A-T, B-T, C-T, D-T, E-F**
Reactive hepatitis, chronic active hepatitis, sclerosing cholangitis, cholangiocarcinoma, avascular necrosis, hypertrophic osteoarthropathy, episcleritis, conjunctivitis.
Erythema nodosum, asculitis, stomatitis and pulmonary vasculitis are other manifestations.

52. **A-T, B-T, C-T, D-F, E-F**
The radiolucent stripe is due to pericolic fat. Mucosal islands are thickened areas seen due to submucosal edema and haemorrhage. But pathologically these are thinned areas, but radiologically appear thick. 15% have acute fulminating attack. 75% have intermittent attacks, 1% have one attack and no subsequent symptoms, 15% have continuous symptoms without remission. 30% have lesions limited to rectum, 30% have pancolitis and 10% have extraintestinal manifestations.

53. **A-T, B-T, C-F, D-F, E-T**
Erythema nodosum, aphthous ulcers and amyloidosis are seen only in Crohn's disease. Pyoderma gangrenosum and sclerosing cholangitis are seen only in ulcerative colitis. Visual symptoms due to episcleritis and iritis, are more common in Crohn's disease. Ankylosing spondylitis can be seen in both patients.

54. **A-T, B-F, C-F, D-F, E-F**
UC—continuous, rectum involved, symmetrical, superficial ulcers, ulcers in inflamed mucosa, normal friability, no cobblestoning, pseudopolyps seen. Rectum involved in 95%.
Crohn's—discontinuous, rectum not involved, asymmetrical, deep and longitudinal ulcers, ulcers in normal mucosa background, increased friability, cobblestoning, no pseudopolyps.

55. **A-T, B-F, C-F, D-T, E-F**
There will be no fecal residue in the portion of the bowel which is colitic. Hence, this is a reliable method, but there may be overestimation, as there might be normal mucosa between the fecal

residue and the colitic segment. In pancolitis, there is no residue. In procolitis, whole colon has residue. Normal mucosa is smooth. In colitis, it becomes indistinct, buzzy, with irregular edges due to ulcers. Mucosal islands are formed due to extensive ulcer. Normal haustra are parallel and 2-4 mm apart running across one-third of the colon. In colitis, the loss of parallel line, with blunting and subsequently loss of haustra. The colonic wall is thickened to more than 3 mm. Colon is dilated more than 5.5 cm. In chronic colitis, 5 cm is upper limit.

56. **A-T, B-F, C-F, D-T, C-F**
Rectal bleeding is a typical presenting feature.
Rectum and sigmoid are the most common sites accounting for 75% of villous adenomas.
Malignant infiltration is seen in 36%. Lacy pattern is seen due to contrast in the interscises.
Causes hyponatremia and hypokalemia.

57. **A-T, B-T, C-T, D-F, E-T**
Majority of the adenomas are tubular adenomas in FAP.

58. **A-T, B-T, C-T, D-T, E-T**
Ulcerative colitis is the most common cause. Other causes include campylobacter, *E. coli*, *Clostridium difficle*, Behçet's, radiation and ischemic colitis.

59. **A-T, B-T, C-F, D-T, E-T**
Giant sigmoid diverticulum is more than 6 cm and often measures up to 25 cm. It is a complication of diverticular disease. There is subserosal perforation and inflammation. This results in air trapping inside the diverticulum, which progressively increases due to a ball valve mechanism. The mucosa is replaced by granulation tissue. There is communication with the lumen in 90% and it fills with barium. It is seen as a large air-filled structure in the mid-pelvis. Infection, infarction, torsion and perforation can occur in this giant diverticulum.

60. **A-T, B-F, C-F, D-T, E-T**
Any large gas or gas fluid containing structure in the lower abdomen and pelvis is the differential for giant sigmoid diverticulum. Volvulus, emphysematous cystitis, giant Meckel's diverticulum, small bowel diverticulum are other differentials.

61. **A-F, B-F, C-F, D-T, E-T**
Clostridium difficle is the cause of pseudomembranous enterocolitis.
Clindamycin, lincomycin, cephalosporins/penicillins are causes
Common in adults. 3.5% mortality. X-ray—Megacolon, thumb-

printing, nodular haustral thickening (specific, but seen only in severe cases. Barium is avoided for fear of perforation. Shows nodular thickening. CT shows specific "Accordion sign" (Trapping of barium between thick folds), Target sign (Enhancing mucosa, hypodense submucosa), stranding ascites, megacolon.

62. **A-T, B-T, C-T, D-T, E-T**
Tuberculosis, actinomycosis, amebiasis, Crohn's, UC, appendicitis, typhlitis. Carcinoma and metastasis are other causes.

63. **A-T, B-T, C-T, D-T, E-T**

64. **A-T, B-F, C-T, D-T, E-T**
Appendicitis, cystic fibrosis, Crohn's disease, lymphoma and lipomatosis of the ileocaecal valve are other causes.

65. **A-T, B-F, C-F, D-F, E-T**
Colonic tuberculosis can be a short segment or a long segment. The most common location of a short segment stricture is the hepatic flexure. Ulceration is circumferential rather than the mesenteric location of Crohn's disease. Anal sinuses and fistulae are more common in Crohn's disease. Inflammatory polyps are occasionally seen. Free perforation is also more common in Crohn's disease.

66. **A-T, B-T, C-T, D-F, E-T**
In the common type of caecal volvulus, the caecum twists on its mesentery, with obstruction at the fixed portion of ascending colon. There is proximal small bowel dilatation.

67. **A-F, B-T, C-T, D-T, E-T**
Majority have 360 degrees rotation. Only 10% have 540 degrees. 50% have 360 degrees. 35% have 180 degrees rotation.

68. **A-F, B-T, C-F, D-T, E-F**
Rigler's sign is seen in pneumoperitoneum. Overlapping of left iliac blade is the pelvic overlap sign. Overlapping the descending colon in the left flank is the left flank overlap sign. Barium enema is not contraindicated and will show a birds beak deformity at the site of twist.

69. **A-T, B-T, C-T, D-F, E-T**
Long, submucosal ulcers produce double tracking.

70. **A-F, B-T, C-T, D-T, E-F**
CT shows the swirling of mesentery and caecum in the right upper quadrant. Smooth surface of coffee bean faces the left lower quadrant. The caecum is anterior to the stomach, unlike the foramen of Winslow hernia which is posterior to the stomach. Barium will show the beaking at the level of ascending colon.

71. **A-T, B-T, C-F, D-T, E-T**
In caecal bascule, there is folding of the right colon but without twisting. The caecum is seen in the midabdomen and it can perforate. In ileosigmoid knotting, a loop of ileum passes around the base of sigmoid colon, below the attachment of the mesocolon and forms a knot, producing a dilated loop of sigmoid on the right side, with retained feces in the proximal colon. There are also features of small bowel obstruction. In transverse colon volvulus, there is severe vomiting due to compression of duodenojejunal junction.

72. **A-T, B-F, C-T, D-F, E-T**
Primary biliary cirrhosis associated with ulcerative colitis in a few cases.

73. **A-T, B-F, C-T, D-T, E-F**
Crohn's disease, high fat, low bulk diet, nitrates, nitrites, alcohol and smoking are other risk factors. 20 years of left colitis.

74. **A-T, B-T, C-T, D-T, E-T**
History of colonic cancer, adenomatous polyp, radiotherapy, cholecystectomy, breast carcinoma, uterine carcinoma and ovarian carcinoma are risk factors.

75. **A-F, B-T, C-T, D-F, E-F**
Seven years for a 1 cm adenoma to develop into cancer.
Right-sided lesions commonly present with iron deficiency anemia and weight loss and left-sided lesions present with obstruction or rectal bleeding. Obstruction is not common in the right-sided lesions.
FOBT has a positive predictive value of only 10%.

76. **A-T, B-T, C-T, D-T, E-F**
Obstruction is a common complication.

77. **A-T, B-T, C-T, D-T, E-F**
Screening for first degree relatives should begin at 40 years. Normal screening begins at 50 years, with FOBT every year and barium enema/sigmoidoscopy every three years.

78. **A-T, B-T, C-T, D-F, E-F**
A—mucosa, B1—muscularis propria, B2—serosa, mesenteric fat, C1—limited to bowel wall + lymph nodes, C2—adipose tissue extension + lymph nodes, D—metastases
TNM staging
T1—submucosa, T2—muscularis propria, T3—subserosa, T4—adjacent organs.

N1—up to 3 pericolic nodes, N2—>4 pericolic nodes, N3—along vessels.

79. **A-T, B-F, C-F, D-F, E-F**
    T2 W images are best for assessing bowel wall anatomy, which is better seen in the lower rectum than the upper rectum. Fatty infiltration is best assessed in T1, because of low intensity tumor within high intensity fat. MRI with body coil does not have significant higher accuracy than CT staging. CT is not useful for assessing depth of invasion inside the wall.

80. **A-F, B-T, C-T, D-T, E-T**
    FDG is not useful in mucosal, submucosal tumours or necrotic tumours.
    After six months following radiation, FDG can differentiate radiation-induced inflammation and tumour recurrence.

81. **A-T, B-F, C-T, D-F, D-F**
    Recurrence is either due to incomplete excision or tumour seeding. It is seen in the tumour bed or in the suture line. It is difficult to differentiate fibrosis and tumour recurrence in CT scan. In MRI, theoretically the fibrosis will have low signal in T1 and T2, but tumour will have high signal in T2. But high signal will be seen in fibrosis in the first year or after radiotherapy. Another problem is tumour surrounded by fibrosis, which will be difficult to diagnose even with biopsy.

82. **A-T, B-T, C-T, D-T, E-T**
    Prerectal space is considered widened if it is more than 1.5 cm at the level of S3-5. The causes are—A normal variant in large, obese patients, inflammatory (ulcerative colitis, Crohn's disease, lymphogranuloma venereum, diverticulitis, abscess), tumours (carcinoma rectum, metastasis to rectum, sacral tumours), enteric duplication cyst, pelvic lipomatosis.

83. **A-F, B-F, C-T, D-F, E-T**
    FAP has autosomal dominant inheritance with complete penetrance. It is composed of thousands of polyps in the colon. It can involve the proximal GIT also. 50% develop polyps by 15 years. When extracolonic findings are present, it is called Gardner's syndrome.

84. **A-F, B-T, C-T, D-F, E-T**
    The apex lies on the left side, under the dome, above the level of T10. Inferiorly, the loops converge on the left side at or below the level of lumbosacral junction.

85. **A-F, B-T, C-F, D-T, E-T**
    FAP—multiple polyps colon, upper GIT, polyps/cancer.
    Gardner's syndrome—FAP + osteomas, desmoid tumors.
    Turcot's syndrome—brain tumours including medulloblastoma.
    Peutz-Jeghers—mucocutaneous pigmentation, hamartomatous polyps, carcinoma gastric, duodenal, colon, breast, ovary, endometrium.
    Ruvalcaba = macrocephaly, abnormal face, pigmented penile macules, developmental delay: Cronkhite Canada syndrome- Juvenile polyps, adenomas, carcinomas
    Cowden's syndrome—ectodermal dysplasia.
    Basal cell nevus syndrome—Basal cell tumours, odontogenic keratocysts.

86. **A-T, B-T, C-F, D-T, E-F**
    Fistulas opening into the anal canal below the anorectal ring are called low level fistulas and those opening above it are called High level. Subcutaneous, submucous and low canal are types of low fistulas and high anal canal and pelvirectal types are high fistulas.

87. **A-T, B-T, C-T,D-T, E-T**
    Lynch syndrome I—High incidence of synchronous and metachronous cancers, adenomas, greater incidence of proximal bowel cancers, younger age.
    II—carcinoma ovary, endometrium, stomach, small bowel, pancreas, ureter and kidneys.
    Streptococcus bovis has a high association with colonic cancer.

88. **A-T, B-F, C-F, D-F, E-F**
    Polyps 1-2 cm have only 5% risk. Pedunculated polyps have malignancy in 10%. Sessile polyps are malignant in 50%.

89. **A-T, B-F, C-T, D-F, E-T**
    Pancolitis has more risk. Left-sided colitis, proctitis have low risk compared to other areas in ulcerative colitis. By 30 years, 11% of ulcerative colitis patients have carcinomas. The cancers in both Crohn's and UC arise early than patients without them. In Crohn's disease, the cancer can arise from strictures, fistulas, inflamed areas and bypassed segments. 70% of cancers in Crohn's arise from colon and only 25% from small bowel, particularly terminal ileum (70%).

90. **A-F, B-F, C-T, D-F, E-T**
    Common condition of colon in western countries. 50% of those above 70 years have this disease. 80% have sigmoid involvement. 12% can have isolated caecal involvement and 17% have diffuse colonic involvement.

91. A-T, B-T, C-T, D-T, E-F, F-F
Pneumoperitoneum is rare. Coloenteric fistula is the most common fistula.

92. A-F, B-T, C-T, D-F, E-T
In polyps—Boweler's hat, the contrast points towards the center of the long axis of colon. In diverticula, it points away from the center of the long axis of colon.
Menicus sign—fades outwards from the lesion in polyps and fades inwards in diverticulum.
Polyps produce filling defect in a barium column, but diverticula will be filled with barium. Fluid levels are seen in erect views and a part of the lesion will be seen outside the bowel lumen.

93. A-F, B-T, C-T, D-T, E-F
A concertina effect otherwise called zig-zag effect is due to thickened circular muscle and shortened taenia, producing alternate, compact, deep haustra. Normal haustra are symmetrical and face each other in the opposite walls. But in diverticular disease, they can indent alternately from one border to another border producing the staggered effect. These are seen in early stages of diverticular disease. In normal persons, the haustral and interhaustral portions contract in alternate fashion, but in diverticulosis, both contract simultaneously producing very high pressure and segmentation, resulting in further diverticulosis. Both phleboliths and diverticula are caused by low fiber in diet and there is a recognised correlation between them.

94. A-T, B-F, C-F, D-F, E-T
Axial images are best for assessment of horseshoe extensions. CT is not useful as MRI in assessing relation to levator. Internal opening is where the fistula opens into the anorectal lumen, and is usually at the site of the crypts. MRI does not directly visualise it, but it can be deduced by its relationship with the bowel lumen and has accuracy of up to 80%, but contrast fistulography will show it in less than 15%. Fistulography is very unreliable because the internal openings cannot be visualised when they are plugged with viscid secretions and the sphincter relation and level of levator plate cannot be assessed.

95. A-T, B-F, C-T, D-T, E-F
Sigmoid is the most common affected segment because it has the narrowest lumen and the most dehydrated stool, due to maximum intrasegmental pressure. There are three taenia in the large bowel, the taenia mesenterica, taenia omentalis and taenia libera. Diverticula are formed, at sites where blood vessels penetrate the

muscularis propria. They usually penetrate on both sides of the taenia mesenterica, mesenteric side of taenia omentalis and taenia libera. Hence, there is no defect between the taenia libera and taenia omentalis, and hence no diverticula. Appearance of diverticula depends on the position and view. A diverticulum inverting into the lumen, resembles polyp. A diverticulum with long neck, resembles a pedunculated polyp and one with large neck resembles sessile polyp.

96. A-T, B-F, C-F, D-F, E-F
The patient with adenoma has 10% risk of developing cancer in 15 years. Five mm is the critical size of intraepithelial neoplasia. 5% of adenomas 5 mm in size, develop into cancer.
Malignancy is seen in 5% of tubular adenomas and 40% of villous adenomas.

97. A-T, B-T, C-T, D-T, E-T
Also used in equivocal cases.

98. A-T, B-T, C-F, D-T, E-F
There is 3% incidence of metachronous cancer. Lymph nodes are of low density in mucinous adenocarcinoma. Colonoscopy misses 12% of colonic polyps, caecum is not visualised in 10-30%.

99. A-T, B-T, C-F, D-T, E-F
Haemorrhage is more common in the right colon, because the neck is larger, hence the blood vessels are exposed along a greater length. Increased density of pericolic fat, soft tissue thickening, streaking, air bubbles and fluid collection are all indicators of inflammation. Stage 0—confined by serosa, I—abscess less than 5 cm and confined to mesocolon, II—abscess 5-15 cm, within pelvis, III—beyond pelvis into peritoneal cavity, IV—fecal peritonitis. Stage 0 is the most common type and IV is the most severe.

100. A-F, B-F, C-T, D-F, E-F
Lymphomas account for only 0.1% of all colorectal tumours. Rectum and caecum are the most common segments of large bowel involved. The most common pattern is nodular, with preservation of mucosa. Other patterns include thickened folds, long strictures and polypoidal mass with involvement of terminal ileum. Irregular excavation of mass is another feature which is more common in lymphoma than carcinoma.

101. A-F, B-F, C-T, D-T, E-T
An irregular base can be seen in both benign and malignant lesions. Polyps between 0.5 -1 cm should be biopsied as malignancy cannot be excluded. Saddle tumour is also called semiannular

tumour. Double contrast is the ideal method, but single contrast can be performed when the patient is too old or infant.

102. A-T, B-T, C-F, D-T, E-F
Cathartics are given before barium to increase the quality of examination. PEG is commonly used. It induces diarrhea. There is no absorption or excretion of electrolytes. Fluid residues are the main disadvantage and this is avoided by using it 12-18 hours before procedure and using stimulants as well to evacuate fluids. Stimulants such as bisacodyl and castor oil, increase peristalsis, causing cramps and fluid depletion. It should be given 6-12 hours before. Hyperosmolar agents cause fluid loss. 2 L of cleansing enema can be used and they should be given 1 hour before procedure. Balloon inflation of colostomy can result in rupture of the colon. Hence, a Foley's inserted through a baby feeding bottle will act as seal. After endoscopic polypectomy, barium enema should be done only after three weeks.

103. A-T, B-T, C-F, D-T, E-T
One-third of cancers have adenomatous polyps within them. Lynch syndrome patients have favourable chromosomal pattern with better prognosis.

104. A-T, B-T, C-T, D-T, E-T
CO_2 and hyperpolarised helium are other agents used.
Single shot half Fourier RARE sequences are used in air insufflated MR colonographs.

105. A-F, B-T, C-T, D-T, E-F
Susceptibility artefacts are not common in RARE sequence.
Heat deposition is more than normal spin echo sequences, but specific absorption rate is not increased. Acquisition time is very fast, resulting in minimal bowel and movement artefacts. Lesions less than 1 cm are difficult to identify and less than 5 mm are not identified.
RARE sequences are better than 3D volumetric images.

106. A-T, B-F, C-T, D-T, E-T
Barium enema—sen 70-90%, false positive rate 5-10%
CT colonography—sen 75-100%, speci-85-100%
MR colonography—sen 90-100%, spec-85-100%.

107. A-T, B-T, C-T, D-T, E-T

108. A-T, B-F, C-T, D-F, E-T, F-F
Angiodysplasia—Degenerative lesion of vessels in caecum, ascending colon, a common cause of GI bleeding. Most common

vascular anomaly of GIT. 2nd common cause of bleeding after diverticular disease. Multifold 25%. 30-40% of obscure GI bleeding. Common in right colon, due to high wall tension in larger right colon > 0.8% prevalence. 90% spontaneously stop bleeding, 1-2% have upper GI lesion. Hegde syndrome AS + Angiodysplasia. Dense, slow emptying vein, vascular tuft and early fillig vein are the 3 angiographic features.

109. **A-T, B-F, C-T, D-T, E-T**
Solitary rectal ulcer is due to prolapse of anterior rectal wall which then undergoes ischemia due to anal sphincter during defecation. The lesion can be ulcerative or polypoid or flat. Single or multiple. Bleeding can be chronic and may require transfusion.
Proctography shows failure of anorectal angle to open when straining and excessive perineal descent.

110. **A-T, B-T, C-F, D-T, E-T**
The two most reliable signs of diverticulitis are identification of a segment of thick-walled diverticula and thickening with preservation of normal layers and enhancement of the bowel wall.

111. **A-F, B-F, C-F, D-F, E-F**
If there is more bowel wall thickening than pericolonic infiltration, it is suggestive of malignancy. There is more pericolonic infiltration and abscess formation in diverticulitis. Saw-tooth type of hypertrophy, seen in sigmoid colon is not usually seen in the right colon. Arrowhead sign is classically seen in acute appendicitis and can be seen in diverticulitis.

112. **A-T, B-F, C-F, D-T, E-F**
In diverticulitis, the bowel is spastic, cone-shaped edge due to narrowing, long segment, intact mucosa, obstruction is variable and there are diverticula.
In carcinoma, the bowel is of normal tone, sharp, shelf like margins, short segment, mucosa destroyed, obstruction is progressive and there are often no diverticula.

113. **A-T, B-T, C-T, D-T, E-T**
Tuberculosis is another cause.

114. **A-T, B-F, C-F, D-F, E-T**
Intersphincteric fistulas do not involve the external sphincter and run completely in the intersphincteric plane. Coronal and axial images·are the best. Intersphincteric type is the most common type.

115. A-T, B-T, C-T, D-T, E-F
PARKS classification of fistula in anos
Intersphincteric—confined to intersphincteric plane, not crossing ext sphincter or levator
Trans-sphincteric—passes through the external sphincter radially.
Suprasphincteric—passes in intersphincteric plane above pubo-rectalis, then going down through levators and ischiorectal fossa to the skin
Extrasphincteric—outside external sphincter along the entire course
Horseshoe extensions are more common in the ischiorectal fossa.

116. A-F, B-F, C-F, D-F, E-F
Supralevator sepsis can arise either as a part of suprasphincteric or extrasphincteric primary tract or upward extension of trans-sphincteric fistula through levators or intersphincteric fistula through intersphincteric plane. Internal opening is not seen in any of the planes, but it can be deduced.
The fistula is seen as bright structure in the STIR images due to pus within them. Axial images are best for assessing inter-sphincteric plane and coronal images are best for levator ani.

117. A-F, B-F, C-T, D-T, E-F
Although the track is visualised in T1W sequences, STIR sequences are the best for assessment of the fistulous tract. T1W sequences are done for delineation of anatomy only and they are not essential. The external opening can be located in anterior perineum, natal cleft or buttocks, the further they are from anal opening, the more likely they are trans-sphincteric.

118. A-T, B-T, C-T, D-T, E-F
Small bowel obstruction can be caused by ileus or adhesions or edematous bowel wall. Pericolonic fibrosis and spasm are other causes of large bowel obstruction. Sigmoid diverticulitis produces sepsis and hence a recognised cause of pseudo-obstruction. There is no increased risk of sigmoid volvulus in sigmoid diverticular disease.

119. A-T, B-F, C-T, D-F, E-T
According to Goodsalls rule, an external opening in relationship to the anterior half of the anus is likely to be a direct type. An opening in the posterior half of the anus with curving tracts is likely to be a horseshoe type fistula. Supralevator fistula can also be formed due to foreign body penetration. MRI is not essential for the diagnosis of fistula, but it is necessary to find the relationship of the fistula to the anal sphincter (since surgery can destroy the sphincter) and if there are any secondary extensions

from the primary tract, which will predispose to relapse of the condition after surgery. According to the cryptoglandular hypothesis of Eisenhammer, infection of anal glands is the primary event, which leads of intersphincteric abscess which extends in all directions and produces fistula in chronic phase when the abscess fails to heal.

120. **A-T, B-F, C-F, D-T, E-T**
In excessive pelvic floor descent, the entire pelvic floor descends during straining, due to pudendal neuropathy. It is associated with chronically elevated intrarectal pressure, intussusception and prolapse. The diagnosis in proctography is made when the anorectal junction is more than 3 cm below the level of ischial spine at rest and descends more than 3.5 cm during defecation.

121. **A-T, B-T, C-F, D-T, E-T**
Proctography shows failure of anorectal junction to open.
This is associated with evacuation failure due to incoordinate puborectalis contraction.

122. **A-F, B-T, C-F, D-T, E-F**
In large bowel obstruction, onset is gradual, abdominal distension more, vomiting uncommon, anemia (hemoconcentration in small bowel obstruction), abdominal mass suggests carcinoma or volvulus and azotemia is infrequent. Strangulation is not common in large bowel obstruction. Third spacing of fluid is also not seen, but it is seen in small bowel obstruction.

123. **A-F, B-F, C-T, D-F, E-T**
Carcinoma is the most common cause of large bowel obstruction. Adhesions are less common in large bowel than small bowel, since it is of larger caliber, thick walled and with appendices epiploicae. If the ileocaecal valve is incompetent, there will be retrograde decompression into the small bowel, with dilatation of large and small bowel loops proximal to the obstruction. In competent ileocaecal valve, there will be no decompression into small bowel, hence the caecum progressively distends due to closed loop obstruction, and when it measures more than 12 cm or if pressure is more than 55 mmHg, it will perforate. In a tumour causing obstruction, the perforation is more common at the site of tumour rather than the caecum. Bacterial production of gas and diffusion of gas from blood are other causes of the distension.

124. **A-T, B-T, C-T, D-T, E-T**
Also seen normally in small intestine and middle and distal part of stomach.

125. A-T, B-T, C-T, D-F, E-T

Inflammation of appendices epiploicae is called appendagitis epiploicae and it can cause obstruction of rectosigmoid. Gallstone is more likely to be lodged in the sigmoid colon which is narrowed by diverticular disease. 70% of faecal impaction occurs in the rectum and 20% occurs in the sigmoid colon. Pancreatitis can cause obstruction due to edema, abscess or phlegmon.

126. A-F, B-T, C-F, D-T, E-F

In carcinoma, rectosigmoid is the most common site to be obstructed, with sigmoid contributing to 65% and rectum to 13% of cases. Almost 50% of splenic flexure tumours obstruct whereas only 6% of rectal tumours cause obstruction. Right-sided tumours are often polypidal and present with anemia or weight loss, but left-sided tumours are often annular constricting and cause obstruction. Caecal caliber is best assessed in the prone or decubitus view, to avoid errors caused by magnification.

127. A-F, B-T, C-T, D-T, E-F

Ogilvies syndrome is acute colonic pseudo-obstruction and is due to interruption of sympathetic innervation with unopposed parasympathetic action, resulting in distension of ascending colon, descending colon, transverse colon and caecum, with sparing of sigmoid colon. Caecum, measuring more than 12 cm, progressive increase over 24 hours and distension for 3 days are signs of impending perforation. Caecum can occasionally reach up to 20 cm, yet not perforate.

128. A-T, B-T, C-T, D-F, E-F

Cardiac disease, inflammation, burns and trauma are other causes of pseudo-obstruction. Carcinoma colon causes true mechanical obstruction.

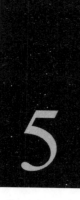

5 Peritoneum, Mesentery, Retroperitoneum

1. **Aorta:**
   A. Calcification is common in women after 60 years
   B. Aorta is wider in the upper part of the abdomen
   C. Aortic bifurcation occurs at L4
   D. There are five pairs of lumbar arteries
   E. Superior and inferior suprarenal arteries arise from aorta

2. **IVC:**
   A. The IVC lies behind the aortic bifurcation
   B. The IVC is formed at level of L5
   C. The IVC has a long intrahepatic portion
   D. The junction of left renal vein and IVC marks the pancreatic uncinate process
   E. Segmental lumbar veins drain the vertebral venous plexus into the IVC

3. **The following nodes drain to the preaortic group of lymph nodes:**
   A. Pararectal   B. Ileocolic
   C. Hepatic   D. Pancreaticosplenic
   E. Colic

4. **Pneumoperitoneum:**
   A. At least 50 ml of air is required for demonstration
   B. After surgery, air remains longer in obese than thin patient
   C. Colonic perforation is more common than peptic ulcer perforation in patients with steroids
   D. Surgical drainage is a frequent cause
   E. Jejunal diverticulosis causes silent perforation

5. **Pneumoperitoneum without clinical signs of perforation occurs in:**
   A. Pneumatosis intestinalis
   B. Peptic ulcer perforation
   C. Pneumomediastinum
   D. Pneumothorax
   E. Infarction of bowel

6. **Fluid levels in intestine are seen in:**
   A. Small bowel obstruction
   B. Laxative abuse
   C. Irritable bowel syndrome
   D. Celiac disease
   E. Gastroenteritis

7. **The following are normal findings in an abdominal X-ray:**
   A. Fluid levels in duodenum
   B. Volvulae conniventes
   C. Gastric rugae
   D. 3 fluid levels in a bowel loop > 2.5 cm
   E. 5 fluid levels in a bowel loop < 2.5 cm

8. **Causes of pneumoperitoneum without peritonitis:**
   A. Jejunal diverticulosis
   B. Embolisation
   C. Steroids
   D. Pneumomediastinum
   E. Endoscopy

9. **Diffuse calcification in abdomen is seen in:**
   A. Tuberculosis
   B. Mucocele of appendix
   C. Serous adenocarcinoma of ovary with pseudomyxoma peritonei
   D. Undifferentiated abdominal cancer
   E. Ovarian cystadenoma

10. **Common causes of calcified abdominal tumours:**
    A. Carcinoma colon
    B. Carcinoma stomach
    C. Lipoma
    D. Desmoid tumour
    E. Gastric leiomyoma

11. **The following are causes of cystic tumours in the peritoneum:**
    A. Leiomyosarcoma
    B. Mesothelioma
    C. Lymphangioma
    D. Teratoma
    E. Hydatid

12. **Signs of pneumoperitoneum:**
    A. Football sign   B. Rigler's triad
    C. Urachus sign   D. Inverted V sign
    E. Tell tale triangle sign

13. **Mesenteric masses:**
    A. Cystic tumours are more common than solid tumours
    B. Benign tumours have predilection for the root of mesentery rather than close to the bowel wall
    C. Malignant primary tumours are more common than benign primary tumours
    D. Secondary tumours are common than primary
    E. Desmoid tumour is the most common primary tumour of mesentery

14. **Loculated cystic masses in mesentery:**
    A. Pseudomyxoma peritonei
    B. Mesothelioma
    C. Leiomyosarcoma
    D. Haematoma
    E. Teratoma

15. **The following are common sites for splenosis:**
    A. Mucosal surface of small intestine
    B. Diaphragm
    C. Morrison's pouch
    D. Greater omentum
    E. Scrotum

16. **Differential diagnosis for omental masses:**
    A. Fibrosarcoma   B. Mesothelioma
    C. Tuberculosis   D. Metastases
    E. Lymphoma

17. **Causes of pseudomyxoma peritonei:**
    A. Mucinous cystadenoma of appendix
    B. Mucinous adenocarcinoma of ovary
    C. Uterus carcinoma
    D. Pancreatic carcinoma
    E. Stomach cancer

18. **Common causes of omental cake:**
    A. Stomach cancer metastasis
    B. Ovarian cancer metastasis
    C. Castleman disease
    D. Colonic cancer metastasis
    E. Kaposi's sarcoma

19. **Mimics of pneumoperitoneum:**
    A. Pulmonary collapse   B. Pulmonary tumour
    C. Chiladitis syndrome   D. Fat
    E. Pneumatosis intestinalis

20. **High density ascites is seen in:**
    A. Myxedema
    B. Tuberculosis
    C. Ovarian tumour
    D. Trauma
    E. Cirrhosis

21. **Peritoneal carcinomatosis:**
    A. Calcification seen
    B. Increased density is seen in peritoneum
    C. Thickened mesenteric vessels are seen
    D. Increased density in abdominal wall
    E. Loculated fluid collection in peritoneum

22. **Mesenteric panniculitis associated with:**
    A. SLE
    B. Lymphoma
    C. Pancreatitis
    D. Hydronephrosis
    E. Rheumatic disease

23. **The following diseases are more common in men:**
    A. Primary biliary cirrhosis
    B. Abdominal aortic aneurysm
    C. Rheumatoid arthritis
    D. Paget's disease
    E. Haemochromatosis

24. **Imaging features of mesenteric panniculitis:**
    A. Common in the right side of the mesentery
    B. Soft tissue nodules are a common feature
    C. High density halo around nodules
    D. Encasement of mesenteric vessels indicates malignancy
    E. Dense stripe is seen in the mesenteric fat

25. **Common causes of bowel wall calcification:**
    A. Rectal stone
    B. Proximal to obstruction
    C. Diverticular stone
    D. Meckel's diverticulum stone
    E. Stone in transverse colon

26. **Abdominal X-ray:**
    A. Caecal fluid levels are abnormal
    B. Critical distension of caecum is 5.5 cm
    C. Critical diameter of transverse colon is 5 cm
    D. Splenic outline is not seen in 40% of normal individuals
    E. Psoas outline is indistinct in 50% of children

27. **Causes of chylous ascites:**
    A. Trauma
    B. Pancreatitis
    C. Tuberculosis
    D. Congenital
    E. Retroperitoneal sarcoma

28. **Features of peritoneal mesothelioma:**
    A. Thickened bowel wall
    B. High density ascites
    C. Uptake by gallium
    D. Ascites is disproportionate to the mass
    E. Invades bowel and bladder

29. **Peritoneal hydatid:**
    A. Always secondary to hepatic hydatid
    B. Peritoneum involved in 13% of abdominal hydatid
    C. In encysted peritoneal hydatid the entire peritoneum is replaced by a multilobulated mass
    D. Ultrasound is the best modality for diagnosing peritoneal seedling
    E. Ultrasound is not useful in diagnosing ruptured cyst

30. **Injections causing calcification:**
    A. Iron
    B. Bismuth
    C. Calcium gluconate
    D. Steptomycin
    E. Penicillin

31. **Common causes of mesenteric metastases:**
    A. Breast
    B. Lung
    C. Leiomyosarcoma
    D. Ovary
    E. Colon

32. **Tuberculosis:**
    A. Peritoneum is involved in 75% of abdominal tuberculosis
    B. Peritoneum is involved by ruptured lymph nodes or fallopian tubes
    C. Dry type of peritoneal tuberculosis has no ascites but abdominal masses are seen
    D. Barium meal is not contributory in diagnosis
    E. Septa within ascites is highly specific for tuberculosis

33. **Drugs that are implicated in retroperitoneal fibrosis:**
    A. Hydralazine
    B. LSD
    C. Amphetamines
    D. Methysergide
    E. Methyldopa

34. **The following features in lymph nodes are in favor of tuberculosis than malignancy or other inflammatory diseases:**
    A. Caesation
    B. Mesenteric nodal enlargement
    C. Calcification
    D. Conglomerate nodes
    E. Retroperitoneal lymph node

35. **Tuberculosis:**
    A. Peritoneal thickening involves mesentery but not omentum
    B. Ultrasound shows stellate bowel loops due to fixity
    C. Bowel wall thickening is eccentric rather than concentric like in Crohn's
    D. Lymphadenopathy is seen in 90% of cases
    E. Pseudokidney sign seen under the liver should raise the suspicion of tuberculosis

36. **The classical sites of intraperitoneal metastasis:**
    A. Posterior border of rectosigmoid
    B. Superior border of sigmoid
    C. Medial border of caecum
    D. Lateral border of ascending colon
    E. Lateral border of descending colon

37. **Peritoneal tumours:**
    A. Lipoma is the most common benign tumour in the mesentery
    B. In mesothelioma the amount of ascites is less in comparison to peritoneal metastasis
    C. Metastasis in the left inframesocolic space, extends up to the lesser sac
    D. Hematogenous metatasis are more common in the mesenteric border of the bowel
    E. Enhancing nodules in peritoneum and omentum with ascites is indicative of metastasis

38. **Common causes of calcified lymph nodes in abdomen:**
    A. Silicosis
    B. Kaposi's sarcoma
    C. Chronic granulomatous disease
    D. Tuberculosis
    E. Cirrhosis

39. **The following are features of peritoneal metastasis:**
    A. Thick bowel wall
    B. Loculated ascites
    C. Stellate mass in mesentery
    D. Ascites, with no fluid in cul de sac
    E. Omental cake

40. **Peritoneal lesions:**
    A. Enteric cyst has no muscle lining in its wall
    B. Enteric cyst is caused by migration of diverticulum into mesentery
    C. Acute thrombus within mesenteric vein is hyperdense in plain CT
    D. In hypoalbuminemia, high density is seen in both mesenteric and retroperitoneal fat due to edema
    E. Lymphangioma has fat density within it

41. **Retroperitoneal fibrosis is associated with:**
    A. Oribital pseudotumour
    B. Reidel's thyroiditis
    C. Abdominal aortic aneurysm
    D. Carcinoid syndrome
    E. Crohn's disease

42. **Mesenteric panniculitis:**
    A. Onset in children
    B. Males are commonly affected
    C. Resection is the treatment of choice
    D. Malignant stage of the disease is called retractile mesenteritis
    E. Autoimmunity is the cause of panniculitis

43. **Causes of retroperitoneal fibrosis:**
    A. Renal obstruction   B. Actinomycosis
    C. Road traffic accident D. Pancreatitis
    E. Renal tumour

44. **Retroperitoneal fibrosis involves:**
    A. Mediastinum   B. Mesentery
    C. Perirenal space D. Periduodenal space
    E. Pelvis

45. **Femoral hernia:**
    A. More common in women
    B. Highest risk of strangulation among all hernias
    C. The femoral canal is lateral to the femoral vein and artery
    D. Arises in the medial inguinal fossa
    E. Runs perpendicular to the inguinal ligament

46. **Lymphoma—the following are features of Hodgkin's and not seen in non-Hodgkin's:**
    A. Extranodal presentation
    B. Disseminated at presentation
    C. Mediastinal nodes
    D. Mesenteric nodes
    E. Noncontiguous spread

47. **Staging of lymphoma:**
    A. Involvement of two lymph node regions in the abdomen is stage I
    B. Extranodal sites are classified as IV
    C. Bulky disease is when the mediastinum measures more than 5 cm
    D. Presence of constitutional symptoms warrants A subtype
    E. The prognosis depends on site of involvement in NHL

48. **Lymphoma staging:**
    A. Skeletal survey with plain films is essential once diagnosis is suspected
    B. Head CT should be done only if there is clinical suspicion
    C. Chest, abdomen and pelvis CT are done in all cases
    D. If the patient presents with bone involvement, further staging is not required
    E. Splenectomy has to be done for complete staging

49. **Peritoneal hydatid:**
    A. The ectocyst is hypoechoic in ultrasound
    B. Floating membranes indicate rupture
    C. CT shows high density in cyst
    D. Treatment is peritoneal lavage
    E. Diagnosis is confirmed by serological assay

50. **Plain X-ray of abdomen:**
    A. Fluid level in caecum is seen in less than 10% of normal population
    B. The psoas outline is seen in less than 50% of population
    C. The bladder outline is not seen in 40% of population
    D. The spleen is seen in only 40% of population
    E. The colonic haustra are not routinely seen

51. **Gastrointestinal radiology:**
    A. Pneumoperitoneum tamponades the cysts in pneumatosis cystoids intestinalis
    B. Any air in peritoneum, after three days of laparatomy should be viewed with suspicion

    C. It may take up to 24 days for postsurgical pneumoperitoneum to be resorbed

    D. 500 ml of intraperitoneal air is required for demonstrating Rigler's sign

    E. Visualisation of at least 3 diaphragmatic slips indicates pneumoperitoneum

52. Peritoneum:
    A. 75 ml of fluid is normal in the peritoneal cavity
    B. Clinical examination will reveal ascites only when it is 500 ml
    C. Ultrasound can detect less than 1 ml of ascites
    D. Loculated ascites has irregular borders
    E. Presence of septa within a fluid rules out hemoperitoneum

53. Adrenal calcification is seen in:
    A. Addison's disease
    B. Conn's disease
    C. Pheochromocytoma
    D. Haemorrhage
    E. Myelolipoma

54. Calcified abdominal nodes are seen in:
    A. Amyloidosis
    B. Sarcoidosis
    C. Castleman's disease
    D. Whipple's disease
    E. *Mycobacterium avium intracellulare*

55. Plain film signs of ascites:
    A. Lateral displacement of ascending and descending colon
    B. Medial displacement of liver margin
    C. Separation of loops
    D. Thick flank stripe
    E. >2 mm distance between properitoneal fat stripe and gut

56. Peritoneal carcinomatosis:
    A. More common in the pelvic peritoneum
    B. Does not occur without ascites
    C. Usually grows outwards towards abdominal wall rather than into the peritoneal cavity
    D. Chylous ascites occurs in peritoneal carcinomatosis
    E. In omental cake, there is never fluid anterior to the omentum between it and the abdominal wall

57. Herniography:
A. Normally contrast does not pass into the obturator canal
B. Obturator hernia is one of the least common hernias to strangulate
C. Obturator hernia is best seen on the prone views
D. Direct inguinal hernia is always seen medial to the lateral umbilical fold in the medial inguinal fossa only
E. The neck of direct inguinal hernial sac is usually narrower than indirect inguinal hernia

58. Abnormal bone scan uptake in ascites:
A. Uremia
B. Infection
C. Cirrhosis
D. Cardiac failure
E. Malignant fluid collection

59. Peritoneal tumours:
A. History of asbestos exposure is seen in 95% of those with peritoneal mesothelioma
B. 90% of peritoneal mesothelioma have ascites
C. Scalloped liver surface is highly indicative of peritoneal mesothelioma
D. In pseudomyxoma peritonei, the ascites is echogenic with starburnt appearance
E. Echogenic foci in ascites of pseudomyxoma is mobile and is due to small cysts

60. Retroperitoneal tumours:
A. Malignant fibrous histiocytoma is the most common type
B. Solid component is always seen in liposarcomas
C. Lymphangiomas encase blood vessels without compressing them
D. Floating aorta sign is highly specific for lymphoma
E. Neurofibroma is the most common tumour that extends along the sympathetic ganglia

61. Lymphoma:
A. Ultrasound is the best modality for staging abdominal lymphomas, especially those involving porta nodes
B. Gallium scanning is not useful if the lesion is more than 5 cm
C. Gallium scanning is best for Hodgkin's than non-Hodgkin's lymphoma
D. Lymphangiography is not useful for evaluation of nodes above the L2 level
E. There is no significant benefit of lymphangiography over CT

62. **Herniography:**
    A. Medial umbilical fold separates the supravesical fossae
    B. Lateral umbilical fold separates the supravesical and medial inguinal fossae
    C. Deep inguinal ring is situated in the external oblique aponeurosis
    D. Median umbilical fold is a remnant of obliterated urachus
    E. The inferior epigastric artery is the component in lateral umbilical fold

63. **Herniography:**
    A. The inferior epigastric artery is medial to the deep inguinal ring
    B. The transversalis fascia forms the posterior boundary of inguinal canal
    C. Conjoint tendon is situated anteriorly to the inguinal canal
    D. The roof of inguinal canal is formed by external oblique aponeurosis
    E. Inguinal ligament is situated superior to the inguinal canal

64. **Retroperitoneal tumours:**
    A. Neurofibromas have high signal in T2 similar to cystic lesions
    B. Ganglioneuroma is most likely neurogenic tumour to calcify
    C. Myxoid component of a tumour enhances on contrast
    D. A tumour with high cellular content is low in both T1 and T2
    E. Myxoid liposarcoma has the worst prognosis amongst liposarcomas

65. **Retroperitoneal tumours:**
    A. Extensive necrosis is typical of retroperitoneal leiomyosarcoma
    B. Paragangliomas are avascular tumours arising from ganglion cells
    C. Extra-adrenal paragangliomas are more malignant than adrenal neoplasms
    D. Fluid-fluid levels are seen in paragangliomas
    E. Hemangiopericytoma is the most hypervascular tumour in retroperitoneum

66. **Retroperitoneal tumours:**
    A. Lymphomas are hypointense in T1 and hyperintense in T2
    B. Anterior displacement and rotation of right branch of portal vein is a specific indicator of retroperitoneal origin
    C. Anterior displacement of renal vein is reliable indicator
    D. Obliteration of psoas stripe is very sensitive for diagnosis of retroperitoneal origin of masses
    E. Separation of bowel loops is very suggestive of retroperitoneal mass

67. **Retroperitoneal tumours with myxoid stroma:**
    A. Liposarcoma
    B. Malignant fibrous histiocytoma
    C. Lipoma
    D. Schwannoma
    E. Lymphangioma

68. **Retroperitoneal lymph node with hypodense center:**
    A. Whipple's disease
    B. Lymphoma
    C. Tuberculosis
    D. Embryonal carcinoma metastasis
    E. Cervical carcinoma metastasis

69. **Lymph node enlargement in abdomen and pelvis:**
    A. External iliac node > 15 mm
    B. Inguinal lymph node > 12 mm
    C. Common iliac node > 10 mm
    D. Internal iliac node > 8 mm
    E. Obturator node > 9 mm

70. **Lymph node enlargement in abdomen and pelvis:**
    A. Perirectal lymph node > 6
    B. Porta hepatis > 10
    C. Para-aortic nodes from celiac axis to renal artery > 10
    D. Para-aortic nodes from renal artery to aortic bifurcation > 10
    E. Gastrohepatic ligament > 8

71. **Lymph nodal assessment in tumours:**
    A. STIR sequences are the most useful in the diagnosis
    B. Oval nodes are more likely to be abnormal than round nodes
    C. Fast spin echo images are good for identification of subtle nodes
    D. MRI is useful for characterizing lymph nodes
    E. Ultrasmall super paramagnetic iron oxide particles are useful as lymphographic agents

72. **Desmoid tumours:**
    A. Inflammatory in origin
    B. Seen in up to 50% of those with familial adenomatous polyposis
    C. Obstructs ureters and blood vessels
    D. A well-defined nodule cannot be desmoid, since it produces extensive fibrosis
    E. Fat can be seen within the mass

73. **Common locations of desmoid tumour:**
    A. Paraspinal muscles
    B. Mediastinum
    C. Retroperitoneum
    D. Pelvis
    E. Thigh

74. **Lymphoma:**
    A. Herpes virus is a common cause of lymphoma etiogenesis
    B. Increased risk of lymphoma in those with collagen vascular disorders

C. Hodgkin's disease has typical bimodal distribution
D. Mediastinal lymphomas peak in 60-70 years
E. Bacterial infections can predispose to production of lymphoma

75. **The following are considered bad risk factors in lymphoma:**
    A. Age less than 20 years
    B. Involvement of spleen
    C. High LDH
    D. Involvement of more than one extranodal site
    E. Involvement of liver

76. **Lymphomas:**
    A. Primary involvement of extranodal site occurs in 40% of cases of lymphomas
    B. Primary involvement of extranodal site, automatically upgrades the stage of lymphoma to stage IV
    C. Extranodal involvement is more common in Hodgkin's than non-Hodgkin's disease
    D. Retroperitoneal nodes are more commonly involved in Hodgkin's than non-Hodgkin's disease
    E. Porta hepatis and splenic hilar nodes are more commonly involved in non-Hodgkin's disease

77. **Lymphoma:**
    A. GIT is the primary site of involvement in lymphoma in 30% of patients
    B. GIT is the second most common site of extranodal spread after bone marrow
    C. Involvement of GIT from a mesenteric nodal disease is more common than primary involvement
    D. Liver and spleen can be involved in primary lymphoma of gastrointestinal tract
    E. Involvement of lymph nodes beyond the locoregional nodes, excludes the diagnosis of primary gastrointestinal lymphoma

78. **Aortocaval fistula:**
    A. Continuous abdominal bruit is a characteristic feature
    B. The density of suprarenal part of IVC is used for assessment of fistula
    C. Equal and rapid enhancement of both aorta and IVC
    D. Normally the peak enhancement of entire IVC occurs till 90 sec
    E. Dilated renal veins are present

79. **Causes of early contrast opacification of IVC in contrast enhanced CT scans:**
    A. Right heart failure   B. Aortocaval fistula
    C. IVC obstruction   D. Leiomyosarcoma of IVC
    E. Carcinoid syndrome

80. Herniography:
A. Contrast is injected through the iliac fossa
B. The bladder should always be emptied before the procedure
C. Aortic aneurysm is a contraindication
D. To confirm intraperitoneal position of dye, the table should be tilted head down 10%
E. Procedure abandoned if contrast enters bowel

81. Herniography:
A. 10 ml of contrast is enough
B. Prone images are not necessary
C. AP and 45 degree oblique views are routinely done
D. Tangenital views—for anterior abdominal wall hernias
E. Valsalva's manoeuvre is a helpful technique during herniography

82. Herniogram:
A. Cranial angulation is useful for differentiating femoral and inguinal hernia
B. Small bowel is commonly punctured in the iliac fossa approach
C. Small bowel puncture requires admission and treatment
D. Adhesions secondary to previous surgery will cause high failure rate
E. All the patients should be monitored in the deparment for half an hour after the procedure

83. Indirect inguinal hernia:
A. Caused by persistent processus vaginalis
B. Always arises from the lateral inguinal fossa
C. Enters inguinal canal at the superifical inguinal ring
D. Passes through defect in transversalis fascia
E. Runs parallel to inguinal fossa

84. Left-sided IVC:
A. Caused by persistent left subcardinal vein
B. Crosses at the level of left renal vein
C. Associated with horseshoe kidney
D. The left IVC never extends proximal to the left renal vein
E. The left gonadal and suprarenal vein drain into the left-sided IVC

85. The following are recognised causes of peritoneal fibromatosis:
A. Aortic aneurysm   B. Estrogen therapy
C. Gardner's syndrome   D. Familial adenomatosis polyposis
E. Cronkhite Canada syndrome

86. Causes of enhancing lymph nodes:
A. Castelman's disease   B. Sarcoidosis
C. Tuberculosis   D. Renal metastasis
E. Testicular metastasis

ANSWERS

1. **A-T, B-T, C-T, D-F, E-F**
Calcification is common in men before 60 years and in women after that.
There are four pairs of lumbar arteries. The middle suprarenal artery rises from the aorta. The superior suprarenal artery rises from inferior phrenic artery and inferior suprarenal artery from renal artery.

2. **A-T, B-T, C-F, D-T, E-T**
The IVC lies behind right common iliac artery, aortic bifurcation, small bowel loops, mesenteric root, duodenal 3rd part and pancreatic head.
It pierces the diaphragm at T8.

3. **A-T, B-T, C-T, D-T, E-T**
Celiac, superior mesenteric and inferior mesenteric are the preaortic group of lymph nodes situated close to the respective arteries. Gastric, hepatic and pancreaticosplenic drain into celiac. Mesenteric, Ileocolic, colic and pararectal drain into superior and inferior mesenteric nodes.

4. **A-F, B-F, C-F, D-F, E-T**
About 1-2 ml of air is enough to be demonstrated in erect or lateral decubitus films. Peptic ulcer perforation is more common than colonic perforation.

5. **A-T, B-T, C-T, D-T, E-F**
There is a silent phase in peptic ulcer perforation, where there are no clinical signs of peritonitis.

6. **A-T, B-T, C-F, D-T, E-T**
Irritable bowel syndrome has no pathologic appearances in imaging.

7. **A-T, B-F, C-T, D-F, E-T**
Gastric rugae in supine film and fluid levels in erect film are normal. up to 5 fluid levels, mainly colonic, in bowel loop < 2.5 cm is normal. > 2 fluid levels in dilated small bowel loop > 2.5 cm is abnormal.

8. **A-T, B-T, C-T, D-T, E-T**

9. **A-T, B-T, C-F, D-T, E-T**

10. **A-T, B-T, C-T, D-F, E-T**
Mucinous adenocarcinomas (stomach, colon) and mucoceles are common causes.

11. A-T, B-T, C-T, D-T, E-F
Hydatid cyst is infection.

12. A-T, B-F, C-T, D-T, E-T
Football sign—air outlining entire abdominal cavity. Rigler's sign-air on both sides of bowel wall (Rigler's triad is seen in gallstone ileus (pneumobilia, stones and dilated bowel loops). Tell tale sign is air in between three loops of bowel. Outlining of medial umbilical ligaments, both lateral umbilical ligaments (inverted V sign) and middle umbilical ligament (urachus sign) are other signs.

13. A-T, B-F, C-F, D-T, E-T
In the mesentery, secondary tumours are common than primary, benign common than malignant, cystic common than solid. Desmoid tumour is the most common primary tumour in mesentery.

14. A-T, B-T, C-T, D-T, E-T
Lymphangioma is the most common cause. Mesenteric cyst is another common cause.

15. A-F, B-T, C-T, D-T, E-F
Splenosis is autotransplantation of splenic tissue within peritoneal cavity due to trauma or splenectomy. The common places are serosal surface of small intestine, serosal surface of large intestine, greater omentum, parietal peritoneum, mesentery, porta hepatitis, paracolic gutters and pelvis. These lesions have all characteristics of spleen in all imaging modalities. They show uptake of heat damaged RBCs labelled with technetium.

16. A-T, B-T, C-T, D-T, E-F
Infections, benign and malignant tumours are seen.

17. A-T, B-T, C-T, D-T, E-T
Also in bile duct tumours, urachal duct and omphalomesenteric duct tumours.

18. A-T, B-T, C-T, D-T, E-F
Tuberculosis is another common cause.

19. A-T, B-F, C-T, D-T, E-T
Subphrenic abscess, subdiaphgramatic fat and diaphgramatic irregularity are some of the other causes. Chiladitis syndrome is interportion of bowel loops between liver and diaphragmatic dome.

20. A-F, B-T, C-T, D-T, E-F
Appendicial tumour is another recognised cause. Exudative ascites has high density.

21. **A-T, B-T, C-T, D-T, E-T**
Nodular lesions can be seen throughout the peritoneum. Calcification is common in serious cystadenocarcinoma. High density is seen in the mesenteric fat.

22. **A-T, B-T, C-T, D-F, E-T**
Mesenteric panniculitis is chronic nonspecific inflammation of the mesentery. It is very commonly associated with malignancy and inflammatory conditions. Granulomatous diseases, malignancies including gastrointestinal carcinomas and vasculitis are other causes.

23. **A-F, B-T, C-F, D-T, E-T**

24. **A-F, B-T, C-F, D-F, E-T**
It is more common in the jejunal mesentery, so predominantly seen in the left side. Soft tissue nodules are seen due to inflammation, and are surrounded by low density fat halo of normal mesentery. High density stripe can be seen and indicates infiltration of mesenteric fat with macrophages. The inflammatory mass encases the mesenteric vessels.

25. **A-T, B-T, C-T, D-T, E-F**
Schistosomiasis, ischemic colitis, hemangioma and mucinous adenocarcinoma are other causes.

26. **A-F, B-F, C-F, D-T, E-T**
Caecal fluid levels seen in 10% of normal individuals.
Critical diameter of transverse colon is 5.5 cm and that of caecum is 9 cm.

27. **A-T, B-F, C-T, D-T, E-T**
Tumours causing obstruction to lymphatic drainage are common · causes.

28. **A-T, B-F, C-T, D-T, E-T**
Peritoneal mesothelioma is associated with asbestos exposure. Peritoneal nodular masses are seen, which may be a large conglomerate mass, but the ascites is of small quantity and of normal water density. Mesentery, peritoneum, omentum and bowel wall are thickened with stellate configuration of neurovascular bundles. Bowel, bladder, liver and pancreas are invaded.

29. **A-T, B-T, C-T, D-F, E-F**
Peritoneal hydatid is almost always secondary to hepatic hydatid, the usual mode of dissemination, being a surgery for hepatic hydatid. The other mode of spread is spontaneous rupture of hepatic hydatid. Ultrasound and CT are both useful for diagnosing

rupture when the communication is wide. CT is the best for diagnosing peritoneal seedling.

30. **A-F, B-T, C-T, D-F, E-T**
Quinine is a common cause.

31. **A-T, B-F, C-F, D-T, E-T**
Ovary is the most common cause.

32. **A-F, B-T, C-F, D-T, E-F**
Peritoneum is involved in only 30% of abdominal tuberculosis. It can spread by blood/ruptured lymph nodes/perforated bowel lesion/fallopian tube. There are three types, wet—with ascites, dry—with lymph nodes and adhesions, fibrotic fixed type—with abdominal masses. Barium meal can show separation of bowel loops/adhesions/masses/obstruction. Septae within ascites is seen in most of exudative ascites and is not specific for tuberculosis.

33. **A-T, B-T, C-T, D-T, E-T**
Methysergide, ergotamine, phenacetin, amphetamines, LSD, methyldopa and hydralazine are drugs causing retroperitoneal fibrosis.

34. **A-T, B-T, C-T, D-T, E-F**
Mesenteric lymph nodes are more in favour of tuberculosis. Retroperitoneal lymph nodes can be involved in other metastatic or lymphomatous lesions. Conglomerate nodes are due to periadenitis and are highly suggestive of tuberculosis. Caesation and calcification are also more in favour of tuberculosis.

35. **A-F, B-T, C-F, D-F, E-T**
Peritoneal thickening involves both the omentum and the mesentery. Bowel wall thickening is concentric. Lymphoma is the closest mimic. Crohn's is more eccentric towards the mesenteric border and malignancy is variegated. Lymphadenopathy is seen in 30%. Pseudokidney is due to bowel wall thickening and in this location could be due to cancer or a thickened pulled up caecum in tuberculosis.

36. **A-F, B-T, C-T, D-T, E-F**
Anterior border of sigmoid and medial border of distal ileum are other most common locations.

37. **A-F, B-T, C-T, D-F, E-T**
Fibromatosis is the most common benign tumour of the mesentery, followed by lipoma. Metastasis takes two routes for spread within the ascitic fluid. Those in the right inframesocolic compartment spread along the leaves of the mesentery to the medial caecum

and then spill into the pelvis. Those in the left inframesocolic compartment spread along the leaves of the sigmoid mesocolon and spill into the pelvis from where they can pass to the right paracolic gutter, right subhepatic space and into the lesser sac. Peritoneal metastases are common in the antimesenteric border, since the tumour embolises to the most distal radicles of blood vessels supplying the bowel.

38. **A-T, B-F, C-T, D-T, E-F**
Histoplasmosis is another known cause.

39. **A-T, B-T, C-T, D-T, E-T,**
Other findings include smudged omentum, discrete nodules, cysts, mixed cystic and solid lesion, fine linear strands, focal mass in mesentery.

40. **A-T, B-T, C-T, D-F, E-T**
Enteric cyst has a mucosal lining, but there is no reduplication of bowel wall and there is no muscle lining. Enteric duplication cyst has a bowel wall and muscle lining. In hypoalbuminemia, the retroperitoneal fat is spared and high density is seen only in the mesenteric fat.

41. **A-T, B-T, C-T, D-T, E-T**
Sclerosing cholangitis, mediastinal, orbital fibrosis are associated.

42. **A-F, B-T, C-F, D-F, E-T**
It typically starts in mid or late adulthood, with a slight male predominance. Resection is not helpful. It is believed to be autoimmune or idiopathic. A predominant inflammatory or fibrofatty disease is called mesenteric panniculitis and a predominant fibrotic disease is called retractile mesenteritis.

43. **A-T, B-T, C-T, D-T, E-F**
Causes of retroperitoneal fibrosis are idiopathic, abdominal aortic aneurysm, inflammatory (Crohn's, Ulcerative colitis, pancreatitis, diverticulitis, actinomycosis, urine extravasation secondary to trauma or obstruction), malignancy (lymphoma, metastasis from colon and breast carcinoid), drugs, surgery, trauma associations included other sclerosing conditions like Reidel's thyroiditis, orbital pseudotumour, mediastinal fibrosis and sclerosing cholangitis.

44. **A-T, B-T, C-T, D-T, E-T**

45. **A-T, B-T, C-F, D-T, E-T**
It has a very narrow sac and is very common in females. The femoral canal is medial to the femoral vein. The hernia is best seen in straight views.

46. **A-F, B-F, C-T,D-F, E-F**
    Hodgkin's lymphoma usually has nodal presentation, spreads contiguously, localized at presentation, mediastinal lymph nodes/ spleen involvement are common. Involvement of mesenteric lymph nodes, Waldeyer's ring, liver, GIT, marrow, CNS and skin are uncommon. In non-Hodgkin's, extranodal pattern is common, spread is hematogenous and noncontiguous, disseminated at presentation. Mediastinal lymph nodes and spleen are uncommon. Involvement of liver, Waldeyer's ring, mesenteric nodes, GIT, marrow, CNS, skin can be seen.

47. **A-F, B-T, C-F, D-F, E-F**
    Cotswold's staging of lymphoma
    I—one lymph node group, II—two or more groups on one side of diaphragm, III—lymph nodes on both sides of diaphgram, IV— extranodal.
    A—absence of constitutional symptoms, B—presence of constitutional symptoms
    X-bulky disease, mediastinum > 10 cm of mass more than 1/3rd thoracic diameter
    The prognosis depends on the bulk of the tumour and pathology than the site in NHL.

48. **A-F, B-T, C-T, D-F, E-F**
    Skeletal survey is unnecessary. Staging CT of chest, abdomen and pelvis are performed. Brain and spine are performed only if there are clinical symptoms. Splenectomy is no longer done for staging purposes.

49. **A-T, B-T, C-F, D-F, E-T**
    Pericyst and endocyst are hyperechoic and ectocyst is hypoechoic. Floating membranes is due to detachment of ectocyst from pericyst. CT shows low density in the cyst.
    Treatment for disseminated hydatid cyst, is albendazole, for three weeks, with three weeks gap and for three cycles.

50. **A-F, B-T, C-T, D-F, E-F**
    Fluid level in caecum is normally seen in 20% of population in erect films.
    Colonic haustra are normally seen as are multiple fluid levels. The psoas outline is seen only in 48%, the spleen in 58% and bladder in 60% of normal population.

51. **A-T, B-T, C-T, D-F, E-T,**
    It may take 1-24 days for reabsorption of air subsequent to laparotomy or laparoscopy, more in obese individuals. However, any air after three days of surgery, should be viewed with

suspicion. At least 1L of intraperitoneal air is required for demonstrating Rigler's sign, which is visualization of both surfaces of bowel. Visualization of 3 diaphragmatic slips, arching parallel to the diaphragmatic dome is indicative of pneumoperitoneum.

52. **A-T, B-T, C-T, D-T, E-F**
    Hemoperitoneum can be a clear fluid or filled with debris, septations or a heterogeneous mass with cystic areas.

53. **A-T, B-T, C-T, D-T, E-F**
    Idiopathic, haemorrhage, tuberculosis, pheochromocytoma, neuroblastoma, adenoma, Addison's and cysts are the common causes of adrenal calcification.

54. **A-T, B-T, C-T, D-F, E-F**
    TB, histoplasmosis, paracoccidioidomycosis, lymphoma after treat, metastasis from mucinous tumours, are other causes.

55. **A-F, B-T, C-T, D-T, E-F**
    The ascending and descending colon are displaced medially. The liver is displaced medially (Hallmer's sign). Bowel loops are placed centrally and separated by fluid.
    The abdomen is bulging and grey. > 3 mm distance between the fat stripe and gut.

56. **A-T, B-F, C-F, D-T, E-F**
    Peritoneal carcinomatosis can occur without ascites. Detection of lesions without ascites will be difficult. Usually grows towards the peritoneal cavity. Ascites can be clear or with septations or debris or chylous or haemorrhagic. Omental cake can be adherent to the parietal peritoneum or it may be free floating with fluid anterior to it.

57. **A-F, B-F, C-F, D-F, E-F**
    Normally contrast can pass into obturator canal. Obturator hernia has a narrow sac and is very prone for strangulation. It is best seen in supine views. Direct inguinal hernia is always medial to the lateral umbilical fold, but it can be seen either in the medial inguinal fossa or supravesical fossa. The neck of direct hernia is always wider than that of indirect hernia.

58. **A-T, B-T, C-F, D-F, E-T**

59. **A-F, B-T, C-F, D-T, E-F**
    History of asbestos exposure is seen in 65% of cases. Scalloped liver surface is highly suggestive of pseudomyxoma peritonei, also seen in ovarian carcinoma. Echogenic foci within pseudomyxoma peritonei is not mobile.

60. A-T, B-F, C-T, D-T, E-F
Most of the liposarcomas have solid and fatty components. A well-differentiated liposarcoma can have purely fatty components without any solid component. Differentiation from a benign lesion often requires a biopsy. Lymphangiomas, ganglioneuromas and lymphomas extend between structures without compressing them. Floating aorta is encasement of aorta and anterior displacement from the spine, which is seen peculiarly in lymphoma and not in other malignant neoplasms. Ganglioneuroma is the most common tumour that extends along the sympathetic chain.

61. A-F, B-T, C-F, D-T, E-T
CT or MRI are the ideal methods for staging of lymphomas. Ultrasound does not have a primary role in staging, since it is not sensitive or accurate. It can be used for confirming the nature of a suspected lesion in CT scan. Gallium scanning is very sensitive, but not useful if more than 5 cm, below the diaphragm. High sensitivity is seen in Hodgkin's lymphoma and histiocytic non-Hodgkin's lymphomas. Lymphangiography is the best in demonstrating the internal lymph nodal architecture. But it demonstrates abnormalities in nodes less than 1 cm, in less than 10% of cases. Lymphangiography is also not useful for lymph nodes outside the retroperitoneum.

62. A-F, B-F, C-F, D-T, E-T
From medial to lateral there are two supravesical fossae, two medial inguinal fossae and two lateral inguinal fossae. Median umbilical fold—obliterated urachus (between two supravesical fossae). Medial umbilical fold—obliterated umbilical artery (between supravesical and medial inguinal). Lateral umbilical fold—inferior epigastric artery (between medial and lateral inguinal fossae). The deep inguinal ring is in the transversalis fascia.

63. A-T, B-T, C-F, D-F, E-F
Posterior wall—transversalis fascia laterally, conjoint tendon medially. Anterior wall— external oblique aponeurosis. Superiorly—internal oblique and transverses. Inferiorly—inguinal ligament.

64. A-T, B-T, C-T, D-T, E-T
Ganglioneuromas have a heterogeneous signal in MRI depending on the content. Myxoid elements are low in T1 and very high signal in T2. Cellular components are low in both T1 and T2. Myxoid liposarcomas have intermediate prognosis, better than poorly differentiated and worse than well differentiated.

65. A-T, B-F, C-T, D-T, E-T
Paragangliomas and hemangiopericytomas are very vascular. Haemorrhage inside tumour will produce fluid-fluid level.

Although necrosis is seen in many tumours, it is very extensive in leiomyosarcoma. Necrosis is low signal in T1 and high in T2, but does not enhance, unlike myxoid stroma.

66. **A-F, B-T, C-T, D-F, E-F**
Lymphomas are hypointense in both T1 and T2, because of their intense cellular nature. Anterior displacement of IVC, adrenals and duodenum are other reliable signs. Psoas stripe is not very sensitive. It might not be obliterated in large masses with fatty component. It is also not very specific. Separation of bowel loops indicates mesenteric rather than retroperitoneal disease.

67. **A-T, B-T, C-F, D-T, E-F**
Myxoid stroma is high signal in T1 and T2. It is also seen in other neurogenic tumours.

68. **A-T, B-T, C-T, D-T, E-T**
Also in pyogenic infection, and other metastasis.

69. **A-F, B-F, C-F, D-F, E-F**
Inguinal lymph node > 10, common iliac > 9, external iliac > 10, internal iliac > 7, obturator node > 8 mm.

70. **A-F, B-F, C-T, D-F, E-T**
Gastrohepatic ligament >8, porta hepatis >8, portocaval >10, celiac axis to renal artery >10, renal artery to aortic bifurcation >12, perirectal node—visualization is enough.

71. **A-T, B-F, C-F, D-F, E-T**
Enlarged lymph nodes are seen as low signal lesions in T1 and intermediate to high signal in T2 and STIR. Fast spin echo and turbo spin echo images are not very useful since the signal approaches that of fat. Round nodes > 8 mm are likely to be pathological than oval nodes. MRI is not capable of characterizing lymph nodes yet.

72. **A-F, B-F, C-T, D-F, E-T**
Desmoid is infiltrating fibroblastic proliferation. It is not inflammatory or neoplastic. Seen in 10-20% of people with FAP. It is seen as a well-defined discrete mass in the early stages. Later, it produces ill-defined soft tissue infiltration of mesenteric fat. Later, a soft tissue mass with engulfed mesenteric fat is seen. It produces obstruction of gastrointestinal tract or genitourinary tract or vasculature.

73. **A-T, B-F, C-T, D-T, E-F**
It is also seen in anterior abdominal wall muscles and mesentery.

74. A-T, B-T, C-T, D-F, E-T
Herpes viruses are recognised causes in development of lymphoma. Epstein-Barr virus is a type of herpes virus and is the most common viral agent responsible for the production of many types of lymphoma. Infections, especially bacterial, are recognised causes of producing mucosal associated lymphomas. *Helicobacter pylori* is a known cause of gastric lymphoma. Hodgkin's disease has a bimodal distibution, the first peak in 20-30 years and the second peak after 60 years. Mediastinal disease is more common in young age between 25-35 years. Immunosuppression associated with collagen vascular diseases and other diseases are predisposing factors for development of lymphoma.

75. A-F, B-F, C-T, D-T, E-F
Age more than 60 years, Stages 3 and 4 are other poor prognostic features for lymphomas.

76. A-T, B-F, C-F, D-F, E-T
Involvement of extranodal sites can occur secondarily to lymphoma elsewhere or might be the primary manifestation of lymphoma. Primary and secondary extranodal lymphomas are more common in the non-Hodgkin's type than the Hodgkin's. If only a primary extranodal site is involved, with regional lymph nodes the stage is only I or II but with added E stage, but does not upgrade it to stage IV. Retroperitoneal nodes are more often involved in Hodgkin's than non-Hodgkin's, but mesenteric, splenic hilar and porta hepatitis nodes are more common in non-Hodgkin's lymphoma.

77. A-T, B-F, C-T, D-F, E-T
Gastointestinal tract is involved secondarily in both Hodgkin's and non-Hodgkin's, more more common in the non-Hodgkin's type. GIT is the most common site of extranodal involvement, being involved in 10% of adults and 30% of children. Certain diagnostic criteria should be met before a diagnosis of primary lymphoma of gastrointestinal tract is made. The lymphomatous lesion should involve a primary gastrointestinal tract organ, such as stomach or intestine, with only regional lymph nodes involved, without involvement of liver or spleen and normal WBC count.

78. A-T, B-F, C-T, D-F, E-T
The infrarenal IVC is opacified by contrast which returns from the lower limbs after passing through abdominal aorta and lower limb arteries and the density increases slowly up to 90 sec. The suprarenal portion of IVC is opacified by contrast returning from the renal veins and it opacifies earlier, with maximum density at

20 seconds. So suprarenal IVC density cannot be used to assess fistula. The fistula between aorta and IVC will be suspected when there is rapid early simultaneous enhancement of aorta and infrarenal IVC. The IVC will be dilated and the underlying abdominal aortic aneurysm will be seen.

79. **A-T, B-T, C-F, D-F, E-T**
Early contrast opacification in right heart failure and carcinoid syndrome is due to associated tricuspid regurgitation. In aortocaval fistula, there is direct communication between the aorta and IVC.

80. **A-T, B-T, C-T, D-F, E-F**
Herniography is contrast visualisation of the peritoneal coverings. The contrast can be injected through the subumbilical region or in the iliac fossae. The bladder should be emptied to avoid puncture and aortic aneurysm should be excluded. The table can be tilted head up 10 degrees to confirm intraperitoneal location of the contrast. If the needle has punctured, the bowel and contrast has opacified the bowel, the needle is withdrawn a few centimeters and abandoning procedure is not required.

81. **A-F, B-F, C-T, D-T, E-T**
50 ml of contrast is normally given. Prone images are necessary. Valsalva's manoeuvre may be necessary to visualise the hernia, which may manifest only with increased intra-abdominal pressure.

82. **A-T, B-F, C-F, D-T, E-T**
Small bowel is commonly punctured in the subumbilical puncture and large bowel in the iliac fossa puncture. Small bowel puncture does not usually require any admission, but large bowel perforation is serious due to impending peritonitis and the patient has to be admitted and treated.

83. **A-T, B-T, C-F, D-F, E-F**
Enters inguinal canal through deep inguinal ring. Direct inguinal hernia passes through defect in transversalis fascia. Runs perpendicular to the inguinal fossa.

84. **A-T, B-T, C-T, D-F, E-F**
Normal IVC is formed by joining of posterior cardinal vein, right supracardinal vein and right subcardinal vein. The left subcardinal vein and supracardinal vein normally disappear. Left-sided IVC is formed when there is persistent subcardinal vein on the left side. The left-sided vein usually crosses over to the right side to join the normal right-sided IVC at the level of left renal vein. Occasionally, there may be continuation of hemiazygos vein above the level of left renal vein. The left gonadal and suprarenal vein,

drain as usual to the left renal vein, and not into the left-sided IVC. Only the left common iliac vein drains into the left-sided IVC.

85. **A-F, B-T, C-T, D-T, E-F**
Aortic aneurysm predisposes to retroperitoneal fibrosis due to leakage of ceroid.

86. **A-T, B-T, C-T, D-T, E-F**
Tuberculosis, thyroid metastasis, Kaposi's sarcoma, angio-immunoblastic lymphadenopathy are other causes.

6 *Acute Abdomen*

1. **Acute cholecystitis:**
   A. 90% have stone in the cystic duct
   B. Ultrasound has 95% specificity
   C. CT and MRI are more sensitive for diagnosing wall thickening in cholecystitis
   D. Plain X-ray reveals stones in 45-50% of cases
   E. Immediate cholecystectomy is the treatment for cholecystitis

2. **Emphysematous cholecystitis:**
   A. Calculus is seen in majority of the cases
   B. Associated with diabetes mellitus in 75%
   C. More common in females
   D. Mortality higher than in acute cholecystitis
   E. Acoustic shadowing is seen behind the gas

3. **Causes of right upper quadrant pain and fever but no Murphy's sign:**
   A. Cholangitis   B. Pneumonia
   C. Pancreatitis   D. Gangrenous cholecystitis
   E. Perforated duodenal ulcer

4. **Features of gangrenous cholecystitis:**
   A. Intraluminal membranes
   B. Irregular wall thickening
   C. Pericholecystic fluid
   D. Sonographic Murphy's sign
   E. Immediate surgery is mandatory

5. **Acute cholecystitis:**
   A. Murphy's sign has a high positive predictive value for acute cholecystitis
   B. Gallstones with Murphy's sign is indicative of acute cholecystitis
   C. Increased omental blood flow is seen in pericholecystic abscess
   D. Intramural edema is highly suggestive of acute cholecystitis
   E. Cystic duct dilatation is highly predictive of acute cholecystitis

6. **Causes of microabscesses in liver:**
   A. *Candida*
   B. Tuberculosis
   C. Atypical mycobacteria
   D. Cryptococcosis
   E. Histoplasmosis

7. **Predisposing factors for liver abscess:**
   A. Biliary stricture
   B. Trauma
   C. CBD stones
   D. GI inflammation
   E. Surgery

8. **Differential diagnosis of emphysematous cholecystitis:**
   A. Cholecystoenteric fistula
   B. Bowel
   C. Intramural cholesterosis
   D. Porcelain gallbladder
   E. Gangrenous cholecystitis

9. **Causes of AIDS cholangitis:**
   A. CMV is the most common cause
   B. Cryptosporidiosis is a recognised cause
   C. Both the intrahepatic and extrahepatic ducts are dilated in the earlier phases
   D. Mucosal thickening in earlier stages due to edema
   E. Strictures are similar to sclerosing cholangitis

10. **Pyogenic liver abscesses:**
    A. Mortality of 10%
    B. Cryptogenic liver abscess is the most common cause in community settings
    C. Sepsis the most common cause in elderly
    D. Majority are produced by *E. coli*
    E. Polymicrobial infection is a significant cause

11. **Acute cholecystitis:**
    A. Impacted stone in the neck of gallbladder correlates strongly with acute cholecystitis
    B. Harmonic images reduce side lobe and revertebration artefacts
    C. Harmonic images increased detection of acoustic shadowing
    D. Generalised symmetric gallbladder wall thickening is specific for intrinsic biliary disease
    E. Increased flow in fundus of gallbladder signifies acute cholecystitis

12. **Cholangitis:**
    A. Normal biliary system is against diagnosis
    B. Pain, fever, biliary dilatation in ultrasounds warrant direct ERCP
    C. Drainage of infected system is mandatory
    D. Undiagnosed CBD stones are the most common cause
    E. The triad of right upper quadrant pain, jaundice and fever is almost always seen

13. **Liver abscess:**
    A. A solitary abscess is most likely cryptogenic
    B. Microabscesses are those less than 5 mm
    C. 25% of abscesses are hyperechoic in ultrasound
    D. Rim enhancement is seen in 75% of CT examinations
    E. There is reversal of flow in the portal vein near the abscess

14. **The following are indications of catheter drainage of liver abscess:**
    A. Lesion more than 5 cm
    B. Unilocular
    C. No communication with biliary tree
    D. Communication with gastrointestinal tract
    E. Well-defined walls

15. **Predisposing factors for liver abscess:**
    A. Subphrenic abscess
    B. Pneumonia
    C. Proctitis
    D. Colonic cancer
    E. Endocarditis

16. **Acute acalculous cholecystitis:**
    A. 10% of cholecystitis
    B. Seen in critically ill patients
    C. Mortality and morbidity are low
    D. Gallbladder wall thickening without gallstones is specific
    E. Scinti scans are highly accurate

17. **Liver abscess:**
    A. An abscess of biliary tract origin involves the right lobe preferentially
    B. Portal origin liver abscess involves both lobes
    C. Appendicitis is the most common factor for liver abscess development
    D. A cluster of abscesses is common with coliform organisms
    E. Miliary pattern is common with *Staphylococcus*

18. **Acute acalculous cholecystitis:**
    A. CT scan is the most useful investigation for diagnosis
    B. Murphy's sign is negative
    C. Progressive thickening of gallbladder wall is indicative
    D. Pericholecystic fluid is a useful sign
    E. Increased density is seen in pericholecystic fat

19. **Scintigraphy in acute cholecystitis:**
    A. Scintigraphy has similar accuracy as sonography
    B. False positive scintigraphy is seen in hepatic dysfunction
    C. False negative studies are rare
    D. Scintigraphy should always be done if sonography is negative
    E. Scintigraphy has 75% accuracy

20. **Causes of generalised gallbladder wall thickening:**
    A. Congestive cardiac failure
    B. Benign ascites
    C. Hepatitis
    D. Cirrhosis
    E. Hereditary spherocytosis

21. **CT target sign is seen in:**
    A. Ulcerative colitis
    B. Pseudomembranous colitis
    C. Graft-versus-host disease
    D. Shock bowel
    E. Typhlitis

22. **CT of GIT:**
    A. Mesenteric fat shows attentuation values between −15 and −40 HU
    B. 1000 ml of barium is given the evening before CT
    C. The normal wall thickness of colon should be less than 7 mm
    D. CT is a reliable method of diagnosing ulcerative colitis
    E. Fibrosis produces high density in the mesentery

23. **Ulcerative colitis:**
    A. CT scan shows pseudopolyps
    B. Mural stratification helps in distinguishing ulcerative colitis and granulomatous colitis
    C. Mean colonic thickeness in ulcerative colitis is less than in Crohn's disease
    D. Colonic wall is smooth unlike granulomatous colitis
    E. Rectal narrowing is a hallmark of ulcerative colitis

24. **Causes of separation of bowel loops in Crohn's in barium:**
    A. Mesenteric lymph nodes
    B. Creeping fat
    C. Abscess
    D. Bowel wall thickening
    E. Phlegmon

25. **Associated features to be evaluated in colitis:**
    A. Osteomyelitis
    B. Avascular necrosis
    C. Sacroilitis
    D. Hydronephrosis
    E. Sclerosing cholangitis

26. **Crohn's:**
    A. Mesenteric lymph nodes more than 1 cm, indicates lymphoma or carcinoma
    B. Hypervascular mesentery (COMB SIGN) rules out lymphoma
    C. Abscesses are seen in 15%
    D. CT is better than fistulography for demonstraton of full extent of tracts
    E. Phlegmon produces smudging of mesentery

27. **Crohn's disease:**
    A. Bowel wall enhancement correlates with the disease activity
    B. Bowel wall stratification is preserved in chronic stage of Crohn's disease
    C. Mural stratification indicates medical therapy will be successful
    D. Homogeneous thickening indicates irreversibility
    E. Cobblestoning is seen in thin section CT

28. **The following fistulae are seen in Crohn's:**
    A. Colobronchial
    B. Pancreaticoduodenal
    C. Enterospinal
    D. Enterocutaneous
    E. Gastrocolic

29. **Amoebic liver abscess:**
    A. Spreads to the liver from colonic wall through the liver capsule
    B. Trophozoites are seen adjacent to the outer wall
    C. 85% of lesions are solitary
    D. Gallium scan finding of cold center and hot rim is specific for amoebic liver abscess
    E. Left lobe lesions extend into the pericardium

30. **The following are typical findings of amoebic liver abscess in ultrasound:**
    A. Subcapsular location
    B. Posterior acoustic enhancement
    C. Round shape
    D. Homogeneous low level internal echoes
    E. Wall echoes

31. **The following bowel layers are thickened in ulcerative colitis:**
    A. Mucosa   B. Muscularis mucosa
    C. Submucosa   D. Lamina propria
    E. Serosa

32. **Mural stratification of bowel wall in CT is seen in:**
    A. Ulcerative colitis
    B. Crohn's disease
    C. Radiation
    D. Mesenteric venous thrombosis
    E. Graft-verus-host disease

33. **CT features of ulcerative colitis:**
    A. Dilated colon
    B. Luminal narrowing
    C. Mural thickening
    D. Mural thinning
    E. Pneumatosis

34. **AIDS colitis:**
    A. Cytomegalovirus is the only known pathogen
    B. CD4 count is less than 200
    C. Proximal ascending colon is the most common site
    D. Submucosal low density is a common feature in CT
    E. Ascites

35. **Enterohaemorrhagic colitis:**
    A. E 015:H7 is the most common organism
    B. Fever is absent
    C. Fecal leucocytes seen
    D. Right side of colon is always involved
    E. Improperly cooked beef is the most common mode of infection

36. **Causes of typhilitis:**
    A. Aplastic anemia
    B. AIDS
    C. Multiple myeloma
    D. Tuberculosis
    E. Leukemia

37. **Typhlitis:**
    A. Ileum is involved
    B. CT is the study of choice
    C. Neutropenia is the underlying cause
    D. Bacteria alone are isolated from the bowel
    E. Perforation is common

38. **Common features of graft-versus-host disease:**
    A. Abdominal cramps   B. Diarrhoea
    C. Intestinal haemorrhage D. Perforation
    E. Submucosal fat deposition

39. **The following features should be evaluated in CT scan of colitis:**
    A. Presacral space
    B. Mesenteric fat density
    C. Retroperitoneal fat homogenity
    D. Extraluminal contrast collection
    E. Splenic abnormalities

40. **Colitis:**
    A. Ascites indicates chronic cause of colitis
    B. Submucosal fat deposition indicates subacute or chronic stage
    C. Lymph nodes are seen in presacral space in chronic ulcerative colitis
    D. The fat density in presacral space is 50 HU more than retroperitoneal fat
    E. Mural stratification is a characteristic feature of ulcerative colitis

41. **Pseudomembranous colitis:**
    A. Vancomycin is a causative drug
    B. Accordion pattern is a specific CT feature
    C. Toxic megacolon is an important complication
    D. Subcutaneous edema occurs
    E. Pseudomembranes are seen in contrast enhanced images

42. **Causes of ascites in colitis:**
    A. Ulcerative colitis
    B. Crohn's disease
    C. Ischemia
    D. Pseudomembranous colitis
    E. AIDS

43. **Indications for CT in acute pancreatitis:**
    A. Establishing and confirming diagnosis
    B. Sudden deterioriation following initial response
    C. Patients presenting with clinically suspected severe acute pancreatitis
    D. Patients unresponsive to 48 hours of conservative treatment
    E. Development of fever

44. **Causes of acute pancreatitis:**
    A. ERCP
    B. Hypocalcemia
    C. Hyperlipidemia
    D. Trauma
    E. Steroids

45. **Acute pancreatitis:**
    A. 80% of pancreatitis are mild
    B. Interstitial edema is the pathological hallmark of mild acute pancreatitis
    C. Ultrasound is the modality of choice for management
    D. MRI is useful for assessment of pancreatic necrosis
    E. Ultrasound is used for assessment of disease severity

46. **Staging of acute pancreatitis:**
    A. Single pancreatic fluid collection is stage E
    B. CTSI of 10 has mortality of 80%
    C. CTSI of 2 has 0% mortality
    D. Necrosis involving 40% of pancreatic parenchyma is given 2 points
    E. Stages A and B pancreatitis have good prognosis

47. **Features of acute pancreatitis:**
    A. Serum amylase > 500 IU
    B. The splenic artery is the most frequently involved artery in complication
    C. Isolated superior mesenteric vein thrombosis occurs in 30%
    D. Complications of acute pancreatitis occur in 20%
    E. Mortality is 10%

48. **CT scan for pancreatic necrosis:**
    A. Normal pancreas shows values up to 150 HU after contrast administration
    B. Necrosis of the head is the most dangerous type
    C. Central pancreatic necrosis warrants distal pancreatectomy
    D. CT has a specificity of 100% in all cases of pancreatic necrosis
    E. CT has false negative rate of 20% when less than 30% of pancreas is necrosed

49. **Fluid collection in pancreatitis:**
    A. 50% develop collection
    B. 50% resolve spontaneously
    C. 20% develop pancreatic ascites
    D. Pseudocyst takes 4 weeks to develop
    E. Pseudocyst does not have a capsule

50. **CT of acute pancreatitis:**
    A. Free fluid is more common in greater than lesser sac
    B. Increased attenuation suggests haemorrhage
    C. Pancreas is enlarged with homogeneously decreased density
    D. Calcification is rarely seen
    E. Normal pancreas has density of 60-80 HU

51. **Imaging features of mesenteric ischemia:**
    A. The most common location of superior mesenteric artery embolus is distal to the middle colic artery
    B. In thrombosis of superior mesenteric artery, the ileocolic artery is the most common vessel involved
    C. Portal hypertension is a predisposing factor for superior mesenteric vein thrombosis
    D. In nonocclusive mesenteric ischemia, slow flow is seen in angiography
    E. Barium is not done in acute mesenteric ischemia

52. **Infected collections in pancreatitis:**
    A. Majority of infection is polymicrobial
    B. The mortality rate of pancreatic abscess is more than of infected pancreatic necrosis
    C. Pancreatic abscesses are never formed before 4 weeks
    D. Presence of gas inside collection is specific for infection
    E. 70% of abscesses have gas

53. **Infected collections in pancreatitis:**
    A. Abscess develops in 10% of patients
    B. Infected necrosis requires surgery
    C. Tissue aspiration is required for diagnosing infected necrosis
    D. Mortality for infected necrosis is 70%
    E. Abscesses show wall enhancement

54. **Complications of pseudocyst:**
    A. Jaundice   B. Gastric obstruction
    C. Invasion of spleen   D. True aneurysm
    E. Venous occlusion

55. **Vascular complications of pancreatitis:**
    A. Pseudoaneurysm is most common in splenic artery
    B. Gastroduodenal artery is involved in 22% of cases
    C. Pancreatic veins are the most common involved in venous occlusion
    D. Colour doppler or contrast CT should be done before draining a collection
    E. Perigastric collaterals indicate venous occlusion

56. **Pancreatic necrosis:**
    A. C reactive protein is the most reliable method for detection of pancreatic necrosis
    B. Develops after 6 days
    C. Morbidity is 95% in those with necrosis >30%
    D. 10% of patients with acute pancreatitis develop necrosis
    E. 30% mortality

57. **Ischemic bowel:**
    A. The patient is relatively well in colonic ischemia
    B. Barium enema is diagnostic in chronic ischemia
    C. Collaterals can maintain the viability of only short segments of bowel for only short time
    D. Acute mesenteric ischemia occurs in older age group than colonic ischemia
    E. Nonocclusive mesenteric ischemia involves the small bowel and right side of colon

58. **Severe acute pancreatitis:**
    A. Vessel necrosis is seen in pathological specimens
    B. 90% of pancreatitis is caused by gallstones
    C. Mortality of 60%
    D. More than 5 Ransen's criteria should be seen in 48 hours for diagnosis
    E. APACHE II more than eight criteria indicates severe pancreatitis

59. **The following are typical plain X-ray findings of acute mesenteric ischemia:**
    A. Normal in 70% of cases
    B. Obliteration of volvulas conniventes
    C. Stiff fixed bowel loops
    D. Pseudo-obstruction
    E. Fluid levels

60. **Acute pancreatitis:**
    A. CT should be done every 7-10 days for patients with Grades D and E pancreatitis
    B. CT should be done before discharging patients with acute pancreatitis
    C. CT evidence of improvement is later than that of clinical improvement
    D. Pancreatic body is the most common involved part in focal pancreatitis
    E. Phlegmon is the term for ill-defined inflammatory masses

61. **High risk factors for development of acute mesenteric ischemia:**
    A. Ischemic heart disease
    B. Hypotension
    C. Digitalis
    D. Sepsis
    E. Inflammatory bowel disease

62. **Mesenteric ischemia:**
    A. Air in mesenteric vessels is the most specific CT sign of mesenteric ischemia
    B. There is enhancement of the superior mesenteric venous wall in thrombosis
    C. Bowel wall thickening with edema is high specific for ischemia in the clinical context
    D. The pain in chronic mesenteric ischemia is characteristically seen 1-2 hours after meal and is localised to the epigastric region
    E. Doppler of mesenteric vessels should be done in empty stomach for better visualisation of the vasculature

63. **Colonic ischemia:**
    A. Most common subtype is colonic gangrene
    B. Plain film is normal in 80% of cases
    C. Thumbprinting is due to submucosal edema and haemorrhage
    D. Haustral pattern is preserved unlike inflammatory bowel disease
    E. Barium enema is contraindicated in ischemia colon

64. **Colonic ischemia:**
    A. Thumbprinting is seen in 75% of barium enemas
    B. Transverse ridges are produced due loss of haustra
    C. Ischemia is sequelae of obstruction but not a cause
    D. Ulceration is seen only after one to three weeks
    E. Strictures in colonic ischemia are reversible

65. **Ischemia:**
    A. The most common cause of mesenteric ischemia is thrombus in the superior mesenteric artery
    B. Ischemia is the second most common cause of colitis in elderly after inflammatory bowel disease
    C. The most common vascular disorder of GIT is acute mesenteric ischemia
    D. Polycythemia rubra vera is a risk factor for colonic ischemia
    E. Oral contraceptives increase the risk of colonic ischemia

66. **The following are considered risk factors for colonic ischemia:**
    A. Amyloidosis
    B. Diabetes
    C. Radiation
    D. Shock
    E. Digitalis

67. **Fluid collection in pancreatitis:**
    A. Enhancement of pseudocyst wall has shown to have correlation with severity of disease
    B. Spontaneous resolution of pseudocyst less than 5 cm
    C. 30% of pancreatitis gets infected
    D. Septic complications account for 80% of deaths in pancreatitis
    E. The infective organisms spread hematologically

68. **Chronic mesenteric ischemia:**
    A. At least two mesenteric arteries are involved
    B. MRI done postprandially, shows decreased oxygen in mesenteric veins
    C. Median arcuate ligament can compress celiac artery to produce pain worse in inspiration
    D. Two-thirds of elderly patients have stenosis of mesenteric arteries
    E. Mimicked by chronic mesenteric venous thrombosis

ANSWERS

1. **A-T, B-F, C-F, D-F, E-F**
   About 90% have stone in cystic duct and 10% are acalculous cholecystitis. Ultrasound has 95% sensitivity and only 80% specificity. CT and MRI are less sensitive than ultrasound. Plain X-ray shows stones in 10-15% of cases. Immediate cholecystectomy is not done, unless the patient has gangrene or perforation.

2. **A-F, B-F, C-F, D-T, E-F**
   Calculus is not common and seen in only 35% of cases. Diabetes mellitus is associated in 38% of cases. More common in males with a ratio of 7:3. Mortality is higher than acute cholecystitis due to gangrene, perforation and peritonitis. Reverberation artefacts producing dirty shadowing is seen distal to the bright gas.

3. **A-T, B-T, C-T, D-T, E-T**
   Liver abscess is another common cause.

4. **A-T, B-T, C-T, D-F, E-T**
   Intraluminal membranes are due to sloughed mucosa and fibrinous exudate. Murphy's sign is negative due to loss of innervation. Immediate surgery of percutaneous treatment is mandatory.

5. **A-T, B-T, C-T, D-T, E-F**
   Pericholecystic abscess elicits inflammatory response involving the omentum which seals the abscess, and thus an increased omental flow is seen in Doppler.

6. **A-T, B-T, C-T, D-T, E-T**
   Microabscesses are seen as small enhancing hypodensities.

7. **A-T, B-T, C-T, D-T, E-T**
   Underlying malignancy is another common cause.

8. **A-T, B-T, C-T, D-T, E-F**
   Emphysematous cholecystitis has bright gas in the wall and inside the lumen. Cholecystoenteric fistula has gas inside the gallbladder, but not in the wall.
   Bowel adjacent to gallbladder can be differentiated by changing the position and rescanning. Intramural cholesterosis will produce bright shadows which are focal and not generalised. Gangrenous cholecystitis has pericholecystic fluid collection and membranes and no gas.

9. **A-T, B-T, C-F, D-T, E-T**
   In early stage, there is only mucosal edema, but in later stages, both the intra- and extrahepatic ducts are dilated.

10. **A-F, B-T, C-T, D-T, E-T**
Mortality is 2%, especially in elderly, who have underlying malignancy and generalised sepsis.

11. **A-T, B-T, C-T, D-F, E-T**
Generalisd gallbladder wall thickening is nonspecific and seen in a lot of conditions.
Normally, flow can be seen in cystic artery in Doppler. Increased flow in the fundus signifies hyperemia and indicates acute cholecystitis. But this sign is not sensitive as it is detected in late stages. No flow will be seen in gangrenous cholecystitis.

12. **A-T, B-T, C-T, D-T, E-F**
The clinical triad is called Charcot's triad and seen in only a few cases.

13. **A-T, B-F, C-T, D-F, E-T**
Microabscesses are those which are less than 2 cm. 50% of the abscesses are anechoic in ultrasound, 25% are hypoechoic and 25% are hyperechoic. Rim enhancement is seen in only 6-10% of cases of liver abscess.

14. **A-T, B-F, C-F, D-T, E-F**
Well-defined lesion < 5 cm, unilocular, no communication with biliary tree or bowel, are managed by aspiration alone. Lesions more than 5 cm, ill-defined, multilocular, with communication to gut or biliary tree require catheter drainage.

15. **A-T, B-T, C-T, D-T, E-T**
Appendicitis, diverticulitis, necrotic colonic cancer, perforated ulcer, osteomyelitis, trauma and pancreatitis are other predisposing factors.

16. **A-T, B-T, C-F, D-F, E-F**
Mortality and morbidity is quite high.
Gallbladder thickening is not specific for acalculous cholecystitis. Scinti scans are not accurate as biliary stasis can produce similar finding and is not specific.

17. **A-F, B-F, C-F, D-T, E-T**
The most common cause of abscess is biliary origin. Biliary origin abscesses are seen bilaterally. Portal origin abscesses are preferentially seen in the right lobe, due to streaming of mesenteric flow into the right branch of the portal vein. Diffusely scattered abscesses are seen in immunocompromised patients.

18. **A-T,. B-T, C-T, D-T, E-T**
CT is more useful since it will show pericholecystic fluid collection and increased density in pericholecystic fat.

19. **A-T, B-T, C-T, D-T, E-F**
    Scintigraphy and sonography has similar accuracy of about 90%.
    False positive studies are seen due to hepatic dysfunction and
    sludge in gallbladder blocking uptake of isotope.
    False negative studies are rare, making it very sensitive.

20. **A-T, B-T, C-T, D-T, E-F**
    Gallbladder wall thickening is a very nonspecific finding and seen
    in a lot of systemic conditions. In the presence of ascites, a thicke-
    ned gallbladder is said to be suggestive of benign disease, whereas
    a normal gallbladder wall is indicative of malignant ascites.

21. **A-T, B-T, C-T, D-F, E-T**
    Target sign, is alternate high and low density in bowel wall post-
    contrast, due to submucosal edema, inflammation or fat. Crohn's
    and ischemia are other causes.

22. **A-F, B-T, C-F, D-F, E-T**
    Mesenteric fat normally shows values between –75 and –125 HU.
    1000 ml of 2% barium given the day before, will opacify the colon.
    1000 ml is given one hour before procedure to opacify the stomach
    and duodenum. Although CT shows some features for ulcerative
    colitis, it is not sensitive or specific enough for making diagnosis.
    The thickness of bowel in distended state should never be more
    than 4 mm. Edema, haemorrhage, fibrosis, cellular infiltrate and
    fluid are causes of high density in the mesentery.

23. **A-T, B-T, C-T, B-T, E-T**
    When the pseudopolyps are large, they can be visualised in CT
    scans. Although mural stratification is nonspecific, it is found more
    often in ulcerative colitis than in granulomatous colitis. Mean
    colonic thickness in UC is 7 mm, whereas in Crohn's it is 11 mm.
    Colonic wall is smooth and regular in UC, whereas in
    granulomous colitis, it is irregular.

24. **A-T, B-T, C-T, D-T, E-T**
    Creeping fat is fibrofatty proliferation of mesentery and is the most
    common cause of separation of bowel loops.

25. **A-T, B-T, C-T, D-T, E-T**
    These are non-GIT complications.

26. **A-T, B-T, C-T, D-T, E-T**
    Mesenteric involvement, produces the comb sign, which indicates
    vascular dilation, wide spacing and tortuosity. It rules out
    lymphoma and metastasis which are avascular.

Mesenteric lymph nodes, up to 8 mm can be seen in mesenteric involvement, but large nodes, more than 10 mm indicate development of lymphoma or carcinoma.

Abscesses are seen in 15%. Clinically they may be masked by steroids and barium is not specific.

Fistulography is difficult if there is edema of the tract, and it is painful in anorectal region, making MR and CT better.

Phlegmon is ill-defined inflammatory mass, and produces smudging of mesentery.

27. **A-T, B-F, C-T, D-T, E-F**
Bowel wall stratification is seen in the acute phase only and medical therapy at this stage will reduce the inflammation and edema and will prevent luminal narrowing.
In chronic stage, the bowel wall becomes homogeneously thickened and causes irreversible narrowing.

28. **A-T, B-T, C-T, D-T, E-T**
Enteroenteric, enterocolic and colocolic are common fistulas.

29. **A-T, B-T, C-T, D-F, E-T**
The most common mode of spread is through the portal circulation from the gastrointestinal tract into the right lobe of the liver which is affected in more than 75% of cases. Gallium scan finding of cold center with hot rim is not specific and is also seen in pyogenic liver abscess. Right lobe liver abscess. can extend into the peritoneum or pleural cavity producing consolidation.

30. **A-T. B-T, C-T, D-T, E-F**
The typical location is right lobe, subcapsular, touching the capsule. It is round or oval. There is characteristic absence of wall echoes.

31. **A-F, B-T, C-T, D-T, E-F**
Submucosa is infiltrated by fat. Lamina propria is thickened by round cells.
Muscularis mucosa hypertrophies. All these changes result in wall thickening and luminal narrowing. In Crohn's disease, any part of the bowel can be thickened from esophagus to rectum.

32. **A-T, B-T, C-T, D-T, E-T**

Layer	Bowel layer	CT	MR
Inner	mucosa, muscularis, propria	soft tissue	hypo
Middle	submucosal fat	low	hyper
Outer	muscularis propria	soft tissue	hypo

Also.seen in pseudomembranous colitis, edema and ischemic colitis.

33. **A-T, B-T, C-T, D-T, E-T**
Mural thinning, dilatation, perforation and pneumatosis are seen in toxic megacolon.

34. **A-F, B-T, C-T, D-T, E-T**
Cryptosporidiosis is also a known cause. Colitis can also occur with normal immunity in HIV. Caecum and proximal ascending colon commonly affected. Pancolitis can occur.
Edema causes submucosal low density. Mural thickening and soft tissue stranding are seen. Pneumatosis can occur.

35. **A-T, B-T, C-F, D-T, E-T**
Fever is absent or low grade. Fecal leucocytes are not seen.
Right side of colon is affected and distal extension can be variable.

36. **A-T, B-T, C-T, D-F, E-T**
Typhlitis is inflammation of caecum. Bone marrow transplantation is another cuase.
Immunosuppression is the most common cause.

37. **A-T, B-T, C-T, D-F, E-T**
Caecum and ascending colon are inflamed in typhlitis, but ileum can also be involved occasionally. Since the bowel is friable and prone for perforation, colonoscopy and barium are contraindicated. Because of neutropenia, bacteria, virus and fungi proliferate in the submucosa. Perforation and abscess are common.

38. **A-T, B-T, C-T, D-F, E-T**
Vomiting and nausea are also seen. Perforation is very rare.
Submucosal fat deposition occurs in chronic GVHD.

39. **A-T, B-T, C-T, D-T, E-F**
Bowel wall thickness, homogeneity and contrast enhancement, mesenteric perirectal, retroperitoneal and omental fat density and masses, abscess, fistulae, sinus tracts, fatty chanes in liver, spinal and ligamentous ossification have to be assessed.

40. **A-F, B-T, C-T, D-F, E-T**
Ascites indicates acute colitis, not chronic disease.
Submucosal fat infiltration is a feature of chronic disease, especially chronic ulcerative colitis. Increased density in fat is due to inflammation and edema and is characterised by stranding. The fat density is 20 HU more than normal fat.

41. **A-F, B-T, C-T, D-T, E-F**
Vancomycin and metronidazole are used for treatment. Accordion pattern is produced by contrast accumulating between thickened haustra which are arranged in parallel rows like accordion. Toxic megacolon, perforation, pericolitis and abscess are complications.

Ascites and pleural effusion can occur. Pseudomembranes cannot be visualised in CT. Wall thickening, mucosal and serosal enhancement are characteristic.

42. **A-F, B-F, C-T, D-T, E-T**
Usually ascites is not seen in chronic inflammatory bowel disease and less frequently in acute inflammatory bowel disease.

43. **A-T, B-T, C-T, D-F, E-T**
Other indications are—Patients unresponsive to 72 hours of conservative treatment. Patients developing clinical signs of complication such as fever, pain, hypotension, falling hematocrit.

44. **A-T, B-F, C-T, D-T, E-T**
Gallstones and alcoholism are the two common causes.
Hypercalcemia is a cause and hypocalcemia is a sequelae of acute pancreatitis.

45. **A-T, B-T, C-F, D-T, E-F**
Ultrasound—for gallstone, pancreatic collections, not for pancreatic parenchyma
CT—diagnosis, staging, complications. It is the modality of choice for assessment.
MRI—pancreatic necrosis, vascular complications.
ERCP—patency of biliary and pancreatic system, sphinecterotomy, connection of ductal system with collections.
MRCP—for ductal system.
Angiography—vascular complications.

46. **A-F, B-F, C-T, D-F, E-T**
CT staging of acute pancreatitis
A—Normal Pancreas (0); B. Pancreatic enlargement focal/diffuse (1); C-Peripancreatic inflammation (2); D-Single fluid collection (3) E-Multiple fluid collections/single abscess (4).
Necrosis; <30%, -(2), 30-50% (4), >50% (6)
CT sensitivity index 1-2-0% mortality 0-4% morbidity, 7-10-17% mortality, 80% morbidity.

47. **A-T, B-T, C-F, D-T, E-T**
Splenic artery is involved in 50% of complications. Amylase > 500—95% chance of pancreatitis; 250-500—repeat amylase; SMV thrombosis < 5%.

48. **A-T, B-F, C-T, D-F, E-T**
Central pancreatic necrosis, in between the head and tail, is the most lethal, as it is associated with pancreatic ductal disruption, fistula formation and warranting distal pancreatectomy for the

isolated pancreatic duct in tail. CT has specificity of 100% for necrosis more than 30% of gland, but 50% for less than 30%. False negative rate 20% for necrosis less than 30% and 10% for necrosis > 30%.

49. A-T, B-T, C-F, D-T, E-T
Almost 7% develop pancreatic ascites. Pseudocysts have well-defined non-epithelialised wall or capsule. 50% develop pseudocyst.

50. A-F, B-T, C-F, D-T, E-F
Free fluid is common in the lesser sac rather than the ascites in the greater sac.
Pancreas is enlarged but with heterogeneous low density due to inflammation, edema and necrosis. Calcification is a feature of chronic pancreatitis.

51. A-T, B-F, C-T, D-T, E-T
The most common site of thrombosis of superior mesenteric artery is the proximal 2 cm of the artery. Portal hypertension, hyper-coagulability, surgery, trauma and tumours are common causes of superior mesenteric vein thrombosis which has better prognosis than arterial thrombosis. Arterial flow will be slow and veins will not be visualised. In nonocclusive disease, there is low flow in the mesenteric circulation, which is seen in congestive cardiac failure due to constriction of visceral vessels. There is high incidence of aortic reflux, slow flow, narrowed origins of main branches, irregularities, spastic intestinal arcades and impaired filling.

52. A-F, B-F, C-T, D-F, E-T
Majority of infections are gram negative. One-third are polymicro-bial. Mortality rate of infected pancreatic necrosis is twice that of pancreatic abscess. Gas is seen only in 30-40% of infected collection and is not very specific. It may also be due to enteric fistula.

53. A-F, B-T, C-T, D-T, E-T
Abscesses develop in 3%. Infected necrosis requires surgical debridement, and abscess requires percutaneous drainage. Tissue aspiration, gram stain and culture are required for diagnosing infection. Mortality for abscess is half of that of infected necrosis. Sterile necrosis has mortality of 14%.

54. A-T, B-T, C-T, D-F, E-T
Pseudoaneurysm is a complication.

55. A-T, B-T, C-F, D-T, E-T
Splenic artery (42%), gastroduodenal artery—22%, pancreatic arteries—-25% of pseudoaneurysms. Splenic vein is the most

common vein involved in occlusion resulting in perigastric collaterals. Retroperitoneal haemorrhage is a sequelae of the pseudo-aneurysms when they rupture.

56. **A-T, B-F, C-T, D-F, E-T**
C reactive protein has a sensitivity of 95% for diagnosing acute pancreatic necrosis.
30% develop pancreatic necrosis. Normally, it develops in 96 hours.
Mortality is 30% and morbidity 95% in those with pancreatic necrosis > 30%.

57. **A-T, B-T, C-T, D-F, E-T**
In acute mesenteric ischemia, the patient is over 50 years, with an obvious precipitating cause, serious ill clinical status, severe abdominal pain with fewer clinical symptoms, angiography being diagnostic. Colonic ischemia is seen above 50 years, with no obvious precipitating cause, with the patient being relatively well, rectal bleeding and diarrhea, barium enema or colonoscopy being procedures of choice. Acute mesenteric ischemia can be due to superior mesenteric artery embolus or thrombus, superior mesenteric vein thrombosis and nonocclusive mesenteric ischemia.

58. **A-T, B-T, C-F, D-F, E-T**
Extensive peripancreatic fat necrosis, vessel necrosis, pancreatic ductal necrosis, turbid haemorrhagic ascites are pathological features. Mortality is 30%. More than 3 Ransen's criteria and more than 8 APACHE II criteria.

59. **A-T, B-T, C-T, D-T, E-F**
Ileus, thick wall, thick folds, colon cut off sign, pneumatosis and portal venous gas are other findings.

60. **A-T, B-F, C-T, D-F, E-F**
CT should be done before discharge in patients with Grade 4 or 5. Pancreatic head is commonly involved in focal pancreatitis, incidence being 18%. Phlegmon is a term which is not used now. Ill-defined inflammatory masses made up of pancreatic fluid, edema, inflammation, haemorrhage.

61. **A-T, B-T, C-T, D-T, E-F**
Congestive cardiac failure, myocardial infarction and arrhythmia are other predisposing factors for acute mesenteric ischemia.

62. **A-T, B-T, C-F, D-F, E-F**
Air in mesenteric fat, edema, portal venous gas, nonenhancement of vessels, filling defects and bowel wall thickening are other features of bowel wall ischemia. In SMV thrombus, the wall is enhanced since it is supplied by vasa vasorum. Pain in chronic

mesenteric ischemia occurs within 15 minutes after eating. Often, Doppler is done postprandially to provoke the symptoms. Angiography shows reduction of at least two-thirds circumference of at least 2 or 3 major arteries.

63. **A-F, B-T, C-T, D-F, E-F**

There are many subtypes of colonic ischemia such as ischemic colopathy, reversible ischemic colitis, chronic ulcerative ischemia colitis, gangrene, ischemia colitis stricture, fulminant universal ischemic colitis. Thumbprinting is scalloped indentations on the bowel gas pattern and is nonspecific. Haustral pattern is lost. Barium enema is very useful in diagnosis of colonic ischemia. Pneumatosis in wall and portal venous gas are other findings.

64. **A-T, B-F, C-F, D-T, E-T**

Transverse ridges are seen perpendicular to the long axis of the bowel and are seen secondary to bowel wall thickening. This can be detected in plain film or in barium. Ischemia causes obstruction in 20% of cases. Stricture develops after 3 weeks and produces obstruction. These are reversible and can be irreversible.

65. **A-F, B-F, C-F, D-T, E-T**

There are four kinds of mesenteric ischemia. Superior mesenteric artery embolus accounts for 50% of cases. Superior mesenteric artery thrombus is only 15% of cases. The other conditions are superior mesenteric vein thrombosis (15%) and nonocclusive mesenteric ischemia (30%). Ischemia is the most common cause of colitis in elderly. The most common vascular disorder of GIT is colonic ischemia.

66. **A-T, B-T, C-T, D-T, E-T**

Inferior mesenteric artery ligation, or thrombosis or embolism, strangulated hernia, congestive heart failure and collagen vascular disease are other recognised causes of colonic ischemia.

67. **A-F, B-T, C-F, D-T, E-F**

There is no correlation between enhancement of pseudocyst and severity of disease.
12% is the infection rate. Infective organisms spread from colon.

68. **A-T, B-T, C-F, D-T, E-T**

Chronic mesenteric ischemia is commonly caused by atherosclerosis and affects at least two of the three arteries. Mesenteric stenosis is seen in more than two-thirds of elderly patients. Patients have characteristic pain, which is worse postprandially and in epigastric region. Median arcuate ligament can compress the superior part of celiac artery to produce abdominal pain, which is worse in expiration.

Biliary Tree

7

1. **Cystic artery can arise from the following arteries:**
   A. Gastroduodenal artery
   B. Retroduodenal artery
   C. Middle hepatic artery
   D. Left hepatic artery
   E. Right gastric artery

2. **Percutaneous transhepatic cholangiogram (PTC):**
   A. Antibiotics should be given for three days after the procedure
   B. Patient should not breathe once the needle is in the liver
   C. More the number of passes, more the complication
   D. The maximum number of passes acceptable is ten
   E. If duct is not entered with first attempt, it should be introduced deeper in the same plane

3. **Biliary techniques:**
   A. T tube cholangiography is mainly done to assess if there are any remnant calculi
   B. T tube cholangiography should ideally be performed on the day after surgery
   C. Contrast injected into the biliary system can reflux into the vein
   D. Biliary duct should be canalized before pancreatic duct in ERCP
   E. In preoperative cholangiogram, the sphincter of Oddi is narrowed due to anesthesia

4. **The following are contraindications for ERCP:**
   A. Acute cholecystitis
   B. HIV positive patient
   C. Pseudocyst of pancreas
   D. Pyloric stenosis
   E. Esophageal varices

5. **The following findings indicate that T tube cholangiogram is satisfactory:**
   A. No spasm of sphincter of Oddi
   B. CBD < 12 mm
   C. Contrast reflux into stomach
   D. No filling of hepatic veins
   E. Visualization of terminal duct

6. **The following are contraindications for use of buscopan:**
   A. Myasthenia gravis
   B. Thyrotoxicosis
   C. Pyloric stenosis
   D. Cholecystitis
   E. Subacute small bowel obstruction

7. **Biliary tree:**
   A. The length of common bile duct depends on the insertion of the cystic duct
   B. The CBD diameter is proportional to the age of the patient
   C. The CBD caliber increases postcholecystectomy
   D. The common hepatic duct is roughly considered to be enlarged if it is more than the size of the endoscope
   E. The walls of cystic duct are echogenic

8. **Biliary tree:**
   A. In PTC, the left biliary system is punctured via segment IVa
   B. The right biliary system is punctured via segment VIII
   C. The middle third of the common bile duct creates an impression on the posterior aspect of the second part of the duodenum
   D. The distal third of the bile duct is anterior to the right renal vein
   E. The gallbladder creates an impression in the anterior aspect of first part of duodenum

9. **Biliary tree:**
   A. The cystic duct has no muscles in the wall
   B. The spiral valves of Heister regulate the flow of bile
   C. Accessory bile ducts are seen in 20% of population
   D. The cystic artery invariably arises from the right hepatic artery
   E. Biliary lymphatics drain to the liver

10. **Causes of high density within the gallbladder in CT scan:**
    A. Cystic artery embolisation
    B. Hemobilia
    C. Cholecystitis
    D. ERCP
    E. Adenomyomatosis

11. **Common causes of distension of gallbladder without wall thickening:**
    A. Diabetes mellitus
    B. Cholecystitis
    C. Hepatitis
    D. Postprandial
    E. Carcinoma pancreas

12. **The following stones are considered suitable for chemical dissolution:**
    A. Hypodense stones
    B. Isodense stones
    C. Rim calcification
    D. Laminated calcification
    E. Homogeneous hyperdense

13. **Gallbladder:**
    A. Gallbladder is seen in the interlobar fissure
    B. The normal density of gallbladder lumen is 50-60 HU
    C. The density of gallbladder lumen is high after intravenous contrast
    D. In renal failure, the luminal density is low
    E. Milk of calcium bile is denser than normal bile but less dense than blood

14. **Gallbladder:**
    A. Ectopic gallbladder is most common in the anteroinferior quadrant of the liver
    B. In cirrhosis the gallbladder is placed more anteriorly than normal
    C. Wandering gallbladder is often present as a mass in the head of the pancreas
    D. An abnormally placed gallbladder is never seen above the superior surface of the liver
    E. The gallbladder is situated in the left side in polysplenia

15. **Cholecystitis:**
    A. Gallbladder is contracted in chronic cholecystitis
    B. Sandwich appearance in gallbladder wall indicates gangrenous cholecystitis
    C. Pericholecystic collection can be excluded by absence of blood vessels coursing through it
    D. In cholecystitis, the gallbladder measures more than 6 cm and the wall thickness is more than 5 mm
    E. CT has 100% sensitivity for detection of gallstones

16. **Biliary scintigraphy:**
    A. In acute cholecystitis, the gallbladder is visualized after morphine is administered IV
    B. CCK increases tone of the sphincter of Oddi and contraction of gallbladder (CCK-cholecystokinin)
    C. Ejection fraction of gallbladder is calculated after administering morphine
    D. If bowel is not visualized in 6 hours, no further imaging is required
    E. TBIDA is not useful when there is elevated bilirubin

17. **Cholesterol gallstones:**
    A. Occur in hemolytic anemia
    B. No acoustic shadowing in ultrasound
    C. Dissolved by chenodeoxycholic acid
    D. Associated with Crohn's disease
    E. Isodense to bile on CT

18. **False negative ultrasound for cholelithiasis:**
    A. Contracted GB   B. Bowel gas
    C. Stone in neck   D. Cystic duct stone
    E. Small stone

19. **Gallbladder:**
    A. Xanthogranulomatous cholecystitis is associated with lymphadenopathy
    B. In porcelain gallbladder the calcium is seen in the mucosal layer
    C. Cholesterosis is not seen in ultrasound
    D. Intramural diverticula are seen in adenomyomatosis
    E. Cholecystitis can occur in the cyst duct remnant after cholecystectomy

20. **Mirizzi's syndrome:**
    A. Caused by impacted stone in the neck of gallbladder
    B. Common bile duct is dilated
    C. Intrahepatic ductal dilatation is seen
    D. Cholecystobiliary fistula is seen
    E. Can erode into the hepatoduodenal ligament

21. **Features indicative of CBD stone:**
    A. Pancreatitis
    B. Obscured bile duct
    C. Sludge within CBD
    D. Recent history of jaundice
    E. CBD > 3 mm

22. **Complications of calculus:**
    A. Cholangiocarcinoma
    B. Pancreatitis
    C. Gastric outlet obstruction
    D. Fistula
    E. Cirrhosis

23. **Choledocholithiasis:**
    A. Migration of stone from gallbladder is related to the size of the stone
    B. Once a stone migrates from the gallbladder into the CBD, it does not grow
    C. Secondary calculi are those which migrate from the gallbladder
    D. Oval stones are less likely to impact in the ampulla of Vater
    E. Traumatic stricture is a predisposing factor for bile duct stone formation

24. **Sclerosing cholangitis is associated with:**
    A. Hashimoto's thyroiditis
    B. Pancreatitis
    C. Diverticulitis
    D. Primary biliary cirrhosis
    E. Crohn's disease

25. **Sclerosing cholangitis:**
    A. Common in females
    B. 20% of those with inflammatory bowel disease develop sclerosing cholangitis
    C. Liver function tests are normal
    D. Intrahepatic ductal calculi seen
    E. Echogenic portal triads in ultrasound

26. **Risk indicators for CBD stone:**
    A. Elevated serum amylase
    B. Elevated serum bilirubin
    C. Elevated transaminase
    D. Dilated ampulla
    E. Thickened wall of CBD

27. **Sclerosing cholangitis:**
    A. Saccular outpouchings in bile ducts is pathognomonic of sclerosing cholangitis
    B. Beaded appearance is a classical feature
    C. Gallbladder irregular
    D. Pruned tree appearance indicates development of cholangiocarcinoma
    E. Has predilection for bifurcation

28. **Sclerosing cholangitis:**
    A. 50% show nodular irregularities in bile ducts
    B. Portal hypertension is a complication
    C. The extrahepatic ducts show enhancement in all the cases
    D. HIDA scan will show retention of contrast
    E. Gallbladder is not visualised in 30%

29. **Risk factors for development of cholangiocarcinoma:**
    A. Liver fluke
    B. Hepatitis B
    C. Choledochal cyst
    D. Sclerosing cholangitis
    E. Primary biliary cirrhosis

30. **Features of cholangiocarcinoma developing in sclerosing cholangitis:**
    A. Marked ductal dilation upstream
    B. Intraductal mass > 5 mm
    C. Progressive changes with 1.5 years
    D. Increased echogenicity of the walls
    E. Hepatic metastases

31. **Causes of secondary sclerosing cholangitis:**
    A. AIDS   B. Floxuridine
    C. Bacterial   D. Neoplasm
    E. Liver abscess

32. **Recurrent pyogenic cholangitis:**
    A. Cryptosporidiosis is the cause
    B. Most common in medial segments of left lobe
    C. Complicates Caroli's disease
    D. Calcium bilirubinate stones seen in majority
    E. Dilated intrahepatic ducts with normal common bile duct

33. **Gallbladder carcinoma:**
    A. Calcification occurs in mucinous types
    B. Intraperitoneal seeding is more common than hematogenous spread
    C. Spread is most common through the ducts
    D. Polypoid tumour is the most common type
    E. Direct invasion of liver is common in the anteromedial aspect

34. **Complications of recurrent pyogenic cholangitis:**
    A. Pancreatitis   B. Splenomegaly
    C. Hepatic atrophy   D. Pneumobilia
    E. Strictures

35. **Predisposing factors for cholangiocarcinoma:**
    A. ADPKD (autosomal dominant polycystic liver kidney disease)
    B. Alpha one antitrypsin deficiency
    C. Caroli's disease
    D. Thorotrast
    E. Ascariasis

36. **Inflammatory bowel disease and cholangiocarcinoma:**
    A. Multicentric tumours are more common
    B. Predominantly in intrahepatic ducts
    C. Latent period of 25 years
    D. Associated with gallstones
    E. More common in ulcerative colitis than Crohn's disease

37. **Common complications of cholangiocarcinoma:**
    A. Cirrhosis
    B. Peritonitis
    C. Abscess
    D. Portal vein invasion
    E. Hepatocellular carcinoma

38. **Sclerosing cholangitis:**
    A. Typically presents with recurrent jaundice and fever
    B. Cannot be diagnosed by liver biopsy
    C. Increased mitochondrial antibody
    D. Affects intrahepatic ducts only
    E. Occurs in Crohn's disease

39. **Cholangiocarcinoma:**
    A. Polypoid type is the most common pattern of tumour
    B. Most common type is the Klatskin type
    C. Most common in 6th and 7th decades
    D. In infiltrating type, the strictures are more often short than long
    E. Intraductal tumour mass is seen in 45%

40. **Cholangiocarcinoma:**
    A. The tumour is avascular
    B. Polypoid tumour is seen in 100% of ultrasound as isoechoic mass
    C. Exophytic tumour is seen in 60% of ultrasound scans
    D. Infiltrating tumour is seen as high echogenic lesion
    E. Prestenotic dilatation is seen in 100% of cases

41. Intrahepatic cholangiocarcinoma:
A. Second most common hepatic malignancy
B. Diffuse infiltration of liver is in favour of metastasis rather than cholangiocarcinoma
C. Diffuse type is best visualised in CT than ultrasound
D. Lymph nodal spread does not occur
E. Satellite nodules are seen in 65%

42. Associations of gallbladder carcinoma:
A. Gallstones
B. Familial polyposis coli
C. Caroli's
D. Clonarchis sinesis
E. Porcelain gallbladder

43. Gallbladder carcinoma:
A. Cystic duct is the frequent location
B. Gallbladder polyp > 2 cm is malignant
C. Porcelain gallbladder is associated with gallbladder carcinoma and is not a predisposing cause
D. The gallbladder will not be visualised in oral cholecystography
E. Dilatation of biliary tree is uncommon

44. Ascariasis:
A. Diagnosed by plain film
B. Causes fleeting pulmonary opacities
C. Causes portal hypertension
D. Presents with jaundice
E. Occurs following larval penetration of skin

45. Gallbladder carcinoma:
A. Invasion of hepatoduodenal ligament produces ductal dilataion
B. Lack of definition of gallbladder wall indicates extension to liver
C. Hepatic hilar nodes are involved in early stages of gallbladder tumour spread
D. Anaplastic type is the most common subtype of gallbladder carcinoma
E. Thickened, irregular wall is highly specific for gallbladder carcinoma

46. Findings of emphysematous cholecystitis:
A. Gas in wall of gallbladder
B. Gas in portal vein
C. Gas in lumen of gallbladder
D. Gas in intrahepatic bile ducts
E. Gas in peritoneum

47. **Intrahepatic cholangiocarcinoma:**
    A. Increased uptake in gallium scan
    B. Early peripheral enhancement like hemangioma
    C. Centripetal filling similar to hemangioma
    D. The contrast clears fast from the center of the lesion than the periphery
    E. The periphery of the tumour is hypointense in T2

48. **Sclerosing cholangitis:**
    A. More common in total colitis
    B. Does not involve cystic duct
    C. Intermittent jaundice is earlier feature
    D. More than 50% have gallstones
    E. Commonly occurs before evidence of colitis

49. **High density bile is seen in:**
    A. Hemorrhagic cholecystitis
    B. Hemobilia
    C. Gangrenous cholecystitis
    D. Milk of calcium bile
    E. Perforated gallbladder

50. **Causes of fixed filling defect in gallbladder:**
    A. Neurinoma
    B. Stone
    C. Polyp
    D. Cholecystitis
    E. Sludge

51. **Nonvisualisation of gallbladder in ultrasound:**
    A. Congenital   B. Perforation
    C. Chronic cholecystitis   D. Carcinoma
    E. Eating before scan

52. **Nonvisualisation of gallbladder in oral cholecystography:**
    A. Pharyngeal pouch
    B. Gastric ulcer
    C. Crohn's disease
    D. Cystic duct obstruction
    E. Hiatal hernia

53. **Causes of large nonobstructed CBD:**
    A. 60% of postcholecystectomy patients
    B. Intestinal hypomotility
    C. Passage of stone, within a few days
    D. Common duct surgery six months back
    E. Pancreatitis

54. **Percutaneous cholecystostacy:**
    A. Acalculous cholecystitis is a contraindication
    B. Hepatic approach is better
    C. The drain can be removed in 7-10 days
    D. Success rate is better than surgical cholecystostacy
    E. Contraindicated in empyema

55. **Adenomyoma of gallbladder:**
    A. More common in males
    B. Gallstones are seen in up to 75%
    C. Rokitansky-Aschoff sinuses are pathognomonic
    D. Segmental form is often seen in fundus
    E. Adenomyomas are commonly seen in fundus

56. **Causes of small gallbladder:**
    A. Chronic cholecystitis
    B. Pancreatic carcinoma
    C. Cystic fibrosis
    D. Multiseptated gallbladder
    E. Cardiac failure

57. **Diffuse gallbladder thickening is seen in:**
    A. Right heart failure
    B. Lymph nodes in porta hepatis
    C. Venous hypertension
    D. Carcinoma
    E. Perforation GB

58. **Common causes of enlarged gallbladder:**
    A. Pancreatic cancer
    B. Cholecystitis
    C. Hydrops
    D. Pancreatitis
    E. Duodenal carcinoma

59. **Causes of increased echogenicity of fat in the hepatoduodenal ligament:**
    A. Pancreatitis
    B. Appendicitis
    C. Diverticulitis
    D. Perforated peptic ulcer
    E. Cholecystitis

60. **Common causes of mobile mass within ultrasound:**
    A. Stone   B. Polyp
    C. Blood clot   D. Sludge
    E. Adenomyoma

61. Causes of comet tail artefact in the gallbladder:
  A. von Meyenburg's complex
  B. Rokitansky Aschoff sinus
  C. Cholesterosis
  D. Adenomyoma
  E. Polyp

62. Filling defects within the common bile duct are seen in:
  A. Contracted sphincter of Oddi
  B. Mirizzi syndrome
  C. Clonorchis sinensis
  D. Hydatid cyst
  E. Cholangiocarcinoma

63. Common bile duct:
  A. The common bile duct increases in size after a fatty meal
  B. The biliary radicles should be more than 75% of adjacent portal vein radicles to be considered enlarged
  C. The double gun sign is a specific indicator of biliary tract dilatation
  D. The common bile duct is not enlarged in 70% of acute obstruction
  E. Sclerosing cholangitis produces false positive results in biliary dilatation

64. Biliary dilatation:
  A. Cirrhosis produces a false positive diagnosis of biliary obstruction
  B. Infected bile is more common in malignant than benign obstruction
  C. E. coli is the most common infecting organism of biliary tree
  D. The infection is higher in complete obstruction than incomplete obstruction
  E. Ultrasound has a 90% sensitivity for detection of biliary ductal dilatation

65. Causes of periampullary stenosis:
  A. Pancreas divisum   B. Annular pancreas
  C. Stone passage   D. Pancreatitis
  E. Pancreatic cancer

66. Periampullary carcinomas:
  A. 85% are ampullary tumours
  B. Duodenal wall tumours comprise 20%
  C. Cholangiocarcinoma 10%
  D. Carinoids also constitute the differential diagnosis
  E. Pancreatic cancers comprise 5%

67. **Septated gallbladder:**
    A. Duplicated gallbladder have two separate cystic ducts
    B. Bifid gallbladder has transverse septations
    C. Multiseptated gallbladder has no communication between the various compartments
    D. Phyrgian cap is folding of the fundus and there is no septum
    E. Gallbladder diverticulum is due to persistence of the cystohepatic duct

68. **The gallbladder can be identified in the following locations:**
    A. Beneath the right lobe is the most common location
    B. Retrohepatic
    C. Within anterior abdominal wall
    D. Groin
    E. Thorax

69. **Causes of focal gallbladder thickening:**
    A. Ectopic pancreatic rest
    B. Ascaris
    C. Hemangioma
    D. Papilloma
    E. Retention cyst

70. **Locations of ectopic gallbladder:**
    A. Transverse mesocolon
    B. Falciform ligament
    C. Ligamentum venosum
    D. Retrorenal
    E. Intrapancreatic

ANSWERS

1. **A-T, B-T, C-T, D-T, E-F**
   About 45% arise from right hepatic artery. Can also rise from common hepatic artery.

2. **A-T, B-F, C-F, D-T, E-F**
   Antibiotics are given before the procedure and for three days after the procedure. The patient can make shallow breaths when the needle is in the liver. The complication rate is not related to the number of passes. If the duct is not entered in the first attempt, it should be withdrawn and reintroduced in a different direction, till the duct is reached. If after ten attempts, duct is not entered, they are unlikely to be dilated.

3. **A-T, B-F, C-T, D-F, E-T**
   T tube cholangiography can also diagnose any biliary leaks. T tube cholangiography is done 7-10 days after surgery. Pancreatic duct is cannulated before the biliary duct.

4. **A-F, B-T, C-T, D-T, E-F**
   Acute pancreatitis and esophageal obstruction are other contraindications.

5. **A-F, B-T, C-F, D-T, E-T**
   No filling defect should be visualized.

6. **A-T, B-T, C-T, D-F,E-T**
   Prostatitism and closed angle glaucoma are the most common contraindications.

7. **A-T, B-T, C-F, D-T, E-T**
   The CBD normally measures 5 mm and is proportional to the age, with each decade causing 1 mm increase in size. The CBD does not enlarge postoperatively, but stays dilated in the preoperative state. The wall of cystic duct may be echogenic giving confusion with gallstones.

8. **A-F, B-F, C-F, D-T, E-T**
   The left biliary segment is punctured through segment III and right, in segments V, VI.
   The middle third creates a groove in the posterior aspect of first part of duodenum.

9. **A-F, B-T, C-F, D-F, E-T**
   Cystic duct has muscles, which regulates the flow of bile. Accessory ducts are seen in 10% of population. Aberrant hepatic ducts and cystic duct entering the right hepatic duct are other common variants.

The cystic artery rises from the right hepatic artery in 75%. It may rise from the left hepatic artery, common hepatic artery or superior mesenteric artery. Since the biliary lymphatics drain into liver, gallbladder malignancy spreads quite easily to liver.

10. **A-T, B-T, C-T, D-T, E-F**
Debri in cholecystitis, small biliary calculi, milk of bile, empyema and cystic duct obstruction are other causes.

11. **A-T, B-F, C-T, D-F, D-T**
Courvoisier's law states that when gallbladder is distended in a jaundiced patient, it is more likely to be secondary to a carcinoma in pancreatic head rather than a calculus, since the gallbladder is not distended in calculus disease due to cholecystitis and scarring. The exceptions to this rule are recurrent pyogenic cholangitis, calculus in bile duct and cystic duct. The gallbladder is contracted in postprandial state.

12. **A-T, B-T, C-T, D-T, E-F**
Cholesterol stones are the ones which show good results with chemical dissolution. Dense calcified stones do not respond.

13. **A-T, B-F, C-T, D-F, E-F**
The normal density of the gallbladder lumen is 0-20 HU. The density is higher after intravenous contrast, because a small portion can be excreted into the gallbladder. The excretion is increased in patients with renal failure. Milk of calcium bile is made up of calcium bilirubinate and is more denser than blood, >100 HU.

14. **A-T, B-F, C-T, D-F, E-F**
Ectopic gallbladder can be seen in the left lobe/anteroinferior quadrant of liver/in a transverse position /retroplaced. In cirrhosis the right lobe of the liver is atrophied and the gallbladder is placed posteriorly than normal. Wandering gallbladder has a long mesentery and is prone for torsion. In suprahepatic gallbladder, the right lobe is atrophied and there is associated eventeration of the diaphragm. In polysplenia the gallbladder is placed in the center, it is left-sided in situs inversus.

15. **A-T, B-F, C-T, D-T, E-F**
Sandwich appearance caused due to subserosal edema which is surrounded by enhancing mucosa and serosa. This indicates cholecystitis. Differentiation of edema and pericholecystic collection is occasionally difficult. But fluid collection is focal, there is no surrounding enhancing serosa and there are no blood vessels running through it. In cholecystitis, the gallbladder is distended and wall is thickened. CT misses many gallstones.

16. **A-F, B-F, C-F, D-F, E-F**
In acute cholecystis, the gallbladder is not visualized after 60 min. At this point, morphine is given IV. Morphine causes increased tone of the sphincter of Oddi. If gallbladder is till not visualized after 30 min, acute cholecystitis is considered. CCK increases the contractions of gallbladder and relaxes the sphincter and is used for assessing ejection fraction and thereby function of gallbladder. If bowel is not visualized for 6 hours, it indicates obstruction to biliary flow, a 24 hour film is required for excluding biliary atresia. TBIDA is taken by hepatocytes with high extraction rate and hence is useful even when there is high bilirubin, unlike earlier agents.

17. **A-F, B-F, C-T, D-T, E-F**
Pigment stones are seen in hemolytic anemia. Cholesterol stones without calcium are dissolved by chenodeoxycholic acid. Intestinal malabsorption caused by Crohn's disease is a predisposing factor. Slightly hypodense compared with bile.

18. **A-T, B-T, C- T, D-T, E-T**
Stones in neck/cystic duct are missed if not scanned properly.

19. **A-F, B-F, C-T, D-T, E-T**
There is no lymphadenopathy in xanthogranulomatous cholecystitis. A gallbladder with irregular wall and lymphadenopathy raises the possibility of carcinoma than cholecystitis. In porcelain gallbladder, the calcium is seen in muscularis mucosa. In cholesterosis, cholesterol-laden macrophages are seen in lamina propria of gallbladder. In adenomyomatosis, there is outpouching of mucosa into the thickened muscle of gallbladder wall. Calculi can form in the diverticula. Stone formation and cholecystitis occur in the cystic duct remnant and is a frequent cause of pain after cholecystectomy.

20. **A-T, B-F, C-T, D-T, E-T**
Mirizzi's syndrome is caused by a stone impacted in the cystic duct or neck of gallbladder, compressing the common hepatic duct, with proximal dilation of intrahepatic biliary dilatation, without any dilatation of distal common hepatic duct or common bile duct. The stone can erode into the common hepatic duct and then into the hepatoduodenal ligament. Cholecystitis and cholecystobiliary fistula are complications.

21. **A-T, B-T, C-F, D-T, E-F**
CBD dilated more than 6 mm. Shadow of CBD stone obscures the bile duct. Gastric outlet obstruction is Bouveret's syndrome. Secondary biliary cirrhosis is caused by gallstones.

22. **A-T, B-T, C-T, D-T, E-T**

23. **A-T, B-F, C-F, D-T, E-T**
Primary stones are those which migrate from the gallbladder. These often grow in the common bile duct and produce obstruction. Secondary stones are those which are not of gallbladder origin and formed in the common bile duct due to stricture or congenital biliary anomaly or sclerosing cholangitis.

24. **A-F, B-T, C-F, D-F, D-T**
Sclerosing cholangitis is associated with inflammatory bowel disease, cirrhosis, chronic active hepatitis, pancreatitis, retroperitoneal fibrosis, mediastinal fibrosis, Riedel's thyroiditis, Peyronie's disease and orbital pseudotumour. Secondary biliary cirrhosis is a sequelae. Primary biliary cirrhosis is limited to intrahepatic ducts and strictures are less marked.

25. **A-F, B-F, C-F, D-T, E-T**
Males > females, 7:3. 4% of inflammatory disease patients develop sclerosing cholangitis. Liver function tests show obstructive picture. Soft calculi are seen in intrahepatic ducts.

26. **A-T, B-T, C-T, D-F, E-F**

27. **A-T, B-T, C-F, D-F, E-T**
Gallbladder is normal and is not irregular. Pruned tree appearance, can occur in sclerosing cholangitis, itself.

28. **A-T, B-T, C-T, D-T, E-T**
HIDA scan will also show delayed hepatic clearance.
Biliary cirrhosis can cause portal hypertension.

29. **A-T, B-F, C-T, D-T, E-T**

30. **A-T, B-F, C-T, D-F, E-T**
Intraductal mass > 1 cm is suggestive. Increased echogenicity occurs in sclerosing cholangitis.

31. **A-T, B-T, C-T, D-T, E-F**
Congenital abnormality and surgery are causes.

32. **A-F, B-F, C-T, D-T, E-F**
Clonarchis sinesis is considered to be cause of this disease, also called Oriental cholangiohepatitis. *Ascaris* and *E. coli* are also associated. Common in lateral segment of left lobe and posterior segment of right lobe. Dilated intrahepatic ducts, with soft nonshadowing stones in them, failure of branching, and dilated CBD are common features.

33. **A-T, B-T, C-F, D-F, E-F**
Intraductal spread is the least common and invasion of adjacent organs is the most common.
Invasion of liver is more common in the anterolateral aspect of liver. Diffuse or focal thickening of gallbladder is common than polypoid tumour. There are three types of presentation; a large mass replacing the gallbladder fossa (40-75%), polypoidal mass (25%) and mural thickening (least common).

34. **A-T, B-T, C-T, D-T, E-T**
Biloma is another complication. Pneumobilia is associated.

35. **A-T, B-T, C-T, D-T, E-F**
Inflammatory bowel disease is a common risk. Surgery for choledochal cyst and biliary atresia are other recognised risk factors.

36. **A-T, B-F, C-F, D-F, E-T**
The risk of cholangiocarcinoma is increased by ten times in inflammatory bowel disease, more common in ulcerative colitis than Crohn's disease. Latent period is 15 years. The tumours are more often multicentric and gallbladder is involved in 15%. There is no association with gallstones. Extrahepatic ducts are involved more often than intrahepatic ducts.

37. **A-T, B-T, C-T, D-T, E-F**

38. **A-T, B-T, C-T, D-F, E-T**
About 68-89% affects intra- and extrahepatic ducts, 1-25% only extrahepatic.
CBD is almost always involved.

39. **A-F, B-F, C-T, D-F, E-T**
There are three morphologic types: 1. Obstructive type (75%); 2. Stenotic type (10-25%) and 3. Polypoid type (5%). The most common location is the distal CBD. The Klatskin tumour is at the confluence of the right and left hepatic ducts and accounts for 10%. In infiltrating type, the strictures are often long than short. Intraductal tumour mass measuring 2-5 mm is seen.

40. **A-F, B-T, C-F, D-T, E-T**
The tumour is hypervascular with neovascularity. Polypoid tumour is best seen in the ultrasound and exophytic tumour is best seen in CT scans. Infiltrating tumour is not seen as common as the other types and is best seen in ultrasound than CT.
In Klatskin tumour, the right and left hepatic ducts are dilated, but the distal CBD will not be visualised. A mass need not be always seen.

41. **A-T, B-F, C-F, D-F, E-T**
    After hepatoma, intrahepatic cholangiocarcinoma is the most common hepatic malignancy. There is a diffuse type of cholangio-carcinoma. Diffuse type is not seen by CT or ultrasound. Lymph nodal spread occurs in 15%. Satellite nodules are a salient feature.

42. **A-T, B-T, C-F, D-F, E-T**
    Gallstones are seen in majority of the cases, but they are just associations but not etiology for development of cancer. Only 1% of those with gallstones have associated gallbladder carcinoma. Inflammatory bowel disease and chronic cholecystitis are other recognised causes.

43. **A-F, B-T, C-F, D-T, E-F**
    The fundus and body are common locations. Cystic duct is a rare location. Porcelain gallbladder is an association and a cause. Dilatation of biliary tree is seen in 1/3-1/2.

44. **A-T, B-T, C-T, D-T, E-F**
    Plain film can show a soft tissue linear opacity. Group of worms can be seen as a serpigineous soft tissue shadow. Fleeting peripheral pulmonary opacities are produced due to eosinophilia. Ascariasis occurs in humans due to consumption of food contaminated with eggs of *Ascaris lumbricoides*. The larval forms develop in the intestine, travel through blood vessels to the lungs, then slip in to the GIT through the larynx, where the adult forms develop, cause disease and produce eggs which are passed in feces.

45. **A-T, B-T, C-T, D-F, E-F**
    Ductal dilatation in gallbladder carcinoma can be due to several reasons, including intraductal tumour growth, invasion of hepatoduodenal ligament, choledocholithiasis or pericholedochal lymphadenopathy. The lymph node spread is to pericholedochal nodes to postpancreaticoduodenal nodes to celiac nodes to retroperitoneal nodes. Hepatic hilar nodes are not involved. Adenocarcinoma is the most common type of cancer occurring in more than 85%, squamous and anaplastic being uncommon. Thicknened irregular wall is on the presentations of gallbladder carcinoma, but by no means is specific, since it can happen in chronic cholecystitis.

46. **A-T, B-F, C-T, D-T, E-T**

47. **A-T, B-T, C-T, D-F, E-F**
    The tumour shows no uptake in sulfur colloid scan and increased uptake in gallium scan.
    CT—early peripheral enhancement, centripetal filling, early clearing from the rim, (peripheral washout sign). MR—T1—hypo, T2—

hyper in the periphery where the tumour is viable and hypo in center due to fibrosis.

48. **A-T, B-F, C-T, D-F, E-F**
More common in ulcerative colitis than Crohn's. Cystic duct involved in 15%.
Progressive, intermittent jaundice is the main clinical feature.

49. **A-T, B-T, C-F, D-T, E-F**
Vicarious excretion of contrast is another cause.

50. **A-T, B-T, C-T, D-F, E-F**
Impacted stone will cause fixed filling defect.

51. **A-T, B-T, C-T, D-T, E-T**
Postprandial state and chronic—cholecystitis cause contracted GB.
In perforation GB is not visualised after an episode of inflamed GB.

52. **A-T, B-T, C-T, D-T, E-T**
Nonvisualisation of gallbladder.
Gallbladder—cholecystectomy, cystic duct obstruction, chronic cholecystitis.
Failure to ingest contrast.
Failure of contrast to reach gallbladder—vomiting, diarrhea, malabsorption, gastric/esophageal obstruction, ulcer, hernias, diverticulum, ileus, acute pancreatitis, acute peritonitis.
Deficiency of bile salts preventing absorption, including drugs such as cholestyramine.

53. **A-F, B-F, C-T, D-F, E-F**
The caliber of duct increases with age. Seen in 16% of postcholecystectomy patients.
Common duct surgery produces dilation for about two months postsurgery.

54. **A-F, B-T, C-F, D-T, E-F**
Percutaneous cholecystostomy is done in critically ill patients with calculous/acalculous cholecystitis/empyema/perforation. Drain is placed by trocar method/seldinger method for 6-8 weeks. Success rate—95-100%, Surgery has 30% mortality. 6.5-7 F catheter used.

55. **A-F, B-T, C-T, D-F, E-T**
More common in females. Gallstones are seen in 25-75% and cholesterosis is seen in 35%. Hyperplasia of epithelium and muscular tissue, with outpouching of mucosa through the muscular layer is pathognomonic. Segmental form is usually seen in the neck or the distal third. Adenomyomas are seen in the fundus as focal sessile mass.

56. **A-T, B-F, C-T, D-T, E-F**

57. **A-T, B-T, C-T, D-T, E-T**
    Renal failure, AML, sclerosing cholangitis, sepsis and hepatic venous obstruction are other causes of diffuse wall thickening in gallbladder.

58. **A-T, B-T, C-T, D-T, E-T**
    According to Courvoisier's law, if the gallbladder is enlarged in a jaundiced patient, the etiology is likely to be due to an obstructing carcinoma rather than cholecystitis, in which the gallbladder will be contracted due to inflammation.
    But, the exceptions for the gallbladder to be enlarged in present of stones are, cholecystis with stone in cystic duct, double stone in the cystic duct and distal common bile duct and oriental cholangiohepatitis. Acromegaly, alcoholism, appendicitis and diabetes mellitus are other causes of enlarged gallbladder.

59. **A-T, B-F, C-T, D-T, E-T**

60. **A-T, B-F, C-T, D-T, E-F**

61. **A-T, B-T, C-T, D-F, E-F**
    von Meyenburg's complexes are multiple biliary hamartomas.

62. **A-T, B-T, C-T, D-T, E-T**

63. **A-T, B-F, C-T, D-T, E-F**
    The biliary radicles need to be only 40% of the corresponding portal radicles to be considered enlarged. The double gun sign refers to the adjacently placed dilated biliary and portal venous radicles and indicates biliary ductal dilatation. The common bile duct is not enlarged in some cases of obstruction, especially in acute obstruction, sclerosing cholangitis and intermittent obstruction. Thus, sclerosing cholangitis gives a false negative radiological appearance.

64. **A-T, B-F, C-T, D-F, E-T**
    Dilated hepatic artery is a false positive indicator of biliary ductal dilatation and is caused by cirrhosis or hepatic tumour or portal hypertension. Infected bile is twice more common in benign obstruction than malignant obstruction. *E. coli* and *Klebsiella* are the most common organisms in infected bile. The infection is higher in incomplete obstruction than complete obstruction.

65. **A-T, B-F, C-T, D-T, E-F**
    Congenital malformation and ampullary neoplasms are other common causes.

66. **A-F, B-F, C-F, D-T, E-F**
    Pancreatic tumours—85%, cholangiocarcinoma—6%, ampullary tumour—4%.

67. **A-T, B-T, C-F, D-F, E-T**
    Duplicated gallbladder has two separate lumens and two separate cystic ducts. Bifid gallbladder has two separate lumens but one cystic duct. Multiseptated gallbladder have many septations and they communicate with each other through small pores. Phyrgian cap is folding of fundus which has transverse septum.

68. **A-F, B-T, C-T, D-F, E-T**

69. **A-T, B-T, C-T, D-T, E-T**
    All are rare causes of gallbladder wall thickening.

70. **A-T, B-T, C-F, D-T, E-F**
    Beneath the left lobe of the liver is the most common location.

Pancreas

1. Pancreatic ultrasound:
- A. The normal ratio of maximum diameter of vertebral body/ transverse diameter of vertebral body is more than 0.3
- B. The pancreas becomes less echogenic than retroperitoneal fat with age
- C. Pancreas is very hyperechoic in premature infants
- D. Differing echotexture of anterior and posterior aspect of pancreatic body is normal
- E. Tail is best visualized in left lateral decubitus

2. Pancreatic cysts are seen in:
- A. Mucinous tumours
- B. von Hippel-Lindau disease
- C. Tuberous sclerosis
- D. Acinar cell carcinoma
- E. Hemangioma

3. The pancreas is supplied by the following arteries:
- A. Caudal pancreatic arteries from splenic artery
- B. Arteria pancreatic magna from superior mesenteric artery
- C. Dorsal pancreatic artery from celiac artery
- D. Transverse pancreatic artery from splenic artery
- E. Small branches from left gastric artery

4. Endoscopic ultrasound:
- A. Linear array scanners provide complete view of the field sagittal to endoscope
- B. Radial scanners have limited view in comparison to the linear array scanners
- C. Mucosal views are better than endoscopy
- D. Linear and radial array scanners have same accuracy in tumour staging
- E. Mini probes are 20 MHz and can be passed through strictures

5. **Pancreas:**
   A. The pancreas completely lies behind the lesser sac
   B. The superior mesenteric vein and left renal vein pass posterior to the uncinate process of pancreas
   C. The pancreas lies over the levels of L2 and L3
   D. The neck is marked by the presence of gastroduodenal artery
   E. The pancreas becomes more hypoechoic with age

6. **Pancreas:**
   A. The transverse mesocolon is attached to the head, neck and body of pancreas
   B. The pancreatic duct measures 1 mm normally in the head
   C. The pancreatic head has a dual blood supply
   D. The pancreatic head is supplied completely by branches of the celiac axis
   E. The transverse pancreatic artery runs parallel to the pancreatic duct along its entire course

7. **Techniques:**
   A. Ultrasound of gastrointestinal tract is more useful in children than adults
   B. Endoscopic ultrasound of GIT is not useful for performing biopsies in pancreas and biliary tract
   C. MRI is done for evaluation of fistula in ano, if fistulography is not helpful
   D. Good morphologic information is obtained using nuclear medicine scans of GIT
   E. Doppler is not as useful as CT for diagnosis of mesenteric atheroembolic disease

8. **Causes of pancreatic hyperechogenicity in ultrasound and pancreatic insufficiency:**
   A. Diabetes mellitus
   B. Cystic fibrosis
   C. Chronic pancreatitis
   D. Obesity
   E. von Hippel-Lindau disease

9. **Endoscopic ultrasound:**
   A. Pancreatic tail is not visualized in endoscopic ultrasound
   B. Bile duct is visualized through pylorus
   C. Gallbladder has five layers like bowel wall
   D. Common bile duct has three layers only
   E. The ventral aspect of pancreas has a normal hypoechoic area

10. **Pancreas:**
    A. The splenic artery is the only tortous artery in the abdomen
    B. Superior pancreatic duct is called duct of Santorini
    C. The main and accessory pancreatic ductal systems are separate in 20% of people
    D. The CT density of pancreas progressively decreases with age
    E. The inferior mesenteric vein joins the portal vein

11. **Plain film findings of acute pancreatitis:**
    A. Gasless abdomen
    B. Fluid levels in jejunum
    C. No gas in midtransverse colon
    D. Fluid levels in lesser sac
    E. Fluid levels in second part of duodenum

12. **Periampullary carcinoma:**
    A. By definition includes only the tumours arising from the ampulla and pancreatic head
    B. 70% of people have a double barrel opening of common bile duct and pancreatic duct
    C. Sphincter of Oddi has three components
    D. The major papilla is situated in the descending duodenum in 95% of cases
    E. If the major papilla is in the third part of duodenum, pancreatic duct is inferior and medial to the pancreatic duct

13. **Features of ampullary carcinoma:**
    A. Thickening of distal ducts
    B. Papillary projections into the second part of duodenum
    C. Hypointense mass in T1 and T2
    D. Double duct sign
    E. Blunt ending of the distal bile duct

14. **Periampullary cancer:**
    A. Pancreatic cancers are better resectable than biliary ductal cancers
    B. Ampullary and duodenal tumours have worse prognosis than pancreatic cancers
    C. Ampullary cancers are very large at the time of presentation
    D. Lymphatic invasion is least common in ampullary carcinomas
    E. Extraluminal extension is least common in ampullary cancers

15. **Pancreatic intraductal mucin-producing tumours:**
    A. The prognosis is worse than pancreatic adenocarcinomas
    B. The ampulla is very wide
    C. The main pancreatic duct shows a long stricture
    D. Cluster of grapes is a characteristic appearance in branch duct disease
    E. All these lesions are malignant

16. **Intraductal mucin-producing tumours:**
    A. MRCP is better than ERCP
    B. Mural nodules are better seen as filling defects in ERCP
    C. Likely to be malignant if the tumour is larger than 3 cm
    D. If MPD is more than 15 mm, likely to be benign
    E. Segmental dilatation of main pancreatic duct is benign

17. **Causes of pancreatic cysts:**
    A. Papillary carcinoma
    B. Adenocarcinoma
    C. AD polycystic kidney
    D. Melanoma metastasis
    E. Lung metastasis

18. **Pancreatic tumours that are very vascular:**
    A. Adenocarcinoma
    B. Papillary cystic neoplasm
    C. Acinar cell carcinoma
    D. Macrocystic adenoma
    E. Islet cell tumour

19. **Pancreatic anatomy:**
    A. Pancreatic veins more than 5 mm are abnormal
    B. Inferior pancreaticoduodenal is the first branch of superior mesenteric artery
    C. Anterior superior pancreaticoduodenal vein drains into gastrocolic trunk
    D. Posterior superior pancreaticoduodenal vein drains into portal vein
    E. Posterior superior pancreaticoduodenal arcade rises from the gastroduodenal artery

20. **The following findings indicate that the pancreatic adenocarcinoma is irresectable:**
    A. Dilated posterior superior pancreaticoduodenal vein
    B. Peripancreatic lymphadenopathy
    C. Tumour > 3 cm
    D. Alteration in the caliber of vessels
    E. Malignant pleural effusion

21. **Pancreatic calcification is seen in:**
    A. Kwashiorkor
    B. Acute pancreatitis
    C. Hypoparathyroidism
    D. Mucoviscidosis
    E. Gastrinoma

22. **Fatty replacement of pancreas is seen in:**
    A. Malnutrition
    B. Cystic fibrosis
    C. Pancreatic ductal obstruction
    D. Tuberous sclerosis
    E. Influenza

23. **Causes of increased amylase:**
    A. Hepatitis   B. Pneumonia
    C. Renal transplantation   D. Peritonitis
    E. Splenic rupture

24. **Endoscopic ultrasound:**
    A. Has a higher accuracy rate in detecting small pancreatic tumours than MRI
    B. Detection and biopsy of peripancreatic nodes is not possible
    C. Good for assessment of peripancreatic spread of large tumours
    D. Not good for arterial evaluation as CT/MR
    E. Not useful for retropancreatic invasion

25. **MRI of pancreas:**
    A. MRI is good for evaluation of infective collections
    B. There is correlation of over 90 percent for MRCP with ERCP for early diagnosis of ductal abnormalities in chronic pancreatitis
    C. MRI is superior to CT in differentiating chronic pancreatitis from carcinoma
    D. Secretin-stimulated MRI increases ductal delineation
    E. Tissue specific contrast agents like Tesla scan is useful for differentiating chronic pancreatitis from carcinoma

26. **Periampullary carcinoma:**
    A. Four duct sign is a specific finding of ampullary carcinoma
    B. Dilatation of side branches of pancreatic duct is seen only in pancreatic carcinoma
    C. Rat tail shape of distal end of main pancreatic duct is specific for pancreatic carcinoma
    D. The signal intensity of pancreatic carcinoma depends on the desmoplastic response
    E. Pancreatic carcinoma can present with nondilated pancreatic duct and dilated common bile duct

27. **Chronic calcifying pancreatitis:**
    A. Causes biliary obstruction
    B. Does not occur in children
    C. Associated with hypercalcemia
    D. Associated with varices
    E. Associated with cysts

28. Pancreatitis is associated with:
    A. Peptic ulcer   B. Abscess
    C. Pseudocyst   D. Bone necrosis
    E. Hypoparathyroidism

29. Pancreatic calcification is seen in:
    A. Hyperparathyroidism B. Hypoparathyroidism
    C. Sarcoidosis   D. Brucellosis
    E. von Hippel-Lindau disease

30. Common causes of pancreatic metastasis:
    A. Sarcoma
    B. Melanoma
    C. Colon
    D. Liver
    E. Gallbladder

31. Predisposing factors for pancreatic adenocarcinoma:
    A. Smoking
    B. Alcohol
    C. Diabetes
    D. Hereditary pancreatitis
    E. von Hippel-Lindau disease

32. Islet cell tumours:
    A. Venous sampling is done by catheterizing the right branch of portal vein
    B. Samples are obtained at one cm intervals
    C. Collateral channels will produce false localization
    D. Pancreatic head and duodenal lesion can be differentiated
    E. A step of at least two standard deviations above the main portal concentration is essential for localisation

33. Pancreatic cancer:
    A. 45% have disease confined to pancreas at presentation
    B. Extension to posterior structures is more common than anterior extension
    C. The stomach is the most common organ invaded
    D. Lymph nodal spread is seen in 20%
    E. Peritoneal carcinomatosis is seen in 10%

34. Pancreatic cancer:
    A. Extensive desmoplastic response
    B. Vascular tumour
    C. Enhancement excludes pancreatic adenocarcinoma
    D. New onset diabetes is a clinical presentation
    E. It is the most common cause of malignant biliary obstruction

35. **Imaging features in pancreatic cancer:**
    A. Tethering diffusely in peritoneal cavity
    B. Inverted 3 sign in the medial part of duodenum
    C. Extrinsic indentation of greater curvature of stomach
    D. Serration of superior border of transverse colon
    E. Majority of tumours occur in the head

36. **Imaging in pancreatic cancer:**
    A. Double duct sign is specific for pancreatic cancer
    B. Ductal obstruction without mass is seen in 4%
    C. CT has a 99% accuracy rate for assessing nonreactability of tumour
    D. Bile duct dilatation is common than pancreatic ductal dilatation
    E. Pseudocyst is seen

37. **Common radiological features of pancreatic cancer:**
    A. Loss of retropancreatic fat
    B. Thickened Gerotas fascia
    C. Portal vein thrombosis
    D. Thickened wall of superior mesenteric artery
    E. Collateral veins

38. **Pancreatic islet cell tumour:**
    A. Gastrinoma is the most common functioning islet cell tumour
    B. Majority of islet cell tumours are nonfunctioning
    C. Gastrinoma is commonly seen in the tail
    D. Insulinoma is common in the head
    E. VIPomas (vasoactive intestinal peptide) arises from the alpha cells

39. **Islet cell tumours:**
    A. Liver metastasis are hyperechoic
    B. Hypoechoic with hyperechoic halo in pancreas
    C. 70% of gastrinomas are picked up by imaging
    D. Endoscopic ultrasound cannot pick lesions smaller than one cm
    E. Gastrinomas located close to splenic hilum and missed by abdominal scans are best picked by EUS

40. **Causes of increased amylase:**
    A. Duodenal perforation   B. Intestinal obstruction
    C. Mesenteric ischemia   D. Portal vein thrombosis
    E. Pancreatic carcinoma

41. **Intraoperative ultrasound:**
    A. Uses 20 MHz probe
    B. Complete examination of pancreatic tail requires retroperitoneal mobilization
    C. 4 mm is the threshold for detection of islet cell tumours
    D. All insulinomas require distal pancreatectomy
    E. 90% of insulinomas are detected

42. **Uncommon pancreatic tumours:**
    A. Pancreticoblastomas originate in embryonic period
    B. Pancreaticoblastoma is seen before nine years in boys
    C. Acinar cell carcinoma produces tender erythematous subcutaneous nodules and joint swelling
    D. Acanthosis nigricans is a well recognised feature of pancreatic carcinomas
    E. Histiocystic lymphoma is the most common type in pancreas

43. **Cysts in pancreas:**
    A. Pancreatic cysts are seen in 10% of cases of ADPKD
    B. All the cysts in von Hippel-Lindau disease are hemangioblastomas
    C. The most common cystic metastasis of pancreas is from ovarian cancer
    D. 40% of cysts in pancreas are true cysts
    E. Islet cell tumours are never cystic

44. **Macrocystic adenoma:**
    A. 85% of tumours are seen in the tail of pancreas
    B. Positive for CEA
    C. By definition, they are more than 2 cm, and more than 6 in number
    D. The contents are serous
    E. All the tumours are considered malignant and have to be removed

45. **Islet cell tumours:**
    A. PPoma does not produce any symptoms
    B. Islet-related hormones are less malignant than gut-related hormones
    C. Insulinomas can be seen in heterotopic pancreatic rests
    D. Nesidioblastosis produces same symptoms as gastrinoma
    E. Localisation of the pancreatic islet tumour should be done only after biochemical confirmation

46. **Serous cystic lesions:**
    A. Always benign
    B. Seen only in the head of the pancreas
    C. Fibrous scar with calcification is a characteristic feature
    D. A honeycomb or spongy appearance is seen in ultrasound, which is predominantly hyperechoic
    E. High content of glycogen and mucin

47. **Insulinomas:**
    A. More common in females
    B. Majority are seen before 20 years of age
    C. 10% multiple
    D. 40% malignant
    E. C peptide levels are low

48. **Islet cell tumours:**
    A. Majority are hyperdense in unenhanced CT
    B. Calcification is common in malignant
    C. Enhance less than normal parenchyma
    D. Necrosis invariably seen in larger tumours
    E. Liver lesions are hypodense in arterial phase

49. **Islet cell tumours:**
    A. Hyper in both T1 and T2 W images
    B. Invariably hypervascular
    C. A blush is seen in the capillary phase of angiogram
    D. Encasement and venous obstruction suggests malignancy
    E. New vessel formation is seen

50. **Islet cell tumours:**
    A. Venous sampling is not useful in intermittently secreting tumours
    B. Hormonal levels immediately after angiography should be ignored
    C. Mesenteric venous thrombosis is a complication
    D. Higher complication rate in cirrhosis
    E. More useful in gastrinomas than insulinomas

51. **Gastrinomas:**
    A. Most common islet cell tumour
    B. Accounts for 25% of ulcers in jejunum and duodenum
    C. 90% are seen in the gastrinoma triangle
    D. Can arise in lymph nodes
    E. Ovarian gastrinomas are recognized

52. **Gastrinomas:**
    A. Majority are solitary
    B. 1/3rd associated with MEN II syndrome
    C. Majority are large and above one cm
    D. Surgery not useful if associated with MEN
    E. Somatostatinomas do not occur in MEN syndromes

53. Insulinomas:
A. 90% less than 2 cm
B. Multiple lesions are larger than solitary
C. Malignant lesions larger than benign
D. Always arise in pancreas
E. Highest incidence in tail

54. Insulinomas:
A. Surgery is curative in 90%
B. 50% associated with MEN
C. Glucoganomas are malignant
D. VIPOmas produce watery diarrhoea, and are benign
E. Somatostatinomas produce diabetes

55. Islet cell tumours:
A. Majority of functioning tumours are malignant
B. Nonfunctioning tumours are large at presentation than functioning
C. Nonfunctioning tumours common in the pancreatic head
D. PPoma does not produce any syndrome
E. Delta cells produce insulin

56. Ampullary tumour:
A. Associated with familial adenomatous polyposis coli
B. GI bleed is a type of presentation
C. Prominent papilla is often the only endoscopic finding
D. ERCP is the most sensitive imaging modality
E. Double duct sign is invariably associated

57. Ampullary cancer:
A. If the pancreas is invaded more than 2 cm deep, it is T3
B. The tumour surface shows barium filled intersices in barium
C. Indentation is seen in duodenum in barium
D. Dilated distal portion of CBD
E. Associated with CBD calculus

58. Differential diagnosis for ampullary carcinoma:
A. Choledochocele   B. Pancreatic rest
C. Brunner's gland tumour   D. Stone
E. Annular pancreas

59. Islet cell tumours—arterial stimulation and venous sampling:
A. Calcium gluconate is injected into pancreatic arteries for evaluating insulinoma
B. It is more sensitive than venous sampling
C. False negative results are very high, because of selective catheterization

D. Indium 111 octreotide is the most sensitive of all techniques
E. Two-thirds of insulinomas are localized with somatostatin receptor analogues

60. **Common sites of communication of biliary fistula:**
    A. Hepatic artery
    B. Bronchial tree
    C. Colon
    D. Stomach
    E. Portal vein

61. **Causes of cholecystoenteric fistula:**
    A. Acute cholecystitis
    B. Diverticulitis
    C. Peptic ulcer
    D. Pancreatitis
    E. Crohn's disease

62. **Causes of acute pancreatitis:**
    A. Epstein Barr virus
    B. Hypothermia
    C. Shock
    D. Duodenal ulcer
    E. Renal transplant

63. **Drugs known to cause pancreatitis:**
    A. Tetracycline
    B. Erythromycin
    C. Methyldopa
    D. Azathioprine
    E. Omeprazole

ANSWERS

1. **A-F, B-F, C-T, D-T, E-T**
   The AP diameter of pancreatic body/transverse vertebral diameter is usually less than 0.3. It is high in pancreatitis and other pancreatic pathologies. The pancreas becomes more echogneic with age. Differing echotexture can be seen due to asymmetrical lipomatosis. Head is well visualized in right lateral decubitus, body can be seen in upright position.

2. **A-T, B-T, C-F, D-T, E-T**
   Other causes are congenital, traumatic, pseudocysts (pancreatitis), serous cystadenoma, mucinous cystic tumour, papillary cystadenocarcinoma, surgical, AD polycystic kidney disease, enterogenous, dermoid, mucinous ductal ectasia.

3. **A-T, B-F, C-T, D-F, E-F**
   Arteria pancreatica magna—supplies body—from splenic artery
   Dorsal pancreatic artery—from splenic/hepatic/SMA/celiac—supplies posterior portion of pancreas; Transverse pancreatic artery—from dorsal pancreatic A—supplies body and tail
   Branches from dorsal pancreatic A—supply head; Caudal pancreatic arteries—from splenic artery—supplies tail; Short pancreatic arteries—splenic artery—body and tail.

4. **A-F, B-F, C-F, D-T, E-T**
   Linear array, radial array and mini probes are some of the endoscopic scan devices used. Linear array scanners have limited view in a sagittal plane. Radial scanners are better. Both have the same accuracy. Mini probes are very small and can also be passed through achalasia, because it does not interfere with motility unlike the other probes. ENS is better for assessing depth of invasion. Endoscopy gives good mucosal views.

5. **A-T, B-F, C-F, D-T, E-F**
   The pancreas lies over the L1 and L2 vertebral levels. The neck is marked by the presence of gastroduodenal artery anteriorly and formation of portal vein posteriorly. The superior mesenteric vein passes anteriorly and left renal vein passes posteriorly to the uncinate process. The pancreas is usually hyperechoic with liver, and becomes more hyperechoic with age due to deposition of fat.

6. **A-T, B-F, C-T, D-F, E-T**
   The pancreatic duct measures 1 mm in tail, 2 mm in body and 3 mm in head.
   The pancreatic head has a dual blood supply. The superior pancreaticoduodenal artery from gastroduodenal artery, a branch

of celiac axis and inferior pancreaticoduodenal artery, a branch of superior mesenteric artery.

7. **A-T, B-F, C-F, D-F, E-T**
Ultrasound of gastrointestinal tract, is more useful for diagnosis in paediatric diseases such as pyloric stenosis, intussusception and appendicitis. MRI is the ideal modality for imaging fistulae in ano. Nuclear medicine of GIT gives functional details, but morphological details are not obtained. FNAs and biopsies are taken by EUS.

8. **A-T, B-T, C-T, D-T, E-F**
Aging and hereditary pancreatitis are other causes.

9. **A-F, B-T, C-F, D-T, E-T**
Gallbladder and common bile duct have three layers unlike the bowel mucosa
Layer 1—echogenic, mucosa, layer 2—hypoechoic, muscle, layer 3—echogenic, serosa
The ventral component of pancreas has a hypoechoic areas which is due to absence of fat. This can be confused with malignancy, but is usually triangular.

10. **A-T, B-T, C-F, D-T, E-F**
Up to 10% have separate ductal systems, the superior duct of Santorini and inferior duct of Wirsung. CT density progressively decreases due to fat deposition. The inferior mesenteric vein joins the splenic vein.

11. **A-T, B-T, C-T, D-T, E-T**
The absence of gas in midtransverse colon is called Stewart's sign and is due to inflammatory exudates in transverse mesocolon and phrenicocolic ligament. Most of X-ray findings are nonspecific.

12. **A-F, B-F, C-T, D-F, E-F**
Periampullary carcinoma, by definition, includes all tumours which arise within 2 cm of the ampulla, and hence will include ampullary, distal bile duct, duodenal and pancreatic tumours. 60% have a common duct and enter ampulla. 38% have a double barrel opening into ampulla. 2% have separate openings of bile duct and pancreatic duct. Sphincter of Oddi has an ampullary, choledochal and pancreatic component. 75% are in the 2nd part of duodenum, with the pancreatic duct, inferior and medial to bile duct. In 25%, it opens into third part, when the bile duct will be lateral to the pancreatic duct.

13. **A-T, B-T, C-T, D-T, E-T**
Double duct sign is dilated pancreatic duct and biliary duct secondary to ampullary cancers.

14. **A-F, B-F, C-F, D-T, E-T**

    Among the four types of periampullary cancers, ampullary cancers have the best prognosis, followed by duodenal, biliary and pancreatic cancers. Ampullary tumours are very small, manifest early, mainly grow intraluminally, no extraluminal spread, no lymphatic or perineural spread and have better respectability.

15. **A-F, B-T, C-F, D-T, E-F**

    Prognosis is better than pancreatic adenocarcinomas, since they are respectable. Histologically, they can be benign or malignant. The main pancreatic duct is dilated, with wide ampulla. If it involves the branch ducts, they show cluster of grapes appearance.

16. **A-T, B-F, C- T, D-F, E-T**

    ERCP is a good examination, but contrast opacification can be difficult due to abundant mucin production by the tumour. MRCP is good because of inherent contrast between the high signal mucin and the mural nodules. Although there are no classical signs, mural nodules, tumour > 3 cm, MPD > 1.5 cm are likely to be malignant. If the duct is diffusely dilated, it is in favour of malignancy, segmental dilation is likely to be benign.

17. **A-T, B-T, C-T, D-T, E-T**

    Mets from colon, ovary, breast and liver are other recognised causes. Pseudocyst is the most common cause of a pancreatic cyst. Micro- and macrocystic adenoma, papillary cystic tumours, cystic islet cell tumours and mucinous colloid cancers are primary cystic tumours of pancreas. Hydatid, parasites, retention cyst and mucinous ductal ectasia are benign causes.

18. **A-F, B-T, C-F, D-F, E-T**

    Adenocarcinoma is avascular and schirrhous. Microcystic adenoma is vascular, but macrocystic is not. Metastases from hypervascular tumours are other causes.

19. **A-T, B-T, C-T, D-T, E-T**

20. **A-T, B-F, C-F, D-T, E-T**

    Tumour > 3 cm, stranding in the perivascular fat planes and peripancreatic lymphadenopathy are equivocal findings. Lymphadenopathy beyond the peripancreatic chain, malignant ascites, vascular encasement, contiguity more than 50% with vessels, peritoneal deposits and metastases are other indicators of irresectability. Dilated veins are early signs of irresectability, because most of them are due to tumour invasion with collateral dilatation.

21. **A-T, B-T, C-F, D-T, E-F**
Chronic pancreatitis, acute pancreatitis, hereditary pancreatitis, cystic fibrosis, kwashiorkor. Tumours—cystadenoma, cystoadeno-carcinoma, islet cell tumours. Hyperparathyroidism, haematoma, lymphoma, pseudocysts.

22. **A-T, B-T, C-T, D-F, E-T**

23. **A-T, B-T, C-T, D-T, E-F**
Parotid gland lesions such as mumps and trauma are common causes. Perforated peptic ulcer, acute intestinal obstruction, acute biliary obstruction, renal disorders, morphine, hypothermia diabetic ketoacidosis, macroamylasemia, pancreatic carcinoma, mesenteric ischemia, renal transplant, hepatitis, peritonitis. Acute pancreatitis is the most common cause.

24. **A-T, B-F, C-F, D-T, E-T**
Accuracy rate for detection of smaller tumours is greater than CT/MR. It has a sensitivity of more than 95%. It can assess peripancreatic nodes and portal encasement and even biopsy can be taken from these nodes. However, the area evaluated is very limited. It cannot assess the retropancreatic area (blind spot), cannot assess peripancreatic spread of large tumours and cannot assess arterial involvement as good as MRI/CT. It is mainly used as a problem solving tool, especially in equivocal small cases and for equivocal invasion of arteries and veins and for biopsy confirmation.

25. **A-F, B-T, C-F, D-T, E-F**
MRI for pancreas is performed after starvation and administration of glucagon or buscopan. Breath hold axial T1, coronal T2, MRCP images using slab and multi slice acquisition. Breath hold T1 with fat saturation before and after contrast administration are performed with an optional. Manganese DPDP contrast for evaluation of liver metastasis and pancreatic lesions. Because of inability to detect gas and calcification, it is not useful in detecting abscesses. Although ERCP is still the gold standard for the evaluation of chronic pancreatitis, MRCP has a positive correlation of more than 90 percent with ERCP for evaluation of ductal anomalies. Secretin-stimulated MRCP improves ductal delineation, may diagnose papillary stenosis and detects reduced pancreatic reserve. MRI, including tissue specific agents like TESLA scan are not useful in differentiating chronic pancreatitis from carcinoma.

26. **A-F, B-T, C-T, D-T, E-T**
Four duct sign is a specific sign of pancreatic carcinoma. A pancreatic carcinoma can cause dilatation of the proximal end of

common bile duct and pancreatic duct (double duct sign). If there
is a segment of ducts beyond the mass, they can be prominent
and these four ducts will form the four ductal sign. Occasionally,
one of the two ducts can be dilated and the other duct can be of
normal size. The pancreatic mass can be hypo or iso- or hyperintense, depending on the desmoplastic response.

27. **A-T, B-F, C-F, D-T, E-T**
Cystic fibrosis, hereditary pancreatitis occur in children. Venous
thrombosis secondary to pancreatitis can cause varices. Pseudocysts
are associated.

28. **A-T, B-T, C-T, D-T, E-F**
Hyperparathyroidism is associated in 10%. Other complications
are—hypotension, shock, pericardial effusion, hypoxia, ARDS,
pleural effusion, pneumonia, ATN, renal artery/vein thrombosis,
hypocalcemia, hyperglycemia, hyperlipidemia, hypomagnesaemia,
DIC and GI bleeding.

29. **A-T, B-F, C-F, D-F, E-F**
In von Hippel-Lindau disease, there can be cysts, but no calcification. Hereditary pancreatitis, cystic fibrosis, Kwashiorkor, pseudocyst, chronic alcoholic pancreatitis, cystadenomas, cystadenocarcinomas, cavernous lymphangioma and islet cell tumours are
other causes.

30. **A-T, B-T, C-T, D-F, E-F**
Kidneys, lung and breast are other common causes.
Pancreatic metastasis is very rare and is seen just in 3-10% of
autopsy patients.

31. **A-T, B-T, C-T, D-T, E-T**
Two percent of pancreatitis associated with CA; Gastrectomy, VHL,
familial relapsing pancreatitis, Gardner's syndrome, neurofibromatosis, Ataxia telangiectasia, Lynch syndrome are other causes.

32. **A-T, B-T, C-T, D-F, D-T**
The principle of venous sampling is to catheterize the right branch
of portal vein and measure the concentration of the suspected
hormone in portal vein branches and accessible pancreatic veins.
A high concentration in a particular place of portal vein indicates
that the hormone was secreted by the tumour at that location. It
is not possible to exactly pinpoint, but localization is good. It is
not possible to differentiate pancreatic head or duodenal lesion.
Collaterals produced by previous surgery will produce false
localization.

33. **A-F, B-T, C-F, D-T, E-T**
    About 65% of tumours extend beyond pancreas at time of presentation. Posterior extension is common (seen in 95%) than anterior. Duodenum is more commonly involved than stomach or adrenal or spleen or mesentery. Ascites/Metastasis to liver and lung can be seen.

34. **A-T, B-F, C-T, D-T, E-T**
    The tumour is a scirrhous adenocarcinoma and elicits intense desmoplastic response and is avascular. There is no enhancement on contrast administration. New onset diabetes, steatorrhea, paraneoplastic syndromes like acanthosis nigricans and Trousseau's syndrome are recognised clinical presentations.

35. **A-T, B-T, C-F, D-F, E-T**
    Diffuse tethering is seen due to diffuse peritoneal involvement. Inverted 3 sign is seen due to fixed ampulla in the medial part of duodenum (Frostberg's sign). Extrinsic indentation is more commonly seen in the posteroinferior border of antrum. Serration is common in the inferior part of transverse colon and splenic flexure. 60% in head, 26% in body and 12% in tail.

36. **A-F, B-T, C-F, D-F, E-T**
    Double duct sign, is dilatation of common and pancreatic duct. It can be seen in pancreatic and ampullary carcinomas. Dilated ducts without a visible mass can be seen in a small number of cases. CT has an accuracy rate of 85% for assessing nonresectability.
    In 75% both ducts are dilated. In isolated ductal dilatation, pancreatic duct is involved in 2/3rds and bile duct alone in 1/3rd.

37. **A-T, B-T, C-F, D-T, E-T**
    Infiltration of splenic hilum, calcification and invasion of adjacent organs are recognised features.

38. **A-F, B-F, C-F, D-F, E-F,**
    Insulinoma is the most common functioning islet cell tumour. 85% of islet tumours are functioning. Gastrinoma is common in the head. Insulinoma does not have any specific predilection. VIPomas arise from the delta cells.

39. **A-T, B-F, C-F, D-F, E-F**
    Pancreatic lesions are usually hyperechoic with a hypoechoic halo. Only 30% of gastrinomas are picked up by imaging. Transabdominal scans pick lesions more than 1 cm and EUS can detect lesions more than 5 mm. Gastrinomas close to splenic hilum cannot be detected by EUS.

40. **A-T, B-T, C-T, D-T, E-T**
    See answer 23.

41. **A-F, B-T, C-T, D-F, E-T**
Intraoperative ultrasound uses 5-10 MHz probe. It can detect tumours as small as 4 mm and hence it detects 90% of insulinomas. Benign insulinomas require only resection, but malignant ones require distal pancreatectomy.

42. **A-T, B-T, C-T, D-T, E-T**
Pancreaticoblastoma has mixed tissue components and is seen in children. It is a solid tumour and has a good prognosis. It arises commonly from the head, seen as echogenic mass in ultrasound and inhomogeneous solid mass in CT scans. Acinar cell carcinoma is notorious for producing zymogen granules which produce a lot of pancreatic enzymes including lipase, which produces systemic fat necrosis, including subcutaneous nodules, joint symptoms, bone necrosis, eosinophilia and liver metastasis. Acanthosis nigricans is blackish pigmentation, seen predominantly in the axillary region. Lymphomas are very uncommon in pancreas and are often non-Hodgkin's than Hodgkin's.

43. **A-T, B-F, C-F, D-F, E-F**
Cysts are seen in 15% of cases with von Hippel-Lindau disease, and can be either a simple cyst, or serous cystadenoma or hemangioblastoma or adenocarcinoma or islet cell tumour melanoma is the most common metastasis to produce cystic pancreatic lesion, others being lung, breast, prostate and ovary. Serous cystadenocarcinoma, mucinous cystadenoma, mucinous cystadenocarcinoma, microcystic adenoma, mucinous ductactic adenocarcinomas and islet cell tumours are other causes of cystic lesions. True cysts are produced due to sequestration of primitive ducts of pancreas and account for 10-15% of pancreatic cystic lesions.

44. **A-T, B-T, C-F, D-F, E-T**
This tumour is also called mucinous cystic neoplasm, can be benign or borderline or malignant. This tumour is a cystic lesion, uni or multilocular, 1-20 cm in size, filled with mucinous contents, with smooth external surface and smooth or trabeculated internal surface. This tumour is positive for CEA, CA19-9 and mucin. It can produce Zollinger-Ellison syndrome. 85% involve the tail or tail and body. 10-30% involve the head. The tumours less than 3 cm are considered benign and more than 8 cm are considered malignant. It is sometimes difficult to differentiate, even in biopsy and hence surgical excision is carried out. Presence of metastasis is an indication of malignant nature of the lesion. Calcification is seen in 1/6th of cases. The most common differential diagnosis is a serous cystic neoplasm. According to Johnson's criteria,

tumours less than 2 cm and more than 6 in number are likely to be serous cystic lesions, but those more than 2 cm and less than 6 in number are likely to be mucinous cystic lesion.

45. A-T, B-T, C-T, D-F, E-T
Nesioblasts are seen only in embryonic life, but can persist in a very small number of patients beyond fetal life, producing neonatal hypoglycemia. Symptoms resemble insulinoma.

46. A-T, B-F, C-T, D-T, E-F
Serous cystic lesion or microcystic adenoma is a benign tumour that is rich in glycogen, but without mucin, seen in any part of the pancreas without specific predilection. It arises from the centriacinar cell and is negative for CEA. Majority of the cysts are very small and seen as conglomerate lesion. It produces homogeneous solid well encapsulated echogenic mass due to increased number of interfaces between the small cysts. Serous cystadenocarcinoma is very rare.

47. A-T, B-F, C-T, D-F, E-F
Majority are seen after fifty years and in females. Only 10% are malignant. There is high insulin level, high C peptide level and low glucose in the serum.

48. A-F, B-T, C-F, D-T, E-F
The lesions in pancreas are isodense in unenhanced scans and enhance more than the normal parenchymal parenchyma. Calcification is more common in malignant than benign tumours, although it is seen only in 10% of malignancies. Liver lesions are characteristically hyperdense in vascular phase and isodense in the portal phase.

49. A-F, B-T, C-T, D-T, E-T
The islet cell tumours are hypo in T1 and hyper in T2. Capillary blush, tortous feeding vessels, neovascularity, encasement and venous obstruction are seen in malignant subtypes. Occasionally, it can be hypovascular, where it is missed in angiography.

50. A-T, B-T, C-T, D-T, E-F
Injection of contrast can produce a transient elevation of hormone, and hence the findings immediately after injection are largely ignored. Other complications include pneumothorax, biliary peritonitis, haemorrhage and injury to adjacent structures.
It is more useful in occult insulinomas than gastrinomas. It is not very useful if ultrasound, CT, MRI and angiography have been negative.

51. **A-F, B-T, C-T, D-T, E-T**
    Insulinomas are the most common islet tumours. Gastrinoma triangle—superiorly—junction of cystic and common bile duct, inferiorly—junction of second and third portion of duodenum, medially—junction of neck and body of pancreas. Can also be seen in gastric antrum.

52. **A-F, B-F, C-F, D-T, E-T**
    About 60% are multiple. One-third occurs with MEN I syndrome. Majority are small and less than one cm. Surgery is not useful when there is hepatic metastasis or MEN syndrome association.

53. **A-T,-F, C-T, D-T, E-F**
    Multiple lesions are usually smaller. Equal incidence in head, neck, body and tail.

54. **A-T, B-F, C-T, D-F, E-T**
    Insulinomas are easily palpated during surgery which is curative. Less than 5% are associated with MEN syndrome. Glucoganomas are malignant and produce diabetes mellitus. VIPomas produce watery diarrhea, hypokalemia, alkalosis and are malignant. Somatostatinoma—diabetes, gallstones, weight loss, usually benign.

55. **A-T, B-T, C-T, D-T, E-F**
    Majority of functioning tumours are malignant, the exceptions being insulinoma and somatostatinoma. Alpha cells produce glucagons, Beta cells—insulin, Delta cells—somatostatin, PP cells—pancreatic polypeptide.

56. **A-T, B-T, C-T, D-F, E-F**
    Almost 100-fold risk in FAP. Obstructive jaundice is the most common presentation. But tumour necrosis can produce GI bleeding. In majority a tumour can be visualised in endoscopy. But in some, the endoscopy is normal or there can be a prominent papilla with submucosal tumour. Endoscopic ultrasound is the most sensitive imaging modality.
    Double duct dilatation is usually seen. But it is not seen if the tumour is small to compress the ducts, or if there is an accessory pancreatic duct or the main duct drains into the minor papilla.

57. **A-F, B-T, C-T, D-T, E-F**
    T1—confined to ampulla. T2—involves duodenum, T3—pancreas involved, less than 2 cm, and T4—pancreas involved more than 2 cm.

58. **A-T, B-T, C-T, D-T, E-F**
    Stone impacted in ampulla is a cause.

Duodenal carcinoma, leiomyoma and gastrinoma are tumours in similar location.

59. **A-T, B-T, C-T, D-F, E-T**

In arterial stimulation, a secretogogue (calcium gluconate—insulinoma or secretin for gastrinoma) is injected into selective pancreatic arterial branches and the concentration of hormone is measured in the blood which comes into the right hepatic vein. This is more sensitive than just venous sampling, because the secretogogue is injected into arteries, and arterial variation is only minimal in comparison to venous channels. The limitation is placing the catheter only in the right hepatic veins. The pancreatic venous flow has a selective streaming into the portal vein, hence they can go into both right and left hepatic veins. This technique can miss the rise in hormone occurring in the left branch. Indium 111 octreotide is not very sensitive as other techniques. It is useful only in equivocal cases, and to assess extent of disseminated disease. Somatostatin receptors should be expressed for localization by these analogues. Up to 90% of islet tumours express somatostatin receptors.

60. **A-T, B-T, C-T, D-T, E-T**

Duodenum accounts for 70% of fistulae. Other rare locations are pericardium, vagina, ovary, urinary bladder, ureter and renal pelvis.

61. **A-T, B-T, C-T, D-F, E-T**

Chronic cholecystitis, carcinoma or biliary tract and bowel, hydatid and trauma are other reasons.

62. **A-T, B-T, C-T, D-T, E-T**

Gallstones and alcoholism are the most common causes. Other causes are hyperparathyroidism, hyperlipidemia, renal failure, DKA, HIV, mycoplasma, hepatitis, legionella, ascariasis, campylobacter, atheroma, necrotising vasculitis, methyl alcohol, scorpion venom, α_1 antitrypsin deficiency and hereditary.

63. **A-T, B-T, C-T, D-T, E-F**

Metronidazole, pentamidine, frusemide, cimetidine, ranitidine, thianides, sulphonamides, valproate, estrogens, nitrofurantoin, salicylates and paracetamol are other causes.

Spleen

9

1. **Spleen:**
   A. The spleen is considered enlarged if it is more than 14 cm
   B. Accessory spleen is most common in the leinorenal ligament
   C. Accessory spleen can be demonstrated by Tc99m denatured red cells
   D. Spleen has consistent intrasplenic blood supply
   E. The spleen is attached to left kidney by the leinorenal ligament

2. **The following are common causes of nonvisualisation of spleen:**
   A. Splenic infarct
   B. Asplenia
   C. Polysplenia
   D. Wandering spleen
   E. Hereditary spherocytosis

3. **The following are causes of small spleen:**
   A. Polysplenia
   B. Hereditary spherocytosis
   C. Sickle cell anemia
   D. Kala azar
   E. Amoebiasis

4. **The following are common causes of splenic microcalcification (< 10 mm):**
   A. Tuberculosis
   B. Hemangioma
   C. Sarcoidosis
   D. Hydatid
   E. Fungal infection

5. **Common causes of hyperechoic lesions in spleen:**
   A. Fungal infections
   B. Portal hypertension
   C. Lymphoma
   D. Myelofibrosis
   E. Hereditary spherocytosis

6. **Cysts in spleen:**
   A. 80% are pseudocysts
   B. Majority are congenital cysts
   C. Infarct
   D. Hemangioma
   E. Lymphoma

7. **Increased bone scan uptake in spleen is seen in:**
   A. Sickle cell
   B. Lymphoma
   C. Thalassemia
   D. Hemosiderois
   E. G6PD deficiency

8. **The following are causes of splenic artery aneurysm:**
   A. Pancreatitis
   B. Portal hypertension
   C. Splenic metastasis
   D. Trauma
   E. Splenomegaly

9. **Causes of splenic infarction:**
   A. Hodgkin's lymphoma
   B. Pancreatic cancer
   C. Infective endocarditis
   D. SLE
   E. Myeloma

10. **The following cause increased density in spleen, in ultrasound:**
    A. Hereditary spherocytosis
    B. Sickle cell anemia
    C. Thorotrast
    D. Congestive splenomegaly
    E. Hemochromatosis

11. **Lymphoma of spleen:**
    A. Spleen is involved in 90% of lymphoma patients
    B. Splenomegaly in patients with non-Hodgkin's lymphoma indicates splenic involvement
    C. Normal sized spleen in a lymphomatous patient, excludes splenic involvement
    D. Splenic hilar nodes are commonly seen in Hodgkin's than non-Hodgkin's disease
    E. Miliary nodules are seen in 25%

12. **Common causes of splenic calcification:**
    A. Epidermoid cyst
    B. Splenic infarct
    C. *Pneumocystis carinii*
    D. Aneurysm
    E. *Candida*

13. **Hyposplenism:**
    A. Howell Jolly bodies are pathognomonic
    B. Functional asplenia is marked by lack of Tc99 sulphur colloid uptake
    C. Staphylococcus infections are rampant in hyposplenic individuals
    D. Tc99m labeled heat damaged RBCs are taken up in asplenic individuals
    E. Large spleen with functional asplenia is suggestive of sarcoidosis

14. **Splenic lesions:**
    A. Splenomegaly excludes splenic infarction
    B. Spleen is not involved in metastatic spread, protected by reticuloendothelial cells
    C. True cysts are larger than false cysts
    D. Pyogenic abscesses are treated by antibiotics, because of high bleeding from spleen
    E. Sarcoidosis will produce heterogeneous splenomegaly

15. **Causes of microabscesses in spleen:**
    A. Tuberculosis
    B. *Candida*
    C. Aspergillosis
    D. *Cryptococcus*
    E. *Pneumocystis carinii*

16. **The following are causes of splenic abscess:**
    A. Sickle cell disease
    B. Lymphoma
    C. SLE
    D. Hemodialysis
    E. Endocarditis

17. **Causes of necrotic metastasis to spleen:**
    A. Pancreas
    B. Endometrial
    C. Chondrosarcoma
    D. Prostate
    E. Lung

18. **Splenic calcification occurs in:**
    A. Amoebiasis   B. Sickle cell anemia
    C. Hydatid disease   D. Thalassemia
    E. Histoplasmosis

19. **The following are common locations of accessory spleen:**
    A. Gastrosplenic ligament B. Pancreas
    C. Pelvis   D. Phrenicocolic ligament
    E. Left kidney

20. **Spleen:**
    A. In splenic abscess, 80% have underlying splenic disease
    B. Anaerobic organisms are the most common organisms involved in splenic abscess
    C. The typical rim enhancement is not seen in splenic abscess
    D. The most common X-ray finding in splenic abscess is left pleural effusion
    E. Aspergillosis is the most common fungus to affect spleen

21. **Spleen:**
    A. Abscesses in spleen, liver and kidney at same time are more likely to be fungal
    B. Calcification excludes fungal infection and indicates tuberculosis
    C. Bull's eye lesion is an echogenic lesion with a hypoechoic halo
    D. Wheel within wheel appearance has a hypoechoic center
    E. Normal appearance of spleen in imaging does not exclude fungal infection

22. **Spleen:**
    A. The most common pattern of tuberculosis of spleen is miliary disease
    B. In tuberculosis, the ascites is often high density in CT scan
    C. *Mycobacterium avium intracellulare* develops only after AIDS develops
    D. Tuberculosis in AIDS spreads to spleen from gastrointestinal tract rather than hematogenous spread
    E. Spleen is involved in 25% of sarcoidosis

23. **Tuberculosis:**
    A. Splenomegaly is more common in MAI
    B. Hepatomegaly is more common in tuberculosis than MAI
    C. Granulomas are uncommon in MAI
    D. Diffuse jejunal wall thickening is more common in MAI
    E. Low attenuation lymph nodes are more common in tuberculosis

24. **Spleen:**
    A. Cysts are more common in the lower pole than the upper pole
    B. Splenic cyst causes inferior displacement of the splenic flexure
    C. The most common benign tumour of spleen is lipoma
    D. In sickle cell disease, splenomegaly develops only after the age of five
    E. Splenomegaly is not seen in adult life in heterozygous sickle cell disease

25. **Intrasplenic collection in pancreatitis is due to:**
    A. Destructive action of pancreatic enzymes on splenic paren-chyma
    B. Direct extension of pancreatic pseudocyst
    C. Ruptured splenic artery aneurysm
    D. Liquefaction of splenic infarct
    E. Ectopic intrasplenic pancreatic tissue

26. **Differential diagnosis of miliary lesions in spleen (< 8 mm):**
    A. Sarcoidosis
    B. Fungal infection
    C. Lymphoma
    D. Gamma Gandy bodies
    E. Hemosiderosis

27. **Sickle cell disease:**
    A. End stage spleen shows diffusely high signal in MRI due to haemorrhage and hemosiderin
    B. In functional asplenia, the uptake in sulfur colloid is not affected but uptake is seen in bone scan
    C. In splenic sequestration, spleen atrophies
    D. Peripheral hypodense areas in enlarged spleen in homozygous sickle, indicates splenic sequestration
    E. Veno-occlusion produces splenomegaly and infarction in heterozygous sicklers

28. **Splenic artery aneurysms:**
    A. Common in multiparous women
    B. Most common in proximal part of artery
    C. Rupture seen in 40%
    D. Treatment required only if larger than 4 cm
    E. Most common cause of visceral aneurysm

ANSWERS

1. **A-T, B-T, C-T, D-F, E-T**
   Accessory spleens are common in the splenic hilum and the leinorenal ligament.
   Spleen has inconsistent blood supply, which accounts for the heterogeneous enhancement in arterial phase of CT scans. The tail of pancreas, splenic and short gastric vessels are seen in the leinorenal ligament.

2. **A-T, B-T, C-F, D-T, E-F**
   Sickle cell anemia causes infarct and nonvisualisation.

3. **A-T, B-T, C-T, D-F, E-F**
   Kala-azar and amebiasis cause splenomegaly.

4. **A-T, B-T, C-F, D-T, E-T**
   TB, histoplasmosis, infection, phleboliths, Armillifer and brucellosis are common causes of microcalcification.

5. **A-T, B-T, C-T, D-T, E-F**
   Portal hypertension produces Gamma Gandy bodies due to splenic haemorrhage. There are also seen in sic.
   Other causes are tuberculosis, leukemia and other granulomas.

6. **A-T, B-F, C-T, D-T, E-T**
   Up to 80% are traumatic pseudocysts. Pancreatic pseudocysts comprise only 1-5%.
   Hematoma, abscess, fungus, tuberculosis, PCP, hydatid, lymphangioma and metastasis are other causes.

7. **A-T, B-T, C-T, D-T, E-T,**

8. **A-T, B-T, C-F, D-T, E-F**
   Most splenic artery aneurysms are pseudoaneurysms.

9. **A-F, B-T, C-T, D-T, E-F**
   Hemolytic anemias such as sickle cell anemia and infective endocarditis are common causes. Splenic venous thrombosis produces an infarct with enlarged spleen.

10. **A-F, B-T, C-T, D-F, E-T**

11. **A-F, B-F, C-F, D-F, E-T**
    In 30%, spleen is enlarged without splenic involvement and in 30%, the spleen is not enlarged even with splenic infiltration. Hence, neither splenomegaly nor absence of it are specific or sensitive for assessing splenic infiltration with lymphoma. Splenic hilar nodes are common in non-Hodgkin's lymphoma. There are

many forms of splenic involvement—homogeneous splenomegaly/ multiple large nodules/miliary nodules/diffuse infiltration.

12. **A-T, B-T, C-T, D-T, E-F**
Granulomas such as tuberculosis and histoplasmosis are the most common causes.
Haematoma, phleboliths and other cysts are common causes of calcification.

13. **A-T, B-T, C-F, D-T, E-T**
Asplenia may be due to anatomical absence or functional splenia. Lack of Tc99m sulphur colloid uptake is typical. But there is uptake of Tc99m labelled RBCs and In 111 labelled platelets. Howell Jolly bodies, siderocytes, lymphocytosis and monocytosis are the common hematological features. Sarcoidosis, amyloidiosis and sickle cell anemia show functional asplenia with normal or enlarged spleen. Capsulated organisms such as *Pneumococcus, Haemophilus* and *Meningococcus* are the common infectious agents in asplenic patients.

14. **A-F, B-F, C-T, D-F, E-T**
Splenomegaly with infarction occurs in splenic venous thrombosis. Spleen can be involved in metastases, especially from breast, melanoma, lung, colon, kidney, prostate. True cysts are congenital and false cysts are post-traumatic.
Pyogenic abscess are drained percutaneously.
Sarcoidosis produces multiple nodules inside spleen, which will produce heterogeneous patchy pattern.

15. **A-T, B-T, C-T, D-T, E-F**
Lymphoepithelial cysts are seen in HIV.

16. **A-T, B-T, C-F, D-F, E-T**
Splenic trauma, septicemia, immunosuppression, gastric/colonic perforation/subphrenic abscess, pancreatic pseudocyst, IV drug user, chemotherapy, multiorgan failure, direct extension are other causes.

17. **A-T, B-T, C-T, D-T, E-T**

18. **A-F, B-T, C-T, D-F, E-T**
Also seen in brucellosis, PCP, dermoid epidermoid, TB, histoplasmosis, abscess, aneurysm, infarction, haematoma and hemochromatosis.

19. **A-T, B-T, C-T, D-T, E-F**
Splenic hilum is the most common location.

20. **A-T, B-F, C-F, D-T, E-F**

Underlying splenic pathology could be infarct or haematoma or trauma or leukemia.

Staphylococcus, Streptococcus and *E. coli* are more common than anaerobic organisms.

Rim enhancement is seen in spleen as it is seen in other organs. *Candida* is more common than aspergillosis.

21. **A-T, B-F, C-T, D-T, E-T**

Fungal infection in spleen can take many patterns. It can be bull's eye—an echogenic lesion surrounded by hypoechoic band due to inflammatory cells surrounded by fibrosis, or wheel within wheel—a central hypoechogenicity due to inflammatory nidus in center of inflammatory cells, or uniformly hypoechoic or hyper-echoic due to calcification or scarring. Fungal infections can be normal in imaging or cultures. Hence, tissue diagnosis is essential for confirmation and negative imaging does not exclude it.

22. **A-T, B-T, C-T, D-T, E-T**

Tuberculosis of spleen can take the form of an acute inflammatory lesion or miliary or macronodular form. Miliary pattern is the most common and seen as multiple hypoechoic or hypodense lesions. The spleen is enlarged and the ascites is dense. The lymph nodes have hypodense center and show rim enhancement during active disease. Both tuberculosis and MAI develop during HIV. While tuberculosis develops during early stages of HIV, MAI will develop only in later stages.

23. **A-T, B-F, C-T, D-T, E-T**

Splenomegaly is more common in MAI than tuberculosis. Hepatomegaly is also more common in MAI. Segmental ileocaecal thickening is seen in tuberculosis, while diffuse jejunal thickening is a feature of MAI. Small focal splenic lesions are seen in one-third of tuberculosis and only in 7% of MAI.

24. **A-T, B-T, C-F, D-F, E-T**

Cysts can show calcification in plain X-ray. There can be associated basal atelectasis, elevation of left dome of the diaphragm, flaring of ribs and medial displacement of the stomach shadow. The most common benign tumour in spleen is hemangioma. In sickle cell disease, splenomegaly devleops in the first year after the protective action of HbF disappears and splenic function progressively decreases.

25. **A-T, B-T, C-F, D-T, E-T**

Fluid collection in spleen extends from the tail of pancreas, posterolaterally in the anterior pararenal space, along splenic vessels into hilum and parenchyma of spleen. There are associated findings of pancreatitis.

26. **A-T, B-T, C-T, D-F, E-F**
Tuberculosis and metastasis are the most common causes. Gamma Gandy bodies are seen in cirrhosis with portal hypertension and they are larger.

27. **A-F, B-F, C-F, D-T, E-F**
End stage spleen or autosplenectomy is seen in homozygous sicklers. The spleen shows diffuse low signal in MRI due to hemosiderin or calcium. X-ray shows calcification and CT shows small densely calcified lesion. Functional asplenia is due to multiple infarcts. There is no uptake in sulfur colloid scan. Increased uptake is seen in bone scan. Spleen is normal or enlarged. Splenic sequestration is homozygous sicklers. There is sudden trapping of a large amount of blood in enlarged spleen, which results in hypovolemic shock. Imaging shows hypoehcoic or hypodense areas in the periphery of the spleen. MRI shows T1 hyperintensity with dark rim due to subacute haematoma. Splenic vein is patent in Doppler study. Veno-occlusion presents as infarction and autosplenectomy in homozygous cases and infarction with splenomegaly in heterozygous states. There is low uptake in sulfur colloid scan, and focal hypoechoic areas in ultrasound.

28. **A-T, B-F, C-F, D-F, E-T**
Splenic aneurysm—most common visceral aneurysm (60%). 3rd most common intra-abdominal aneurysm after aorta and iliac artery. Pancreatitis, multiple pregnancies predispose. Common in women, 50-60 years, mid and distal part—Incidence 0.02-1% rupture in 5-10%. Operation/Embolisation if more than 2 cm.

10 Liver

1. GIT techniques:
A. 5 MHz probe is used for intraoperative ultrasound
B. In CT arterioportography, the catheter is placed in the portal vein
C. In splenoportography, the contrast is injected into the distal splenic vein, using fluoroscopic guidance
D. Selective portal venous tributaries can be catheterized in portal hypertension
E. Hepatic veins are cannulated by direct puncture of liver

2. Liver:
A. The principal plane of the liver passes 4 cm to the right of midline
B. The principal plane of liver passes through the gallbladder fossa
C. Normal biliary ducts are not visualized in ultrasound
D. The portal veins and hepatic veins have bright walls
E. There is selective uptake of lipiodol in liver secondaries

3. Liver segments nomenclature:
A. I—quadrate lobe
B. IV—caudate lobe
C. VIII—posterosuperior
D. V—anteroinferior
E. II—lateralsuperior

4. Variation of normal hepatic arterial blood supply:
A. 10% have replaced right hepatic artery
B. 10% have accessory right hepatic artery
C. 2.5% have replaced common hepatic arteries
D. 13% have accessory left hepatic artery
E. 12% have replaced left hepatic artery

5. Liver:
  A. The caudate lobe lies within the greater sac
  B. The quadrate lobe lies within the lesser sac
  C. IVC is the most posterior structure in the porta hepatis
  D. The base of the bare area is formed by the inferior vena cava
  E. The liver is the second largest organ in the body after the brain

6. Portal vein:
  A. The portal vein lies posterior to an accessory hepatic artery rising from the SMA
  B. Superior mesenteric vein lies to the left of the mesenteric artery
  C. Gastrocolic trunk, which drains into the SMV is formed by right gastric vein and middle colic vein
  D. IMV is formed by joining of superior rectal, sigmoidal and left colic V
  E. Splenic vein is posteroinferior to the artery

7. Contents of porta hepatis:
  A. Portal vein
  B. Right hepatic artery
  C. Right hepatic duct
  D. Lymphatics
  E. Parasympathetic nerves

8. Hepatic blood supply:
  A. The hepatic artery and portal vein provide 30% and 70% of hepatic blood supply
  B. The hepatic artery lies above the portal vein and to the right of the common bile duct
  C. The caudate lobe receives blood supply only from the left branch of hepatic artery and portal vein
  D. The hepatic artery has two main branches, the right and left hepatic artery
  E. The caudate lobe drains into

9. Hepatic arteries:
  A. The first major branch of hepatic artery is right gastric artery
  B. The right hepatic artery crosses anterior to the common hepatic duct in majority
  C. The anterior segmental branch of RHA has a caterpillar configuration
  D. The RHA loops inferior in the cystohepatic angle
  E. Middle hepatic artery arises usually from the right hepatic artery or left hepatic artery

10. **Vasculature to liver:**
    A. Perfusion defects are seen in 10% of normal individuals
    B. Perfusion defects are common in the right lobe
    C. The perfusion defects are due to aberrant venous drainage by left gastric vein
    D. Riedel's lobe is seen in 5-10% of males
    E. The hepatic veins join IVC at D12

11. **The following organs are directly related to the liver and separated only by peritoneal covering:**
    A. Esophagus
    B. Stomach
    C. Duodenum
    D. Distal IVC
    E. Right kidney upper pole

12. **Hepatic vasculature:**
    A. Hepatic arteries are end arteries
    B. Contribution of the accessory hepatic arteries is not vital
    C. The liver has no lymphatics
    D. In biliary atresia, the bile drains through biliary lymphatics
    E. The liver capsule is supplied from the phrenic nerve branches

13. **Normal portosystemic anastomosis:**
    A. Between branches of right gastric vein and esophageal branches of azygous vein
    B. Paraumbilical vein and superficial epigastric vein
    C. Inferior and middle rectal vein with superior rectal vein
    D. Colic veins with peritoneal veins
    E. Superior mesenteric vein with left renal vein

14. **Dampened hepatic venous Doppler waveform is seen in:**
    A. Cirrhosis
    B. Budd-Chiari syndrome
    C. Hepatocellular carcinoma
    D. Hepatitis
    E. IVC obstruction

15. **Lobar hyperperfusion abnormality in liver is seen in:**
    A. Cirrhosis
    B. Hypervascular gallbladder disease
    C. Portal vein thrombosis
    D. Hepatic vein occlusion
    E. Hepatocellular carcinoma

16. **Causes of scar in a liver tumour:**
    A. Hemangioma
    B. Focal nodular hyperplasia
    C. Cholangiocarcinoma
    D. Hepatocellular carcinoma
    E. Angiosarcoma

17. **Indications of technetium sulphur colloid scan:**
    A. Acute rejection of renal transplant
    B. Lower GI bleeding
    C. Accessory spleen
    D. Gastric emptying
    E. Localising abscess

18. **Sulphur colloid scan:**
    A. The upper size of the particles is 10 microns
    B. Prepared by heating pertechnate and sodium trisulphate
    C. Most common cause of poor preparation is large particle size
    D. The preparation should not be used for more than 12 hours
    E. Imaging is performed 30 min after injection

19. **Hepatic arteries:**
    A. The middle hepatic artery supplies the quadrate and caudate lobes
    B. Normal hepatic arterial pattern is seen in only 50%
    C. 2% have common hepatic arterial origin from the aorta
    D. The left hepatic artery is the major source of blood for the quadrate lobe
    E. The left hepatic artery usually supplies the lateral segments of the left lobe of liver

20. **Sulphur colloid scan:**
    A. 55% localises in spleen
    B. Used to find the sites of erythropoiesis
    C. 10% localises to bone marrow
    D. Decreased splenic activity in hypersplenism
    E. Gelatin is added during preparation to prevent growth of particles

21. **Colloid shift is seen in:**
    A. Cirrhosis
    B. Congestive cardiac failure
    C. Steroids
    D. Hepatitis
    E. Hepatic tumours

22. **Causes of focal hot liver lesion in sulfur colloid scan:**
    A. In caudate lobe in IVC obstruction
    B. Quadrate lobe in SVC obstruction
    C. Caudate lobe in Budd-Chiari syndrome
    D. Hepatocellular carcinoma
    E. Focal nodular hyperplasia

23. **Defects in porta hepatis are seen in sulfur colloid scan:**
    A. Dilated bile ducts
    B. Postsurgical
    C. Focal nodular hyperplasia
    D. Adenomas
    E. Lymphoma

24. **Liver CT:**
    A. Arterial phase images are taken 5 sec after contrast
    B. Portal phase images are acquired 50 sec after contrast
    C. Delayed phase images are acquired after 5 minutes
    D. 120 ml of contrast is ideal for multidetector CT scanner
    E. Portal phase images alone are enough for identifying metastasis in a patient with colonic cancer
    F. Arterial phase is enough for diagnosing islet cell tumour metastasis

25. **Mottled uptake in liver is seen in:**
    A. Lymphomas
    B. Hepatitis
    C. Radiation
    D. Hepatocellular carcinoma
    E. Amyloidosis

26. **Focal defect in sulphur colloid scan is seen in:**
    A. Metastasis
    B. Focal nodular hyperplasia
    C. Pseudotumour
    D. Abscess
    E. Trauma

27. **Focal fatty infiltration:**
    A. Most common in the caudate lobe
    B. Geographical appearance in ultrasound
    C. Blood vessels are displaced inside the lesion but not invaded
    D. Opposed phase imaging MRI can be used to differentiate fatty infiltration and mass
    E. Low echogenic lesion in ultrasound

28. Hypodense mass in porta hepatis is seen in:
   A. Pseudocyst
   B. Enteric duplication cyst
   C. Choledochal cyst
   D. Hepatic artery aneurysm
   E. Portal venous thrombosis

29. Hepatic adenoma:
   A. Haemorrhage is the cause of clinical presentation
   B. Increased incidence in glycogen storage disease
   C. T1 signal is variable
   D. Capsule can be seen
   E. Enhances both in portal and arterial phase

30. Focal nodular hyperplasia (FNH):
   A. The scar enhances in delayed images
   B. Scar is hypointense in T1 and T2
   C. Isointense in equilibrium phase
   D. Generally, smaller than adenomas
   E. Haemorrhage is not as common as in adenoma

31. Hemangioma:
   A. Centripetal filling is due to slow flow in the sinusoids
   B. Peripheral enhancement is due to capsular enhancement
   C. Hyperechogenicity is due to blood within the dilated vascular channels
   D. Acoustic shadowing is due to high density of blood in the hemangioma
   E. Light bulb sign indicates slow flow in the vascular spaces

32. Liver hemangiomas:
   A. The most common liver tumour
   B. More common in males than females
   C. Made up of blood-filled cavernous spaces without any lining
   D. Fibrous septa are seen within the lesion
   E. Fibrinogen levels are low in the serum

33. Grading of injuries:
   A. Devascularisation of one lobe of liver is the most severe injury, grade IV
   B. Lacerations or haematomas less than 3 cm are classified as grade I and managed conservatively
   C. Periportal haemorrhages are considered insignificant in grading liver injuries
   D. Any splenic haematoma less than 5 cm is not graded
   E. Subcapsular haematoma > 3 cm is graded as type III splenic injury
   F. Intraperitoneal haemorrhage in the entire abdomen is graded as type II

34. **Hemangiomas—imaging features:**
    A. A central scar is seen in large tumours
    B. Posterior acoustic enhancement is seen in all hemangiomas more than 2.5 cm
    C. Enlarge during pregnancy
    D. Steroids decrease the size of hemangioma
    E. A giant hemangioma, by definition is more than 5 cm

35. **Liver hemangiomas:**
    A. Early filling is seen in angiography with cotton wool puddling of contrast
    B. Early uptake and early clearance is seen in RBC scans
    C. Hemangioma is never hyperdense in a plain CT scan
    D. The initial peripheral enhancement is always complete and encircling the tumour
    E. T2 value of 80 msec is highly indicative of hemangioma

36. **Imaging protocol for hemangiomas:**
    A. A typical lesion in ultrasound requires no further imaging other than follow-up ultrasound
    B. MRI is the ideal technique for atypical lesions more than 2 cm
    C. RBC scintigraphy is the ideal technique for lesions less than 2 cm
    D. If a typical lesion is diagnosed in CT or MRI, no further imaging is required
    E. Dynamic gadolinium-enhanced MRI is the most sensitive method for differentiating hemangioma and hypervascular liver metastasis

37. **Common causes of very high signal in heavily T2 weighted MRI:**
    A. Pancreatic cancer metastasis
    B. Colonic cancer metastasis
    C. Hemangioma
    D. Islet cell tumour
    E. Mesenchymal hamartoma

38. **HCC:**
    A. Enhancement is typically seen in the arterial phase
    B. The capsule enhances in contrast administration
    C. Opacification of portal vein during arterial phase
    D. Wedge-shaped lesions in liver in arterial phase
    E. Five year survival is 30%

39. **Fat containing tumours in liver:**
    A. Angiomyolipoma   B. HCC
    C. Metastasis   D. FNH
    E. Intrahepatic cholangiocarcinoma

40. MRI:
  A. Halo indicates benign lesion
  B. Halo is caused only due to capsule
  C. Rim enhancement is specific for abscess
  D. The scar of sclerosing HCC enhances
  E. Scar of cholangiocarcinoma enhances more than normal liver

41. Liver tumours:
  A. Metastasis does not show vascular encasement
  B. Intrahepatic cholangiocarcinomas invade blood vessels in liver
  C. Nodule within nodule is characteristic of metastasis
  D. Delayed MR images in HCC show a rim of hypoperfused liver tissue
  E. Necrotic metastasis can show rim enhancement
  F. Small hemangiomas can show uniform high signal in T2, like metastasis

42. Liver tumours:
  A. HCC shows uptake of manganese DPDP
  B. Adenomatous hyperplasia is hypo in T1 and hyper in T2
  C. Regenerative nodules are low signal in both
  D. Adenomatous hyperplasia, regenerative nodules and HCC could not be differentiated based on enhancement characteristics
  E. Confluent fibrosis is hypo in T1 and T2 and does not enhance

43. Predisposing factors for hepatoma:
  A. Galactosemia   B. Alpha one antitrypsin deficiency
  C. Hemosiderosis   D. Cardiac cirrhosis
  E. Anabolic steroids
  F. Cystic fibrosis

44. Liver hemangiomas:
  A. Most common location is centrally in the liver close to the porta hepatitis
  B. Calcification is seen in 45-50% of tumours
  C. Doppler shows a high flow in the periphery of the tumour and extensive central flow
  D. Core biopsy is done with a 20 G cutting needle
  E. Angiography shows large hepatic artery

45. Hepatoma:
  A. 40% incidence in micronodular cirrhosis
  B. 6% incidence in macronodular cirrhosis
  C. 25% present with multiple nodules in liver
  D. 10% are diffusely infiltrative
  E. The main vascular supply is from the portal vein

46. **Hepatocellular carcinoma:**
    A. Most common visceral malignancy
    B. Higher incidence in South East Asia
    C. Occurs earlier than the fibrolamellar type of HCC
    D. Up to 20% incidence
    E. Most common malignant liver tumour in children

47. **Clinical presentations of HCC:**
    A. Hypoglycemia   B. Hypocalcemia
    C. Carcinoid syndrome D. Hypercholesterolemia
    E. Anemia

48. **Causes of portal venous occlusion:**
    A. Pancreatitis
    B. HCC
    C. Metastasis
    D. Crohn's disease
    E. Cirrhosis

49. **Post TIPS (Transjugular intrahepatic portosystemic shunt):**
    A. Stent velocity same at the portal and hepatic ends
    B. Peak velocity more than 150 cm/sec
    C. Portal venous velocity more than 30 cm/sec
    D. Hepatofugal flow
    E. Splenic vein flow

50. **Hepatic calcification is seen in:**
    A. Portal vein thrombosis
    B. Hydatid
    C. Brucellosis
    D. Chronic granulomatous disease
    E. Abscess

51. **HCC:**
    A. Alpha fetoprotein is a screening tool on its own
    B. Spontaneous rupture is seen in 8%
    C. Fat is a significant component of the tumour
    D. Budd-Chiari syndrome is clinical presentation
    E. Calcification is common than in fibrolamellar carcinoma

52. **Features of HCC:**
    A. Portal vein thrombosis is more common than in secondary tumours
    B. Bile duct invasion
    C. Arterioportal shunts
    D. Hepaticojejunal fistula
    E. Invasion of aorta

53. **HCC:**
    A. Lipiodol-enhanced CT shows selective uptake in HCC
    B. HCCs are bright in delayed scans
    C. Mosaic pattern is seen in 65%
    D. Hyperdense lesion excludes HCC
    E. A well-defined lucent halo around the tumour excludes HCC

54. **Ultrasound for HCC:**
    A. Small tumours are homogeneous
    B. Doppler velocity is high as 250 cm/sec
    C. Can be difficult to differentiate from hemangioma
    D. Majority are of mixed echogenicity
    E. Invasion of gallbladder is more common than invasion of liver by gallbladder tumors

55. **Fibrolamellar carcinoma:**
    A. Encapsulated
    B. Central scar is seen in 75-80%
    C. The scar is hypointense in T1 and hyperintense in T2
    D. Arterioportal shunting
    E. Scar calcification is not common

56. **Portal vein thrombosis is associated with:**
    A. Pancreatitis
    B. Hepatocellular carcinoma
    C. Actinomycosis
    D. Umbilical artery catheterization
    E. Schistosomiasis

57. **Portal vein thrombosis is seen in:**
    A. Ascending cholangitis   B. Diverticulitis
    C. Appendicitis   D. Gastric carcinoma
    E. Cholangiocarcinoma   F. Colonic tumours

58. **Portal venous gas is seen in:**
    A. Barium enema
    B. Acute gastric dilatation
    C. Erythroblastosis foetalis
    D. Hepatic embolisation
    E. Toxic megacolon

59. **Histiocytosis of liver:**
    A. Four phases are recognised
    B. Hypoechoic periportal lesions
    C. High signal in T1 in late stages
    D. Chemotherapy improves the disease
    E. Sclerosing cholangitis is end result

60. Primary biliary cirrhosis:
A. Associated with scleroderma
B. Antimicrosomal antibodies are seen in 65% of patients
C. Has specific features on ultrasound
D. Increased incidence of bile duct carcinoma is seen
E. Increased incidence of HCC

61. Infantile hemangioendothelioma:
A. The aorta is large due to increased flow into it
B. Cardiac failure is a presenting feature
C. Multiple lesions indicate Osler-Rendu-Weber syndrome
D. 90% occur in the first six months after birth
E. Majority are solitary

62. Infantile hemangioendothelioma:
A. Enhancement is slow with centrifugal filling in
B. Acoustic shadowing is seen in ultrasound
C. Early uptake and quick clearing are the RBC scintigraphy features of this tumour
D. Large hepatic veins are seen in Doppler
E. Spontaneous involution with time

63. HCC:
A. Threads and streaks is a characteristic angiographic pattern of portal vein invasion
B. MR is hyperintense in T1
C. Capsule is hypointense in both T1 and T2
D. Two layers of capsule can be seen in T1W images
E. Peripheral enhancement mimicking hemangioma is seen

64. Mesenchymal hamartoma:
A. This is an acquired lesion which is always hypo or avascular due to cystic nature
B. Most common age is between 1-3 years
C. High-grade malignant lesion with bad prognosis
D. All the lesions are cystic and presence of solid component should alert to the possibility of malignancy
E. Calcification is seen in 50% of cases due to the hamartomatous nature of the lesion

65. Hepatoblastoma is associated with:
A. Autosomal dominant polycystic kidney disease
B. Beckwith-Wiedemann syndrome
C. Biliary atresia
D. Caroli's disease
E. Gardner's syndrome

66. Hepatoblastoma:
A. Angiography shows spoke wheel pattern of enhancement
B. Peak age is 18-24 months
C. Presence of embryonal hepatocytes indicates bad prognosis
D. Dense coarse calcification is seen due to osteoid formation
E. There is no excretion in the hepatobiliary scan, but uptake is seen in gallium scans

67. The following conditions are associated with development of angiosarcoma of liver:
A. Hemochromatosis
B. Frequent blood transfusions
C. Steroids
D. Vinylchloride
E. Thorotrast

68. Angiosarcoma of liver:
A. Thorotrast infiltration causes diffusely hypoechoic liver
B. Thorotrast is seen in spleen, liver, lymph nodes and peritoneum
C. Thorotrast is not visible in X-rays
D. Rim enhancement is seen in gadolinium enhanced scans
E. The thorotrast is absent in lesions when angiosarcoma arises

69. Hepatoma in children is associated with:
A. HbsAG
B. Tyrosinemia
C. Alpha 1 antitrypsin deficiency
D. Glycogen storage disease
E. Cystic fibrosis

70. Hepatoma in children:
A. Most common paediatric malignancy
B. Common in 12-14 years
C. Fibrolamellar carcinoma does not happen before 20 years
D. Fanconi's anemia is a cause of adenoma in children
E. Neuroblastoma is the most common metastases to children

71. Liver tumours:
A. Biliary cystadenoma has malignant potential
B. Ovarian stroma is seen in bilary cystadenocarcinoma and have good prognosis
C. Presence of lymph nodes occurs in both cystadenoma and cystadenocarcinoma
D. Irregular solid elements are seen in cystadenocarcinoma
E. The treatment is different for cystadenoma and carcinoma

72. **Hepatoma:**
    A. More common in alcoholic cirrhosis than postnecrotic cirrhosis
    B. High incidence in micronodular cirrhosis of hemochromatosis
    C. Chronic hepatitis B is an independent risk factor for hepatoma without cirrhosis
    D. HCC occurring in alcohol-related cirrhosis is macronodular
    E. Thorotrast is a risk factor for hepatoma

73. **Hepatoma:**
    A. Sulfur colloid scan shows colloid shift to spleen and bone marrow
    B. All the tumours are seen as defects in hepatobiliary scans
    C. Tumours less than 3 cm are homogeneously hypoechoic
    D. High signal in ultrasound indicates fatty change for sinusoidal dilatation
    E. Mosaic pattern indicates a nodule within a nodule type of lesion

74. **Hepatoma:**
    A. Basket pattern in Doppler indicates tumour shunting
    B. Hyperintensity in T1 is either due to fat or haemorrhage
    C. Any mass in cirrhotic liver not fulfiling criteria for cyst or hemangioma is likely to be hepatoma
    D. Inoperable small HCCs are managed by percutaneous ethanol injection
    E. Large inoperable tumours are commonly managed by percutaneous ethanol injection

75. **Most common causes of liver metastasis with silent primary are:**
    A. Colon   B. Stomach
    C. Lung   D. Pancreas
    E. Kidney

76. **Liver tumours:**
    A. Alpha fetoprotein is elevated only in 50% of those with HCC
    B. Small hemangiomas show intense arterial enhancement in 25%
    C. Centripetal fllling has 88% sensitivity for diagnosis of hemangioma
    D. In liver, lipiodol is taken only by HCCs .
    E. Hepatic adenoma is a premalignant condition

77. **Liver tumours:**
    A. Lymphomas in liver start from the portal region
    B. Diffusely altered echotexture is a feature of liver lymphoma
    C. Hodgkin's disease commonly presents as a miliary pattern
    D. Spleen is always involved in Hodgkin's disease
    E. Angiography is very vascular

78. **Uncommon liver tumours:**
    A. Undifferentiated embryonal sarcoma is considered as malignant counterpart of mesenchymal hamartoma
    B. Undifferentiated embryonal sarcoma is seen between 6 and 10 years
    C. Mesenchymal sarcoma is predominantly cystic
    D. Epitheloid hemangioendotheliomas are commonly seen in those above 50 years
    E. Capsular retraction is the characteristic feature of epitheloid hemangioendothelioma

79. **Raised alpha fetoprotein is seen in:**
    A. Hepatoblastoma
    B. Anencephaly
    C. Meningomyeocele
    D. Testicular teratoma
    E. Diastomatomyelia

80. **High density liver is seen in:**
    A. Hemochromatosis
    B. Amiodarone
    C. Multiple blood transfusions
    D. Thyrotoxicosis
    E. Steroids

81. **Features of portal hypertension:**
    A. Intrasplenic pressure 20 mmHg
    B. Widened posterior mediastinal shadow
    C. Hepatofungal flow in the short gastric veins
    D. Elevated platelet count
    E. Internal rectal haemorrhoids

82. **Diffuse decrease in liver echogenicity is seen in:**
    A. Acute hepatitis
    B. Fatty infiltration
    C. Lipid storage disease
    D. Primary biliary cirrhosis
    E. Diffuse metastasis

83. **Haemochromatosis:**
    A. Does not occur in women
    B. Associated with chondrocalcinosis
    C. Associated with cardiomyopathy
    D. Increased incidence of HCC
    E. Increased incidence of hemangiomas

84. **Contraindications for liver biopsy:**
    A. Ascites
    B. INR more than 1.2
    C. Platelet count < 150000
    D. Fever
    E. Focal lesion

85. **Differential diagnosis of solitary echogenic liver mass:**
    A. Metastasis
    B. Adenoma
    C. Hemangioma
    D. Lipoma
    E. Hematoma

86. **Haemorrhagic liver metastasis:**
    A. Renal carinoma
    B. Islet cell tumour
    C. Pheochromocytoma
    D. Melanoma
    E. Lung

87. **Bull's eye lesions of liver are seen in:**
    A. Tuberculosis
    B. Sarcoidosis
    C. Candidiasis
    D. Lymphoma
    E. Kaposi's sarcoma

88. **Cystic neoplasms in liver:**
    A. Mesenchymal hamartoma
    B. Metastasis
    C. Undifferentiated embryonal sarcoma
    D. Adenomas
    E. Biliary cystadenoma

89. **Fat containing liver masses:**
    A. Lipoma
    B. Hepatoma
    C. Metastases
    D. Fibrolamellar carcinoma
    E. Mesenchymal hamartoma

90. **Ultrasound liver:**
    A. Hemangiomas are echogenic and show posterior acoustic shadowing
    B. Metastases are usually echogenic
    C. Fatty infiltration is seen as diffuse low-level echogenicity
    D. Acute hepatitis will be seen as diffuse low-level echoes
    E. Ovarian carcinoma metastasis may be mimicked by simple cysts

91. **FNH:**
    A. Have a well-defined peripheral capsule
    B. Decreased uptake in sulfur colloid scan is seen in 40% of cases
    C. RBC scan shows early uptake and late deficit
    D. There is an association with oral contraceptive use and FNH
    E. Increased uptake is seen in gallium scan

92. **FNH:**
    A. A comet tail appearance is seen due to mixed arterial and venous signals in ultrasound
    B. Normal uptake is seen with SPIO (superparamagnetic iron oxide)
    C. Angiography shows a typical spoke wheel pattern of enhancement in 70% of cases
    D. The scar is hyperdense in delayed CT images
    E. The lesion is hyperdense in the portal phase of contrast enhancement in CT

93. **Nodular regenerative hyperplasia of liver is associated with:**
    A. Chronic lymphoid leukemia
    B. Polyarteritis nodosa
    C. Polycythemia rubra vera
    D. Budd-Chiari syndrome
    E. Lymphoma

94. **Cysts of liver:**
    A. 70% of those with multiple liver cysts have polycystic kidney disease
    B. 10% of those with ADPKD have liver cysts
    C. The commonly seen simple liver cyst is lined by hepatocytes
    D. Congenital cysts are commonly seen in the 5th-7th decade
    E. Meyenburg's complexes are formed due to cystic dilatation of aberrant bile ducts

95. **Hepatocellular adenomas:**
    A. Increased incidence in glycogen storage disease
    B. Portal tracts and hepatic veins are seen within this tumour
    C. 80% of these lesions show defect in sulfur colloid scans
    D. Centripetal enhancement is seen in contrast enhanced CT scans
    E. The lesion is characteristically hypoechoic in ultrasound

96. **Hypervascular hepatic lesions:**
    A. Hepatoma
    B. Adenoma
    C. Colonic metastasis
    D. Carinoid metastasis
    E. Focal nodular hyperplasia

97. **Liver metastases:**
    A. Liver is the third most common site of metastatic disease after lymph nodes and lungs
    B. 30-70% of cancer patients have liver metastasis
    C. 30% of colorectal cancer patients may have isolated liver metastasis
    D. Cystic metastasis are commonly seen from ovary
    E. Differentiation of cystic metastasis and benign cyst is achieved by using multiphase liver scans

98. **The following are tumours with high risk of developing liver metastasis:**
    A. Breast
    B. Oesophagus
    C. Large bowel
    D. Prostate
    E. Squamous cell carcinoma of head and neck

99. **Calcified liver metastases are seen in:**
    A. Mucinous adenocarcinoma of ovary
    B. Breast
    C. Malignant mesothelioma
    D. Islet cell tumours of pancreas
    E. Osteosarcoma

100. **Cystic liver metastasis is seen in:**
    A. Pancreatic tumours
    B. Carcinoid
    C. Sarcoma
    D. Colon
    E. Melanoma

101. **Liver metastasis which are hypoechoic in ultrasound:**
    A. Pancreas
    B. Lung
    C. Lymphoma
    D. Nasopharyngeal cancer
    E. Cervical

102. **Echogenic metastasis in ultrasound:**
    A. Hepatoma
    B. Pancreas
    C. Breast
    D. Colon
    E. Lung

103. **CT for liver metastasis:**
    A. Most of the hypovascular metastasis are hypodense in the portal phase images
    B. Rim enhancement is seen in arterial phase of hypovascular metastasis
    C. Hypervascular metastasis are best detected in the portal venous phase
    D. Hypervascular metastasis are isodense during portal phase
    E. Hypovascular metastasis are isodense during arterial phase

104. **Metastasis:**
    A. Metastasis reaching liver via portal veins are usually uniform in appearance
    B. Metastasis have capsule
    C. All metastasis have low signal in T1 and high signal in T2
    D. Enhance less than normal liver in contrast MRI
    E. Metastasis from pheochromocytoma shows intense enhancement in arterial phase

105. **Common causes of diffuse liver metastasis:**
    A. Breast
    B. Kaposi's sarcoma
    C. Melanoma
    D. Lung
    E. Pancreas

106. **The following make liver metastasis unresectable:**
    A. > 2
    B. Extrahepatic disease
    C. Capsular invasion
    D. < 50% normal liver function left after resection
    E. Ascites

107. **CT techniques for liver metastasis:**
    A. CT arterioportography is done with the catheter in the superior mesenteric artery
    B. CT arteriography—catheter is placed in the celiac artery
    C. Delayed iodine scanning is done 24 hours after administration of iodine
    D. CT has a sensitivity of 90%
    E. Delayed filling is seen in 10% of cases like hemangioma

108. **Following are patterns of enhancement in metastasis:**
    A. No enhancement
    B. Peripheral
    C. Mixed enhancement
    D. Peripheral nodular enhancement
    E. Peripheral washout

109. MRI patterns in metastasis:
A. In halo pattern, there is a hypointense rim
B. In doughnut lesion, there is central hyperintensity
C. Target lesions have central hyperintensity surrounded by rind of hypointensity
D. Light bulb pattern is seen in pheochromocytoma metastasis
E. Changing morphology with different sequences

110. Liver metastasis:
A. CT has a sensitivity of 95% for detecting liver metastasis less than 1 cm
B. Lesions less than 1.5 cm are likely to be metastatic in a patient with known tumour
C. Focal fatty change mimicks metastasis
D. Focal steatosis, produced by chemotherapy can be differentiated from metastasis by MRI
E. CT has 94% sensitivity for detecting liver metastasis larger than 1 cm

111. Contrast ultrasound-SH U 508.A:
A. The bubbles have a lipid shell
B. Decreases strength of Doppler signals
C. In pulse inversion imaging, three pulses are sent
D. Normal tissues produce preferential signal that is detected
E. The bubbles are usually broken by the first pulse

112. Contrast ultrasound:
A. In the vascular phase, the bubbles accumulate in the hepatic sinusoids
B. Interval delay flash images are obtained by breaking the bubbles with high mechanical index after four minutes
C. Scanning should be stopped for some time to obtain vascular phase images
D. Postvascular imaging is obtained after four minutes
E. Amount of enhancement in the vascular phase depends on the arterial volume

113. Contrast ultrasound:
A. FNH shows enhancement in all the phases
B. HCC shows enhancement in all the phases
C. Hemangioma shows peripheral nodular enhancement in the vascular phase
D. Metastasis shows no enhancement in all phases
E. Metastasis can show diffuse enhancement in the interval delay flash

114. **MRI contrast for liver:**
    A. SPIO produces T2 shortening
    B. The lesions are seen bright when SPIO is administered
    C. Gadolinium produces T1 and T2 shortening
    D. Gadolinium is taken specifically by reticuloendothelial cells
    E. T1W images are ideal for post-SPIO administration

115. **Gadolinium enhancement—lesions showing early arterial enhancement:**
    A. Colorectal metastasis
    B. Carcinoid metastasis
    C. FNH
    D. Adenoma
    E. HCC

116. **Lesions which appear dark in T2W images after SPIO administration:**
    A. Metastasis
    B. Focal nodular hyperplasia
    C. Adenoma
    D. Hemangiomas
    E. Well-differentiated HCC

117. **Contrast liver:**
    A. Gadolinium BOPTA and EOB DTPA are selectively taken by hepatocytes
    B. Selective uptake is due to BOPTA and EOB DTPA
    C. EOB DTPA shows 50% uptake of dose by hepatocytes
    D. Enhancement persists up to two hours
    E. Metastasis will remain dark and hepatocellular tumours enhance

118. **Liver contrast:**
    A. Ultra small paramagnetic iron oxide particles show shortening of T1 and T2
    B. More uptake of contrast in lymph node and bone marrow
    C. T2 shortening seen after delayed images
    D. Are blood pool agents
    E. Enhancement seen in T1W images, unlike SPIO

119. **Portal venous occlusion:**
    A. Cavernomatous malformation of portal vein is a sequelae
    B. Associated with bowel wall edema
    C. Portal vein is not visible in chronic thrombosis
    D. Causes ascites
    E. Acute appendicitis is a cause

120. **Liver transplant:**
    A. Dilatation of common bile duct is more sensitive than dilatation of intrahepatic biliary radicles for obstructed system
    B. Epithelial cast within biliary tree means the liver has to be retransplanted
    C. Strictures are uncommon in the first two weeks
    D. Stricture is seen in ductal anastomosis site in 15%
    E. Prolonged cold ischemic time is a common cause of stricture

121. **Causes of nonanastomostic stricture postliver transplant:**
    A. Hepatic arterial thrombosis
    B. ABO incompatible donors
    C. Chronic rejection
    D. HCC
    E. Infection

122. **Postliver transplant:**
    A. Anastomostic strictures have worse prognosis than non-anastomostic strictures
    B. Air in biliary tree indicates patent hepaticojejunostomy
    C. Majority of bile leak happens in the third postoperative month
    D. Bilomas need not be aspirated
    E. Most common cause of bile leak is hepatic arterial thrombosis

123. **Postliver transplant:**
    A. Large volume ascites indicates hepatic venous obstruction
    B. Hematomas are common in the subphrenic space
    C. Hematomas should be aspirated immediately to preserve the graft
    D. Septations inside subphrenic fluid is pathognomonic of abscess
    E. Abscess in portal hilar region usually results in pseudoaneurysm formation

124. **Hydatid cysts:**
    A. The most common type of hydatid cyst is the Type I cyst
    B. Type I cyst can be mistaken for simple cyst
    C. Type IV cyst is mistaken for hepatic solid tumour
    D. Type I cyst is hydatid unless proved otherwise, in endemic areas
    E. Type III is the most common of all hepatic hydatid cysts

125. **Manganese DPDP:**
    A. Selectively taken by hepatocytes
    B. T2W images are ideal
    C. Produces low signal in T1W images
    D. Both manganese and DPDP are essential for producing the signal
    E. Lesions are seen as dark against the bright liver

126. Lesions showing uptake with manganese DPDP:
- A. Metastasis
- B. FNH
- C. Carcinoid
- D. Well-differentiated HCC
- E. Adenoma

127. Hydatid cyst of liver:
- A. Type I cyst happens in the older population than other types of cysts
- B. Hydatid sand is seen only in complicated cysts
- C. Pericystic biliary dilation always indicates biliary rupture
- D. Rupture into biliary tree occurs in 10%
- E. Split sign—indicates detachment of endo- and ectocyst

128. Schistosomiasis:
- A. Schistosoma hematobium is the most common organism affecting liver
- B. Thick hyperechoic bands extend from the porta to the periphery of liver
- C. The bands enhance on contrast administration
- D. Increased incidence in HIV infection due to immunosuppresion
- E. A turtle back appearance is seen in CT scan

129. Hepatic artery aneurysm:
- A. Constitutes 20% of visceral aneurysms
- B. Four times increased incidence in the intrahepatic portion of hepatic artery
- C. 66% arise in the right hepatic artery
- D. Frequent in women
- E. Mycotic aneurysms are the most common

130. Hepatic aneurysm:
- A. Jaundice is a component of the classical triad
- B. Rupture has been recognized only into the abdominal cavity
- C. Common hepatic artery should not be embolised because of liver infarction
- D. Embolisation of postgastroduodenal artery segment is avoided
- E. The aneurysm can be embolised if it is in the postgastro-duodenal artery segment

131. Liver intervention:
- A. Resection is the only curative procedure available for hepatic cancers
- B. Resection of colorectal metastasis, will give a survival of 80% at one year
- C. There is no absolute limit on the size of lesion that could be treated with percutaneous ethanol injection

    D. In a single session of percutaneous ethanol injection, not more than 3 lesions are treated   ·

    E. 3 cm is the maximum size for percutaneous ethanol injection

132. **Treatment options for local liver tumour ablation are:**
    A. Microwave coagulation therapy
    B. High intensity focused ultrasound
    C. Cryotherapy
    D. Electrocautery
    E. Hot saline injection

133. **Radiofrequency ablation for liver tumours:**
    A. Immediate coagulation necrosis occurs above 40°C
    B. Preferential cytotoxicity on tumour cells is seen between 41°-45°C
    C. It takes 60 min for cytotoxic effect on tumor cells at 45°C
    D. It takes 240 min for cytotoxic effect on tumour cells at 41°C
    E. The time for cytotoxic effect decreases by half for each degree drop in temperature

134. **Radiofrequency ablation for liver tumours:**
    A. The aim in radiofrequency ablation is to kill the target tumour only
    B. The maximum lesion diameter that can be killed by a single probe is 1.6 cm
    C. Multiple probe electrodes increase the tumour volume that can be destroyed
    D. Saline enhancement increases the tumour volume that can be killed
    E. Cooling the electrodes by saline decreases charring by heat

135. **Common cytotoxic agents used for hepatic chemoembolisation are:**
    A. Cyclophosphamide
    B. Cisplatin
    C. Adriamycin
    D. Mitomycin
    E. Fluorodeoxyuridine

136. **Hepatic arterial embolisation:**
    A. Cannot be done if portal vein is not patent
    B. All cases need prophylactic phytonadione
    C. Child's Type C is a contraindication
    D. Metastasis is not a contraindication
    E. Small lesion is managed first followed by larger ones

137. **Hepatic chemoembolisation:**
  A. Lignocaine injected intra-arterially
  B. Gelfoam is the embolic agent
  C. Lipiodol is an essential component
  D. Follow-up CT scans should begin at 3 months
  E. Antibiotics are not necessary since the tumour undergoes necrosis
  F. If lipiodol uptake is seen in more than 50% of tumour in two weeks, no further treatment

138. **Features of cirrhosis:**
  A. The density of mesenteric fat is lesser than retroperitonal fat
  B. Arterioportal fistulas indicate development of HCC
  C. Regenerating nodules have a predominant portal venous supply
  D. Adenomatous hyperplasia are mainly supplied by hepatic arteries
  E. CT cannot differentiate regenerating nodules and adenomatous hyperplasia

139. **Imaging of cirrhosis:**
  A. The spleen is more darker than normal in SPIO images
  B. A flying bat appearance in sulfur colloid scan indicates severe cirrhosis
  C. Corkscrew appearance of liver in angiography
  D. In wedged hepatic venography the fifth order branches are well visualised
  E. Regenerating nodules produce indentation on the hepatic veins in wedged venography

140. **Plain film findings of cirrhosis:**
  A. Obliteration of the descending aorta shadow
  B. Prominent main pulmonary artery
  C. Posterior displacement of stomach
  D. Chiladitis syndrome
  E. Medial displacement of the right kidney

141. **Plain film findings of cirrhosis:**
  A. Anterior displacement of duodenum indicates lymphadeno-pathy
  B. Soft tissue in anterior or inferior surface of liver indicates hepatoma
  C. Mass adjacent to the descending aorta indicates esophageal tumour
  D. Bilateral enlarged kidneys indicate acute renal failure
  E. Inferomedial displacement of gallbladder indicates shrunken liver

142. **Differential diagnosis for deformed liver:**
    A. Idiopathic portal hypertension
    B. Accessory fissures
    C. Budd-Chiari syndrome
    D. Portal venous obstruction
    E. Sarcoidosis

143. **Ultrasound contrast:**
    A. Demonstrates bleeding points
    B. Particle size of 100 microns does not enter pulmonary circulation
    C. Excreted by kidneys
    D. Produces acoustic shadowing
    E. Resonate with ultrasound beam

144. **Hepatic Doppler:**
    A. If there is no flow in the portal thrombosis, it rules out tumours thrombosis
    B. Flow rate in the portal vein is proportional to the pressure in the portal vein
    C. Portal venous pressure varies with the cardiac cycle
    D. Right portal vein is best imaged from the epicardial regions
    E. Flow in portal vein is typically hepatopetal

145. **Causes of Budd-Chiari syndrome:**
    A. Cirrhosis
    B. Pregnancy
    C. Oral contraceptive pills
    D. Waldenström's macroglobulinemia
    E. Paroxysmal nocturnal hemoglobinuria

146. **Causes of Budd-Chiari syndrome:**
    A. Constrictive pericarditis   B. Adrenal carcinoma
    C. Right atrial tumour   D. Tuberculosis
    E. Radiation

147. **Budd-Chiari:**
    A. In type I, both the IVC and hepatic veins are involved
    B. The caudate lobe is not enlarged
    C. Hepatosplenomegaly
    D. Enlarged middle hepatic vein
    E. Communication between the middle and right hepatic vein

148. **Budd-Chiari syndrome:**
    A. The enhancement pattern is patchy and similar in the early and delayed phases
    B. Flip flop phenomenon is specific for Budd-Chiari syndrome
    C. Hepatic veins are not visualised in CT scans
    D. Paraumbilical vein visualised
    E. Gallbladder wall is thickened

149. **Acute Budd-Chiari syndrome:**
   A. No ascites
   B. Caudate lobe is not hypertrophied
   C. Liver function grossly deranged
   D. Early enhancement of the perpipheral portions of the right lobe of the liver
   E. Delayed enhancement of the caudate lobe, since it is supplied by blood vessels bilaterally

150. **Causes of presinusoidal portal hypertension:**
   A. Veno-occlusive disease
   B. Schistosomiasis
   C. Sarcoidosis
   D. Idiopathic portal hypertension
   E. Vinyl chloride

151. **Causes of cirrhosis:**
   A. Polycystic kidney disease
   B. Type IV glycogen storage disease
   C. Fructose intolerance
   D. Osler-Rendu-Weber disease
   E. Abetalipoproteinemia

152. **Causes of cirrhosis:**
   A. Cardiac failure
   B. Cystic fibrosis
   C. Amyloidosis
   D. Niemann-Pick disease
   E. Intestinal bypass

153. **Drugs causing cirrhosis:**
   A. Methotrexate   B. INH
   C. Paracetamol   D. Alpha methyldopa
   E. Rifampicin

154. **Causes of cirrhosis in children:**
   A. Biliary atresia
   B. Hemochromatosis
   C. Schistosomiasis
   D. Wilson's disease
   E. Abetalipoproteinemia

155. **Causes of micronodular cirrhosis:**
   A. Viral hepatitis   B. Wilson's disease
   C. Alcoholism   D. Hemochromatosis
   E. Biliary obstruction

156. Cirrhosis and nodules:
   A. By definition micronodular cirrhosis is less than 10 mm
   B. In dysplastic nodules, the hepatocyte clusters are more than 1 mm in size
   C. Regenerative nodules are characterised by adenomatous hyperplasia
   D. Cirrhotic nodule is surrounded by fibrous septa
   E. Hepatocellular carcinoma causes nodular changes

157. Associations of cirrhosis:
   A. Gallstone
   B. Pancreatitis
   C. Hypogonadism
   D. Anemia
   E. Peptic ulcer

158. Dysplastic nodules are seen in:
   A. Hepatitis B
   B. Alcoholism
   C. Tyrosinemia
   D. Wilson's disease
   E. Alpha 1 antitrypsin deficiency

159. Budd-Chiari syndrome:
   A. Multiple flow voids will be seen in MRI
   B. Doppler shows high velocity flow in IVC
   C. Reversal of flow in hepatic veins
   D. Hepatofugal flow in portal veins
   E. Low resistive index in hepatic artery

160. Features of cirrhosis:
   A. Atrophied lateral segment of left lobe
   B. Compensatory hypertrophy of right lobe
   C. Caudate lobe/right lobe ratio > 0.65
   D. Quadrate lobe > 30 mm
   E. Enlarged liver in early stages
   F. GB angle is less than 35 degrees

161. Ultrasound features of cirrhosis:
   A. Increased sound transmission
   B. Decreased definition of portal venous walls
   C. Regenerative nodules are hyperechoic
   D. Dilated hepatic arteries
   E. Hepatic venous flow resembles portal vein

162. **CT scan findings of cirrhosis:**
   A. High density in early cirrhosis
   B. Regenerative nodules are hypodense
   C. Hepatic arterial supply to the dysplastic nodules
   D. Hypodense areas adjacent to portal vein
   E. Peribiliary cysts
   F. The right lobe to left lobe length ratio is more than 1:44

163. **Complications of cirrhosis:**
   A. Hepatocellular carcinoma
   B. Spontaneous bacterial peritonitis
   C. Cholangiocarcinoma
   D. Splenic cysts
   E. Peliosis hepatitis

164. **Angiography of cirrhosis:**
   A. Hepato portal shunt
   B. Increased visualisation of peripheral hepatic venous branches
   C. Delayed empyting into veins
   D. Hepatic arteries compressed by nodules
   E. Parenchymal phase is mottled

165. **Sinusoidal causes of portal hypertension:**
   A. Vitamin A overdose
   B. Chemotherapy
   C. Cirrhosis
   D. Noncirrhotic
   E. Alcoholic hepatitis

166. **Prehepatic causes of portal hypertension:**
   A. Congestive cardiac failure
   B. Constrictive pericarditis
   C. Portal venous thrombosis
   D. Tropical splenomegaly
   E. Gastric carcinoma

167. **Recognised extrahepatic causes of portal hypertension:**
   A. Ulcerative colitis   B. Appendicitis
   C. Peritonitis   D. Splenectomy
   E. Chronic pancreatitis

168. **TIPPS:**
   A. Polycystic liver disease is a contraindication
   B. Acites is an indication
   C. Ideal end portal pressure is < 5 mm Hg
   D. Haemoperitoneum is a common complication
   E. Encephalopathy is worsened in 25%

169. **Tc HIDA scan:**
    A. Activity is seen in the bile duct and duodenum in 30-60 minutes
    B. Detects bile leaks better than ultrasound or CT
    C. Best to image at 5-10 minutes for liver SOLs
    D. Negative uptake in gallbladder with acute cholecystitis
    E. GB uptake in chronic cholecystitis is seen in 30-60 minutes

170. **Ultrasound features of portal hypertension:**
    A. Presence of recanalised umbilical vein excludes extrahepatic portal hypertension
    B. Portal vein is abnormal if it is more than 11 mm
    C. Gamma Gandy bodies are hypoechoic and are seen in the left lobe of the liver
    D. Superior mesenteric vein is large if it is more than 12 mm
    E. Bull's eye appearance is seen in ligamentum teres

171. **Hemochromatosis:**
    A. The attenuation of liver is 80-140 HU
    B. Triradiate cartilage is calcified
    C. Arthritis is seen of the distal interphalangeal joint
    D. MRI shows increased T2 for liver
    E. Associated with gonadal atrophy

172. **CT of liver:**
    A. Normal liver parenchyma shows a homogeneous density of 50-70 HU
    B. Caudate lobe is seen between the IVC and porta hepatis
    C. Extra- and intrahepatic cholestatis is readily distinguished on plain scans
    D. Falciform ligament separates right and left lobes
    E. Fatty infiltration decreases liver density in hemochromatosis

173. **Primary biliary cirrhosis:**
    A. Increase in alkaline phosphatase precedes clinical jaundice
    B. Shows dilated ducts in the retrograde studies
    C. Abnormalities rarely seen on ultrasound before symptoms
    D. Hepatic transplantation is the only definitive treatment
    E. Increases risk of gallstone formation

174. **CT of abdominal trauma:**
    A. Haematoma is of higher attenuation than liver
    B. Most bladder ruptures are intraperitoneal
    C. Normal pancreas on CT does not exclude transection
    D. Most liver lacerations require surgery
    E. Pneumoperitoneum is the most common manifestation of bowel injury

175. Abdominal trauma:
  A. Liver is the most frequently injured organ
  B. 20% of blunt abdominal trauma is due to liver injuries
  C. 40% of stab injuries of abdomen involved liver
  D. Splenic laceration is common than liver laceration
  E. Splenic laceration has higher mortality than liver laceration

176. Abdominal trauma:
  A. Presence of hemoperitoneum is an unequivocal indication of surgical intervention
  B. Surgical intervention of liver laceration avoids resection
  C. In 45% of patients, liver and splenic laceration coexist
  D. Coexisting visceral injuries in liver laceration increases the mortality to 15%
  E. Arterial embolisation can be used pre- or postoperatively to control bleeding in abdominal trauma

177. Abdominal injury:
  A. CT is the single greatest factor in deciding on nonoperative management of blunt abdominal trauma
  B. Oral contrast administration is avoided if arteriography or embolisation is indicated
  C. Left lobe of liver is commonly affected than right lobe
  D. Posterior segments are commonly affected
  E. Trauma to left lobe is associated with injuries to retroperitoneum

178. Liver injury:
  A. Liver laceration usually parallels the right and middle hepatic arteries
  B. The most severe hemorrhage is caused by avulsion of right hepatic vein from IVC
  C. Periportal hypodensity is very common finding in hepatic laceration
  D. Hemoperitoneum will occur only if capsule is breached
  E. Gallbladder injury occurs in 2%

179. Abdominal injury:
  A. Injury to bile duct is common at pancreaticobiliary junction
  B. Edema around hepatoduodenal ligament indicates bile duct injury
  C. Follow-up CT has no major value in management of abdominal injury
  D. Grade 3 splenic injury requires surgical intervention
  E. Extravasation of contrast from spleen is an absolute indication of surgery regardless of grade of injury

180. **Bowel injury:**
    A. Intramural air indicates full thickness bowel wall injury
    B. Free retroperitoneal air indicates full thickness bowel wall injury
    C. Mesenteric infiltration is a specific sign of bowel injury
    D. Segmental bowel thickening is the most sensitive sign of bowel injury
    E. Abnormal bowel well enhancement indicates bowel injury only

181. **Contraindications of hepatic chemoembolisation:**
    A. Hepatopetal portal flow
    B. AST > 100 U/l
    C. LDH > 200 U/L
    D. Bilirubin > 2 mg/dl
    E. More than half of liver involved

182. **Complications of hepatic embolisation:**
    A. Splenic infarction   B. Abscess
    C. Biloma   D. Gallbladder infarction
    E. GI bleeding

183. **Complications of hepatic embolisation:**
    A. Postembolisation syndrome has fever
    B. Postembolisation syndrome is seen in 90% of cases
    C. Liver function tests are elevated following the procedure
    D. Pulmonary embolism
    E. Limb ischemia

184. **Radiofrequency ablation for liver tumours:**
    A. Elevation of liver function tests is a common complication
    B. Liver abscess formation is a recognized complication
    C. Tumours 3-4 cm require six overlapping ablations
    D. 12 ablations are required for tumours more than 4 cm
    E. Ultrasound is the best modality for assessing response after radiofrequency ablation
    F. Contrast-enhanced CT scan demonstrates remaining viable tissue after ablation

185. **Radiofrequency ablation for liver tumours:**
    A. RF ablation is more effective in debulking tumours than radiation and chemotherapy
    B. Difficulty in accurate placement of the electrode is a major factor limiting the tumour eradication
    C. Differential blood flow between tumour and normal liver, is another factor limiting the tumour eradication
    D. The complications in RF tumour ablation are lesser than chemoembolisation
    E. It requires fewer sessions to treat hepatocellular carcinoma than percutaneous ethanol ablation

186. **Chronic granulomatous disease:**
    A. Autosomal dominant inheritance
    B. Antibody function is normal
    C. Cell-mediated immunity is abnormal
    D. Liver calcification occurs
    E. Perianal fistula is seen

187. **Liver metastasis with unknown primary:**
    A. Imaging work up will reveal the primary in 40% of cases
    B. No further imaging needs to be done if the biopsy of the liver metastasis is adenocarcinoma
    C. There is a slight improvement in prognosis for those patients treated aggressively following diagnosis of the primary
    D. 80% of metastasis are from adenocarcinoma primary
    E. Median survival for treated adenocarcinoma metastasis is 4 months

188. **Chronic Budd-Chiari syndrome:**
    A. Bicoloured hepatic veins in Doppler is pathognomonic
    B. Homogeneous enhancement in delayed scans
    C. Enhancement radiates from the periphery towards the center
    D. The left lobe of the liver is atrophied
    E. Fibrotic areas do not enhance in early and delayed scans

189. **Doppler findings in portal hypertension:**
    A. The phasic variation of flow in hepatic veins is not affected even in late stages
    B. Decreased flow in the superior mesenteric artery
    C. The lesser omentum to aorta ratio is more than 1.7
    D. Hepatofugal flow indicates splenorenal shunt
    E. The resistive index is increased in hepatic arteries

190. **Abdominal trauma:**
    A. Negative CT excludes splenic trauma
    B. Fresh blood has 35-45 HU density
    C. Mesenteric injury is more common than bowel injury
    D. Subtle lacerations are best seen in arterial phase
    E. Abscess is complication

ANSWERS

1. **A-T, B-F, C-F, D-T, E-F**

   In CT arterioportography, catheter is placed in the superior mesenteric artery and images are acquired in the portal venous phase. In splenoportography, the spleen is punctured.
   Hepatic veins are cannulated either by jugular or femoral venous approach.

2. **A-T, B-T, C-F, D-F, E-F**

   The principal plane passes through the plane of gallbladder and IVC and divides the liver into the right and left lobes. Normal biliary ducts are visualized in high resolution ultrasound. The portal veins have bright wall, but not the hepatic veins.
   The selective uptake of lipiodol is seen in hepatomas and not secondaries.

3. **A-F, B-F, C-F, D-T, E-T**

   I—caudate, II—lateral superior, III—lateral inferior, IV-A— medial superior, IVB—medial inferior, V—anteroinferior, VI—postero-inferior, VII—posterosuperior, VIII—anterosuperior segment.

4. **A-T, B-F, C-T, D-T, E-T**

   About 18.5% have hepatic arteries arising from the superior mesenteric artery. 25% have hepatic arteries arising from left gastric artery. 6% have accessory right hepatic artery.

5. **A-F, B-F, C-F, D-T, E-F**

   The caudate lobe lies within the lesser sac and quadrate lobe in the greater sac.
   IVC is situated posterior to the porta hepatis. The base of bare area is formed by IVC, the sides by superior and inferior coronary ligaments and apex by right triangular ligament.
   The liver is the largest organ in the body.

6. **A-F, B-F, CF, D-T, E-T**

   Normally, portal vein is the posterior structure in the porta hepatis. In the presence of an accessory hepatic artery arising from SMA, it is anterior to the artery. Gastrocolic trunk is formed by union of right gastroepiploic vein, middle colic vein and anterior superior pancreaticoduodenal arcade. Superior mesenteric vein lies to the right of the superior mesenteric artery. This position is reversed in malrotation.

7. **A-T, B-F, C-F, D-T, E-T**

   Common hepatic duct and common hepatic artery pass through porta hepatis.

The portal vein lies posteriorly. Anteriorly, the hepatic artery lies on the left side and common hepatic duct on the right side.

8. **A-F, B-F, C-F, D-F, E-F**
The hepatic artery contributes only 15% of hepatic blood supply. The hepatic artery lies above the portal vein and to the left of the common bile duct. The caudate lobe receives blood from both the branches of hepatic artery and portal vein, which is the reason why this lobe is spared in cirrhosis and drains directly into IVC, accounting for caudate hypertrophy in Budd-Chiari syndrome. The hepatic artery has three main branches, right, left and middle. Riedel's lobe is seen in 5-10% of normal females, and very rare in males.

9. **A-F, B-F, C-T, D-T, E-T**
The first major branch of hepatic artery is the gastroduodenal artery. The right hepatic artery usually crosses posterior to the common hepatic duct, but may be anterior occasionally. The RHA loops so low down, that it can be injured during cholecystectomy. Middle hepatic artery arises from RHA or LHA in 45%. It may also rise in common hepatic, gastroduodenal or celiac arteries.

10. **A-T, B-F, C-T, D-F, E-F**
Perfusion defects are commonly seen in caudate and quadrate lobe. It is due to aberrant venous drainage by left gastric vein and pericardiophrenic veins. These are well seen in triple phase CT scans.
Riedel's lobe is seen in 5-10% of females and rare in males.
The hepatic vein joins IVC at D9.

11. **A-T, B-T, C-T, D-F, E-F**
The right adrenal, upper pole of right kidney and distal portion of IVC, are in relation to the bare area of the liver, hence there are no peritoneal coverings between these.

12. **A-F, B-F, C-F, D-T, E-F**
There are many small anastomosis between branches of hepatic arteries. Contribution of accessory hepatic arteries is vital to the segments which they are supplying. The liver has lymphatics which drain into the preaortic nodes and along celiac axis. The liver capsule is supplied by segmental peritoneal nerves. The sympathetic nerves are from celiac ganglion and parasympathetic nerves from left vagus nerve.

13. **A-F, B-T, C-T, D-T, E-F**
The esophageal branches of the left gastric vein and azygous vein anastomose. These shunts open up in portal hypertension.

14. **A-T, B-T, C-F, D-F, E-T**

    Compression of hepatic veins is another common cause. Diffuse diseases are common cause.

15. **A-T, B-T, C-T, D-F, E-T**

    Portal vein ligation is another cause. Compression by malignant tumours is a well-recognised cause.

16. **A-T, B-T, C-T, D-T, E-F**

    Focal nodular hyperplasia, fibrolamellar carcinoma and adenoma are the most common causes. Also seen in large hemangioma, cholangiocarcinoma, hepatocellular carcinoma and hypervascular metastasis.

17. **A-T, B-T, C-T, D-T, E-T**

    Localises in abscesses due to accumulation in neutrophils and lymphocytes. Uptake by reticuloendothelial cells.
    Also used for assessing esophageal transit time, patency of Denver and Levine peritoneal shunts.

18. **A-F, B-T, C-F, D-F, E-T**

    Sulphur colloid scan is prepared by heating technetium pertechnate and sodium trisulphate for 12 minutes at 90-100 degrees. The upper limit of particle size is 1 microns.
    Usual cause of poor prepration is overheating and alkaline pH. The preparation should not be used more than 6 hours. Imaging is performed 15-30 min after injection.

19. **A-T, B-T, C-T, D-F, E-T**

    The right hepatic artery divides into anterior and posterior segmental branches and also supply the caudate lobe and gall-bladder. The middle hepatic artery, supplies the quadrate and caudate lobe. Left hepatic artery supplies the lateral segments of left lobe, and occasionally a little branch to quadrate lobe.

20. **A-F, B-F, C-F, D-F, E-T**

    Almost 85% localises to liver, 10% to spleen and 5% to bone marrow. In hypersplenism, there is increased splenic activity with colloid shift from liver. Although it localises to bone marrow, the distribution is not an accurate method of determining erythropoiesis.

21. **A-T, B-T, C-T, D-T, E-F**

    Colloid shift is uptake of the Tc 99m sulphur colloid mainly by spleen or bone marrow with reduced uptake in liver, due to liver disease or increased perfusion of spleen and bone marrow. It is also seen in hematopoietic disorders, where increased uptake is seen in bone marrow.

22. **A-F, B-T, C-T, D-F,E-T**
In SVC and IVC obstruction, the quadrate lobe is perfused more than other regions due to collateral flow from the umbilical veins. In Budd-Chiari syndrome, the caudate lobe is the only part spared because of its multiple blood supply. Hepatocellular carcinomas are cold.
FNH and regenerative nodule in cirrhosis show increased uptake.

23. **A-T, B-T, C-F, D-F, E-T**
Porta lymph nodes, metastasis and cyst are other causes.

24. **A-F, B-T, C-T, D-T, E-T**
The phases in liver imaging, are: (1) non-contrast (2) arterial phase—25 sec postcontrast (3) portal phase—50-60 sec post contrast (4) delayed phase—5 min postcontrast. The phases required should be tailored according to the clinical case scenario. If a patient has a known colonic cancer and CT scans are acquired to confirm the presence of metastases, it is enough to obtain only the portal images as the colonic metastases are hypovascular and better seen in portal phase. For metastasis from hypervascular lesions, such as carcinoid and islet cell tumour, the arterial phase images are optimal and a combined arterial phase and portal phase/delayed phase are the best. For hepatomas, dual phase, arterial and portal phase are the best sequences. If a CT scan of abdomen is done for identifying the primary, a single portal phase sequence is all that is needed. The volume of contrast used is 150 ml for single detector and 120 ml for multidetector CT.

25. **A-T, B-T, C-T, D-F, E-T**
Diffuse diseases cause mottled uptake in colloid scan.

26. **A-T, B-T, C-T, D-T, E-T**
Although focal nodular hyperplasia usually causes increased uptake, it may show normal/decreased/no uptake.

27. **A-F, B-T, C-F, D-T, E-F**
Focal fatty infiltration is a high echogenic mass in the liver which can be confused with either hemangioma or hyperechoic metastasis. The lesion is geographical, blood vessels pass through the mass without any displacement or distortion. It is common in the quadrate lobe and adjacent to gallbladder.

28. **A-T, B-T, C-T, D-T, E-F**
Biloma and hepatic cyst are the other reasons.

29. **A-T, B-T, C-T, D-T, E-T**
Hepatic adenomas are benign tumours, which are very prone for haemorrhage and rupture. Oral contraceptives, steroids and glycogen storage diseases are some predisposing causes.
T1 signal depends on presence of haemorrhage.

30. **A-T, B-F, C-T, D-T, E-T**

    Scar is vascular in FNH (unlike fibrolamellar carcinoma or hepatoma) and hence it is hypo in T1 and hyper in T2 and shows delayed enhancement in contrast scans.

Adenomas	*FNH*
Usually > 5 cm	<5 cm
T1-iso, hypo, hyper	iso or hypo
T2-hyper	hyper
Arterial-enhances	enhances
Portal-enhances	enhances
Equilibrium-isointense	isointense
Scar-not seen	seen
	vascular, enhances
Haemorrhage-common	less common
Capsule-common	less common

31. **A-F, B-F, C-F, D-F, E-F**

    Hemangioma produces many salient radiological features in all imaging modalities.

    Ultrasound—hyperechoic—due to cellular interfaces caused by vascular spaces. Acoustic enhancement—due to difference in acoustic impedance between the normal liver and the blood in the sinusoids. The acoustic impedance in the blood within the hemangioma is low compared to the normal liver parenchyma, resulting in better sound penetration and producing better distal through transmission.

    CT—peripheral enhancement due to earlier filling of the feeding vessel. Centripetal filling—due to slow flow and filling of the vascular spaces. The peripheral feeders fill up first, giving the nodular peripheral enhancement, but then the blood circulates slowly in the dilated cavernous spaces and flows from the peripheral sinusoids to the central sinusoids.

    MR—light bulb sign—bright signal in heavily T2 weighted images due to blood products.

32. **A-F, B-F, C-F, D-T, E-T**

    The most common liver tumour is metastases, but hemangioma is the second most common liver tumour, and the most common benign tumour. This is made up of large blood-filled cavernous spaces which have endothelial lining. Fibrous septa separates the lesion into many locules. It is five times more common in females. Platelet levels are low due to sequestration of platelets within the large hemangioma and fibrinogen levels are low due to deposition in clots.

33. A-F, B-F, C-F, D-F, E-T

Mirvis grading of liver injury:

I. Laceration or haematoma < 1 cm or periportal haemorrhage.

II. Laceration or haematoma 1-3 cm.

III. Laceration or haematoma > 3 cm.

IV. Massive haematoma > 10 cm, lobar tissue destruction, devascularisation.

V. Bilobar destruction or devascularisation

Mirvis grading of splenic injuries:

I. Capsular avulsion or laceration or haematoma < 1 cm.

II. Laceration or haematoma 1-3 cm.

III. Laceration or haematoma > 3 cm.

IV. Devascularisation or fragmentation of 3 or more sections.

Grading of hemoperitoneum:

0—None, I—one anatomical space, II—2 or more spaces, III—entire abdomen.

34. A-T, B-T, C-T, D-T, E-F

Central scar in large tumour is a fibrocollagenous scar formed secondary to thrombus or haemorrhgae within the hemangioma. Posterior acoustic enhancement is related to the vascularity and is seen in more than 75% of hemangiomas, and in all hemangiomas more than 2.5 cm. Usually, the hemangiomas are stable, but they can increase or decrease. Hemangiomas are called large when they are more than 5 cm and giant when they are more than 10 cm.

35. A-F, B-F, C-F, D-F, E-T

In angiography there is slow filling and delayed clearance of contrast resulting in cotton wool like puddling of contrast. In RBC scans there is a characteristic delay in uptake with persistent uptake in delayed scans. Hemangiomas are usually hypodense in plain scans, but they can appear hyperdense if the liver is fatty. The initial peripheral enhancement can be completely encircling the tumour, but it is often incomplete and nodular. Sometimes the enhancement is delayed. Then gradual centripetal filling occurs and the lesion is isodense to liver in delayed scans. In small hemangiomas less than 1 cm, the enhancement is immediate and the lesion becomes isodense in 30 seconds. If the scar is large, there may not be a complete central filling in. MRI is low signal in T1 and high signal in T2. The high signal in T2 is very intense seen in heavy T2 weighting unlike other liver tumours. The lesion is well-defined and homogeneously hyperintense when compared with metastasis, which are often inhomogeneously hyperintense with irregular margins. A variety of T2 values have been used for diagnosing hemangiomas including 80, 120 and 180 msec.

36. **A-T, B-F, C-F, D-T, E-T**

    The imaging protocol for hemangioma depends on the first modality in which it is diagnosed. A typical lesion in ultrasound, with no abnormality in liver function test, requires a follow-up ultrasound in 6 months time. If lesion is atypical, and less than 2 cm, MRI is required and if more than 2 cm, RBC scintigraphy is indicated. If lesion is still indeterminate after these tests, angiography or biopsy are performed to confirm the diagnosis. If the lesion is initially diagnosed in MRI or CT, and is typical, no further imaging is required. If it is atypical, the above-mentioned imaging protocol is followed.

37. **A-T, B-F, C-T, D-T, E-F**

    The most common causes of high signal in heavily T2 weighted images are hemangiomas and hypervascular liver metastasis. These include renal carcinoma, pheochromocytoma, sarcoma, islet cell tumour, carcinoid, leiomyoblastoma, uterus and lung cancer metastases.

38. **A-T, B-T, C-T, D-T, E-T**

    The tumour is mainly supplied by hepatic artery and it enhances well in the arterial phase and appears hypodense in the portal phase. Capsule enhances due to rapid washout.

    Opacification of portal vein during arterial phase is abnormal and due to arterioportal shunting. Wedge-shaped defects indicate perfusion defects due to portal vein invasion.

    90% mortality in HCC.

39. **A-T. B-T, C-T, D-F, E-F**

    Lipoma, liposarcoma, focal fatty infiltration, hibernoma and myelolipoma are other causes. Liposarcoma metastasis can contain fat. Adenoma is another tumour which has a lot of fat and glycogen in it. FNH also has fat, but this is not visible radiologically.

40. **A-F, B-F, C-F, D-T, E-F**

    Halo can be seen in HCC and metastasis also. Halo can be due to capsule or edema. Rim enhancement is seen in abscess, HCC and metastasis. Scar of FNH enhances typically. Scar of fibro-lamellar carcinoma does not enhance. Gradual enhancement can be seen in scars of sclerosing HCC and intrahepatic cholangio-carcinoma, but they never enhance more than normal liver enhancement. FNH enhances intensely.

41. **A-T,B-T, C-F, D-F, E-T, F-T**

    Vascular enhancement is seen in HCC and intrahepatic cholangio-carcinoma. Nodule within nodule means altered liver signal with a more abnormal signal within the nodule. It is seen in HCC.

Necrotic metastasis can show rim enhancement like hemangioma, but it will be more of a rind of enhancement than a nodular enhancement and there will be no centripetal filling in. Small hemangiomas show high signal in T2, mimicking metastasis, but they will stay in high signal even in heavy T2 weighting unlike metastasis.

42. **A-T, B-F, C-T, D-T, E-F**
Adenomatous hyperplasia is bright in T1 and T2 due to fat. Regenerative nodules have hemosiderin and are low in both. Enhancement cannot differentiate the various subtypes. Confluent fibrosis can be confusing, can be low in T1, high in T2 and enhance on contrast.

43. **A-T, B-T, C-T, D-T, E-T, F-F**
Chronic hepatitis B and C, cirrhosis caused by alcohol, aflatoxin, oral contraceptives, thorotrast, Wilson's disease, tyrosinosis, von Gierke's disease.

44. **A-F, B-F, C-F, D-T, E-F**
The most common location of hemangioma is in the subcapsular portion of the liver and not in the central porta region. Calcification is seen in 10% of tumours. Doppler shows increased flow in the peripheral feeder, but no flow in the central portions of the tumour. Core biopsy or fine needle aspiration biopsy can be done when the findings in other imaging modalities are inconclusive. Angiography will show normal sized hepatic artery and feeders. There is no tumour neovascularity and no AV shunting.

45. **A-F, B-F, C-T, D-T, E-F**
Micronodular cirrhosis is seen in alcholism and there is 6% incidence. 5% of alcoholics develop HCC. Macronodular cirrhosis is seen in hepatitis B, alcoholism and hemochromatosis. The incidence is 44%.

46. **A-T, B-T, C-F, D-T, E-F**
In west, the incidence is 0.8%, but in South East Asia, Africa, it is as high as 5.5-20%. Occurs in 6th decade in west and two decades earlier in endemic areas. The fibrolamellar carcinoma occurs below 40 years. Hepatoblastoma is the most common tumour in children followed by HCC.

47. **A-T, B-F, C-T, D-T, E-F**
Hypercalcemia is a presenting feature. Hirsutism is also seen. Erythrocytosis is seen due to erythropoeitin production.

48. **A-T, B-T, C-T, D-T, E-T,**
Pancreatic carcinoma and hypercoagulable conditions are other causes.

49. **A-T, B-F, C-T, D-F, E-T**

    Normal stent velocity is between 90-120 cm/sec, should be more than 50 cm/sec. Portal venous velocity is above 30 cm/sec, flow is hepatopetal, flow in splenic vein. There should be no narrowing and there is no turbulence.

50. **A-T, B-T, C-T, D-T, E-T**

    Granulomas, hydatid, tumours, metastases, aneurysm, armillifer, CGD, cysts, haematoma, old liver abscess and portal vein thrombosis are common causes of hepatic calcification.

51. **A-F, B-T, C-T, D-T, E-F**

    Alpha fetoprotein with ultrasound is a useful screening, but alpha fetoprotein alone is not very reliable with low sensitivity and specificity. The lesion shows significant fatty metamorphosis. Budd-Chiari syndrome is produced due to compression or invasion of hepatic veins. Calcification is seen in 3-25%, but it is less frequent than in fibrolamellar carcinoma.

52. **A-T, B-T, C-T, D-F, E-F**

    Portal vein thrombosis can produce collaterals and GZ bleeding. Arterioportal shunting seen as opacification of portal vein in arterial phase.

53. **A-T, B-F, C-T, D-F, E-F**

    Lipiodol is selectively taken up by the HCC because of high vascularity and tumour neovascularity. It is retained for a long time in the tumour because of lack of lymphatics and reticuloendothelial cells. Mosaic pattern is a multiple nodular pattern with differing density values. The lesion is usually hypo- or isodense. It can be hyperdense, especially in fatty liver. There are two growth patterns in HCC. One is encapsulated and the other is infiltrative. In an encapsulated tumour, a well-defined halo can be seen and it does not excluded malignancy.

54. **A-T, B-T, C-T, D-T, E-F**

    The tumours show a large fatty component, which is bright and can be difficult to differentiate from hemangioma when they are small and inflated with fat.
    Invasion of liver by gallbladder tumour is more common than the reverse.

55. **A-T, B-F, C-F, D-F, E-F**

    The fibrolamellar carcinoma is less aggressive than hepatocellular carcinoma, occurs in younger age group and has a better prognosis. Central scar is seen in 40-60%. The scar is not vascular and is hypo in both T1 and T2, unlike the scar of FNH, which is vascular and hypo in T1 and hyper in T2. Scar calcification is seen in up to 55%.

Arterioportal shunting is not as common as in hepatocellular carcinoma.

56. **A-T, B-T, C-F. D-T. E-T**

57. **A-T, B-T, C-T, D-T, E-T, F-F**
Causes of portal vein thrombosis include idiopathic causes, causes secondary to tumor, (hepatocellular carcinoma, cholangio-carcinoma, pancreatic carcinoma, gastric carcinoma), trauma, iatrogenic umbilical vein catheterization, abdominal sepsis, pancreatitis, perinatal omphalitis, appendicitis, diverticulitis, ascending cholangitis, myeloproliferative disorders, clotting disorders (hypercoagulable syndromes), estrogen therapy, severe dehydration, cirrhosis and portal hypertension.

58. **A-T, B-T, C-T, D-F, E-T**
In children the common causes of portal venous gas are NEC, umbilical vein catheterization and erythroblastosis foetalis. In adults, the causes are mesenteric infarction, acute gastric dilatation and barium enema.

59. **A-T, B-T, C-T, D-T, E-T**
Liver pathology

	Proliferative	Granulomatous	Xanthomatous	Fatty infiltration
Ultrasound	Hypo	Hypo	Hypo	Hyper
MR T1	Hypo	Hypo	Hyper	Hyper
CT	Hypo	Hypo	Hypo	Hyper
	Enhances on contrast			

The disease progresses to fibrosis, sclerosing cholangitis and liver failure.
There is a good response to chemotherapy.

60. **A-T, B-F, C-F, D-F, E-T**
Antimicrosomal antibodies are seen in 85-100% of patients. Slight increased incidence of HCCs but less than other cirrhosis.

61. **A-F, B-T, C-F, D-T, E-F**
The aorta is small due to diversion of flow into the hepatic circulation. It is the most common tumour in the first six months and 90% of it occurs in the first six months. Majority of the lesions are multiple and solitary lesions are uncommon.

62. **A-F, B-F, C-F, D-T, E-T**
The imaging features of hemangioendothelioma is the same as hemangiomas, but these are often multiple than solitary. Ultrasound shows multiple well-defined hyperechoic lesions, with acoustic enhancement. RBC scan shows delayed uptake and persistent defect even in delayed scans. Doppler shows large

draining hepatic veins. CT shows multiple well-defined homogeneous hypodense masses, with peripheral enhancement and centripetal filling in. Angiography shows a small caliber of aorta distal to the origin of hepatic artery due to large blood supply to the mass. The feeding arteries are enlarged and tortous, with large draining vessels and large vascular lakes. There is pooling of contrast in the delayed phase.

63. **A-T, B-T, C-T, D-F, E-T**
    Threads and streaks in angiography, is produced due to invasion of portal vein and blood flowing through small portal venous radicles. Capsule is hypointense in T1. In T1, there is an inner layer of hypointense capsule and an outer hyperintense layer of compressed blood vessels and biliary radicles.

64. **A-F, B-F, C-F, D-F, E-F**
    Mesenchymal hamartoma is a developmental lesion, composed of gelatinous mesenchymal tissue and cysts with remnants of hepatic parenchyma. It is common in the first two years, but most common in infancy. It is the second most common tumour in infancy after infantile hemangioendothelioma. The tumour is very large, often more than 15 cm, can be solid (mesenchymal predominant) or multiloculated cystic. Calcification is very uncommon. Ultrasound shows small or large cysts with internal septa. The septa are thick in mesenchymal predominant lesions. CT shows a well-defined mass with central hypodense areas and internal septa. Angiography shows either a hypovascular mass with displacement of vessels or hypervascularity in solid portions. MRI is hypo in T1 and hyper in T2. The stroma is hypointense in T1.

65. **A-F, B-T, C-T, D-F, E-T**
    Familial adenomatous polyposis, Wilms' tumour and hemihypertrophy are other associations of hepatoblastoma.

66. **A-T, B-T, C-T, D-T, E-F**
    Spoke wheel pattern of enhancement similar to focal nodular hyperplasia is seen. This is the most common tumour in children. More common in males (3:2). Pathologically, it can have epithelial or mixed or anaplastic types. Epithelial type can be fetal or embryonal, fetal having good prognosis and embryonal having bad prognosis. There is hepatomegaly. Sulfur colloid and RBC scans show defect. Hepatobiliary scan often excretes, gallium scan shows increased uptake. Ultrasound shows echogenic mass with hemorrhage, calcification and necrosis. Doppler is very vascular. CT is solid and hypodense, enhancing in arterial phase. MRI is hypo in T1 and hyper in T2.

67. **A-T, B-F, C-T, D-T, E-T**
Arsenicals and radiation are other common causes of angiosarcoma.

68. **A-F, B-T, C-F, D-T, E-F**
Angiosarcoma is a very aggressive, vascular tumour, which is derived from endothelium lined cells. The most common cause is thorotrast, which was used as a contrast medium. Thorotrast is seen as metallic density in plain X-rays in the liver, spleen, lymph nodes and can rupture into the peritoneum. The thorotrast will be displaced by nodules of angiosarcoma, when they arise. Ultrasound shows a diffusely echogenic liver, which will show a large tumour. CT scan shows circumferential displacement of thorotrast in the periphery of a nodule. The lesion can be single or multiple and is hypodense. Hyperdense areas of haemorrhage can be seen. Centripetal pattern of enhancement can be seen. MRI shows peripheral enhancement of the lesion which is hypointense in T1 and hyperintense in T2. Angiography demonstrates a moderately hypervascular, with diffuse puddling of contrast, persisting in the venous phase.

69. **A-T, B-T, C-T, D-T, E-F**
Hemochromatosis and cholestatic cirrhosis are other causes.

70. **A-F, B-T, C-F, D-T, E-T**
Hepatoblastoma is the most common paediatric malignancy, followed by hepatocellular carcinoma and undifferentiated embryonal sarcoma. HCC is the most common paediatric malignancy after the age of four. There is a bimodal age distribution, seen in 4-5 years and 12-14 years. Fibrolamellar carcinoma can be seen in adolescents and young adults. Pathologically, the lesion can be multiple, diffuse or infiltrative.

71. **A-T, B-T, C-F, D-T, E-F**
Biliary cystadenoma and cystadenocarcinoma are considered forms of the same disease, with cystadenoma being a benign lesion with malignant potential and cystadenocarcinoma a malignant lesion. Those adenocarcinomas with ovarian stroma, is common in females and arises from pre-existing cystadenoma, have a good prognosis. Those without ovarian stroma, is equally common in males and females, have no pre-existing cystadenoma and have bad prognosis. Ultrasound shows a cystic lesion with septations and mural nodules. The presence of solid irregular components, thick irregular nodular septations, papillary projections, with lymphadenopathy, invasion of adjacent organs and metastasis.

72. **A-F, B-T, C-T, D-T, E-T**

Hepatoma is more common in postnecrotic cirrhosis than alcoholic cirrhosis. Although the most common type of cirrhosis in alcoholism is micronodular, the one leading to hepatoma is macronodular. Thorotrast commonly causes angiosarcoma, but it is a risk factor for hepatoma as well.

73. **A-T, B-F, C-T, D-T, E-T**

Sulphur colloid scan shows a diffuse altered uptake with colloid shift to spleen due to cirrhosis and focal defect of hepatocellular carcinoma. 50% of hepatobiliary scans show defects and 50% show increased uptake due to presence of bile ducts and normal excretion. Small tumours are homogeneously hypoechoic, because they are purely cellular, with hypoechoic halo and occasional posterior acoustic enhancement. Large tumours can be hyperechoic or heterogeneous or mosaic pattern. Diffuse involvement will be seen as diffuse alteration of echotexture.

74. **A-T, B-T, C-T, D-T, E-F**

Doppler can show a basket pattern, which is formed by intra-lesional tangle of vessels and indicates hypervascularity and tumour shunting. HCC is one of the few tumours which has hyperintensity in T1. Hypovascular well-differentiated HCCs and inoperable small HCCs, less than 3 cm are managed by percutaneous ethanol injection. Large inoperable tumours and technically difficult lesions are managed by transarterial embolisation.

75. **A-F, B-T, C-T, D-T, E-F**

Stomach, lung and pancreas are common causes.

76. **A-T, B-T, C-T, D-F, E-T**

Lipiodol can be taken by a lot of vascular tumours, apart from HCCs.

77. **A-T, B-T, C-T, D-T, E-F**

Lymphomas of liver can be secondary or very rarely, a primary. Hodgkin's usually presents as miliary nodules and spleen is always involved. non-Hodgkin's disease can be lymphocytic which is miliary or large cell and histiocytic which are nodular. A large lymphocytic tumour is the most common type in primary Hodgkin's disease. It is seen in middle age. Sulfur colloid scan shows focal defect or inhomogeneous uptake in diffuse disease. Ultrasound can show a focal hypoechoic mass or diffuse alteration of echotexture. Angiography is hypo or avascular. CT can show a solitary large mass or multiple small masses or diffuse infiltration.

78. **A-T, B-T, C-T, D-T, E-T**
Undifferentiated embryonal sarcoma is also called mesenchymal sarcoma and is composed of undifferentiated spindle cells. It is seen between 6-10 years and is the fourth most common hepatic tumour in children. Common liver tumours are hepatoblastoma > HCC > infantile hemangioendothelioma > undifferentiated embryonal sarcoma. Radiological appearances range from a multicystic mass to a inhomogeneously solid neoplasm. Epitheloid hemangioendothelioma is a neoplasm that has epitheloid appearing endothelial cells. These are multiple, peripheral, hypoechoic masses in ultrasound. CT shows multiple nodules which can coalesesce to form a large tumour, with calcification and capsular retraction. There is a hypodense rim in contrast CT and hypointense rim in MRI due to capsule.

79. **A-F, B-T, C-T, D-T, E-F**
In nonpregnant adults—HCC, testicular tumours, cirrhosis, active hepatitis.
In pregnant women—Anencephaly, spina bifida, encephalocele, hydrocephalus, renal agenesis, hydronephrosis, multicystic dysplasia, gastroschisis, omphalocele, twin, millod abortion, wrong dates.

80. **A-T, B-T, C-T, D-F, E-F**
Hemochromatosis, hemosiderosis, iron overload due to multiple blood transfusions, glycogen storage disease and amiodarone are the causes of high density in liver.

81. **A-F, B-T, C-T, D-F, E-T**
Platelet count is low due to chronic liver diseases; Posterior mediastinal widening due to varices.

82. **A-T, B-F, C-F, D-F, E-T**

83. **A-F, B-T, C-T, D-T, E-F**
Men to women 10-1.

84. **A-T, B-T, C-F, D-F, E-F**
Platelet count less than 80000 is a contraindication. Ascites should be drained and coagulopathy corrected.

85. **A-T, B-T, C-T, D-T, E-T**
Hemangioma is the most common cause. Fatty infiltration, focal nodular hyerplasia and hepatoma are less common masses.

86. **A-T, B-T, C-T, D-T, E-F**
Thyroid, choriocarcinoma and colon are other common causes.

87. **A-F, B-T, C-T, D-T, E-T**
Candida is the most common cause. Leukemia and septic emboli are other causes.

88. **A-T, B-T, C-T, D-F, E-T**

89. **A-T, B-T, C-F, D-F, E-F**

90. **A-F, B-F, C-F, D-T,E-T**
Hemangiomas show hyperechogenicity and posterior acoustic enhancement. Metastasis are usually hypoechoic with a halo around them. Fatty infiltration is seen as diffuse hyperechogenicity with loss of definition of posterior structures. Ovarian carcinoma can produce well-defined cystic metastases, which are indistinguishable from simple cysts.

91. **A-F, B-T, C-T, D-T, E-F**
FNH is a benign tumour which contains hyperplastic hepatocytes with bile ductules associated with a central scar, without a peripheral capsule. The presence of a vascular scar and hyperplastic hepatocytes are responsible for the majority of the characteristic imaging findings. Sulfur colloid which is taken by reticuloendothelial cells, shows normal uptake in 50% identical to normal liver, decreased uptake in 40% and peculiary increased uptake in 10% of cases. The RBC scan shows early uptake and late deficit, which contrasts with hemangioma which shows late uptake and persistent deficity. Oral contraceptives do not contribute to the formation of FNH but promote the growth of FNH. There is no increased uptake with gallium scans.

92. **A-T, B-T, C-T, D-T, E-F**
Doppler of FNH shows scattered arterial and venous signals within the tumour producing the characteristic comet tail appearance. SPIO is a paramagnetic agent taken by Kupffer cells in liver, and hence will show normal uptake with FNH, which has normal hepatocytes and Kupffer cells. Angiography shows the hypervascular tumour, which has a centrifugal blood supply producing the spoke wheel pattern. Capillary phase shows intense inhomogeneous stain and venous phase shows large draining veins. The lesion is hyperdense in early arterial phase images and isodense in portal phase images. The scar is usually hypodense or isodense in arterial and portal images, but hyperdense in delayed images. Some authors believe the scar is hyperdense in portal phase itself due to diffusion of contrast from tumour into the scar.

93. **A-T, B-T, C-T, D-F, E-T**
CML, Hodgkin's disease, myeloid metaplasia, multiple myeloma, rheumatoid arthritis, scleroderma and SLE are other associations of NRH. This is just a diffuse nodularity of liver due to multiple regenerative nodules, but not associated with fibrosis. This is

referred by multiple terms including, noncirrhotic nodularities, noncirrhotic portal hypertension, diffuse nodular hyperplasia, nodular transformation of liver, partial nodular transformation, adenomatous hyperplasia and miliary hepatocellular adenomatosis. Ascites, splenomegaly and portal hypertension can be presenting clinical features. Sulfur colloid scan shows patchy diffuse uptake, ultrasound shows multiple nodules of varying echogenicity, MRI shows low signal in T2W images due to iron content in the nodules.

94. **A-T, B-F, C-F, D-T, E-T**
Almost 40% of those with ADPKD have liver cysts. The commonly seen simple liver cyst is a unilocular cyst lined by a single layer of bile duct cuboidal epithelium. This is well-defined, round, hypoechoic with posterior acoustic enhancement. They are hypodense in CT with no contrast enhancement. Polycystic liver disease can produce hepatic fibrosis and portal hypertension.

95. **A-T, B-F, C-T, D-T, E-F**
There is increased incidence of hepatocellular adenomas in those who take oral contraceptives or anabolic steroids and in glycogen storage disease. The lesion is a tumour which is composed or hepatocytes arranged in cords that may form bile but without portal tracts and hepatic veins. It has fat, glycogen and Kupffer cells. RBC scan shows early uptake and late defect. Hepatobiliary scan shows no uptake and no excretion due to paucity of biliary ductules. Ultrasound is very hyperechoic due to fat and glycogen. It is characteristically hypodense in nonenhanced CT scan, hyperdense in arterial phase and centripetal enhancement in portal images. There is no persistence of contrast in delayed images, unlike hemangiomas. Angiography shows a hypervascular lesion with large peripheral vessels, centripetal flow without any AV shunting. MRI is hypo or hyper in T1 and hyper in T2. Normal uptake is seen in SPIO images.

96. **A-T, B-T, C-F, D-T, E-T**
Hypervascular lesions are better see in arterial images. The common hypervascular lesions are hepatic adenoma, focal nodular hyperplasia, hepatoma and metastasis from carcinoid/islet cell tumour/renal cell carcinoma/leiomyosarcoma.

97. **A-F, B-T, C-T, D-T, E-F**
Liver is the second most common organ to be involved in metastatic disease after the lymph nodes. 30-70% of cancer patients have liver metastasis at autopsy. Up to 30% of colorectal cancer patients have isolated liver metastasis, diagnosis of which plays

an important role in management. Cystic metastasis are commonly seen from ovary, pancreas and others. Differentiation of cystic metastasis from simple benign cyst is extremely difficult. The only differentiation feature, is the presence of unsharp margin for the metastasis due to irregularity of interface between the tumour and liver.

98. **A-F, B-T, C-T, D-F, E-F**
Tumours with high risk—large bowel, oesophagus, stomach, pancreas, carcinoids, liver, gallbladder, biliary tree and lung. Intermediate risk—breast, ovary, melanoma and soft tissue sarcoma. Low risk Prostate, kidney, testis, cervix, head and neck, thyroid and bone sarcoma.

99. **A-T, B-T, C-T, D-T, E-T**
Calcified liver metastasis are seen in following primaries: mucinous adenocarcinoma of colon, ovary and pancreas, serous cystadenocarcinoma of ovary, osteosarcoma, chondrosarcoma, neuroblastoma, melanoma, leiomyosarcoma, islet cell tumours or pancreas, embryonal tumour of testis, breast, bronchus, kidney and thyroid.

100. **A-F, B-T, C-T, D-T, E-T**
Mucinous ovarian carcinoma is a common cause. Colonic CA is another primary.

101. **A-T, B-T, C-T, D-T, E-T**

102. **A-T, B-F, C-T, D-T, E-F**
Hypervascular lesions are the most common causes of echogenic ultrasound such as renal carcinoma, thyroid, islet cell tumours, carcinoid, choriocarcinoma, melanoma, pheochromocytoma and breast carcinoma. Calcified metastasis are also echogenic.

103. **A-T, B-T, C-F, D-T, E-T**
The liver receives 70% of blood supply from portal vein and 30% from hepatic artery. During arterial phase, contrast mixes with the blood from hepatic arteries. Since this is only 30% of blood flow, the contrast gets diluted by the portal venous blood contributing 70%. So the liver does not enhance much. Hypovascular lesions, will appear isodense in this phase or may occasionally show rim enhancement. Hypervascular lesions are best seen in this phase, as they will enhance more than the poorly enhancing liver parenchyma. During portal phase, the contrast mixes with portal blood and the liver enhances uniformly. The hypervascular metastases will be seen as isodense lesions during portal phase,

but the hypovascular metastases stand out as hypodense lesions against the enhancing liver.

104. A-F, B-F, C-F, D-T, E-T
Metastasis reaching through hepatic arteries are uniform, not portal vein. There is no capsule for metastasis. Hemorrhagic metastasis are high in T1 and T2. Melanoma is bright in T1 and T2. Calcification will produce low signal in T2 also.

105. A-T, B-T, C-T, D-T, E-F

106. A-F, B-T, C-F, D-F, E-F
Up to 4 metastatic lesions can be resected. Capsular invasion and ascites do not preclude metastasis. < 30% liver function left after resection.

107. A-T, B-F, C-F, D-T, E-F
CT arteriography is done with the catheter in the hepatic artery CT arterioportography is done with the catheter in the superior mesenteric or splenic artery and obtaining images in the portal phase. Delayed iodine scanning is done after 4-6 hours of contrast administration. Delayed filling similar to hemangioma is seen in 5%

108. A-T, B-T, C-T, D-T, E-T
Metastasis can enhance in any pattern.

109. A-F, B-F, C-T, D-T, E-T
There are many patterns of enhancement.
Halo—hypointense center surrounded by hyperintense rim, due to edema or viable tumour. Central hypointensity is usually due to necrosis.
Doughnut pattern—hypointense lesion with central more hypointense region, seen in large lesions, prone for necrosis.
Target lesion is a central hyperintensity surrounded by a rind of hypointensity.
Light bulb is due to very high signal in T2 images, due to cystic metastasis, pheochromocytoma, carcinoid and islet cell tumours.

110. A-F, B-F, C-T, D-T, E-T
CT and MRI have a sensitivity of 85-90% for detecting liver metastasis. The sensitivity is 95% for lesions above 1 cm and 45% for lesions less than 1 cm. With the advent of multiphase CT, many smaller lesions have been identified and incidental discoveries lead to diagnostic dilemma. Small lesions seen in patients without a known primary are almost always benign, but in patients with known malignancy, 10% will be metastatic disease. Focal fatty infiltration may mimic metatasis and the best way of differen-

tiating it is by using chemical shift MRI, using in phase and out of phase images, where fat will suppress in opposed phase images.

111. **A-T, B-F, C-F, D-F, E-T**
SHU508A is the commonly used ultrasound contrast agent. It is a microbubble which increases Doppler signal from vessels. In pulse inversion imaging, two pulses 180 degrees out of phase are sent in. In normal tissues, no net signal is produced. The bubbles produce asymmetrical echoes, which are detected. The quality can be improved by breaking the bubble with the first pulse.

112. **A-F, B-F, C-F, D-T, E-T**
There are three phases, vascular, interval delay flash and post-vascular. Initially, baseline images are obtained. IV administration of contrast. Vascular phase—accumulation depends on arterial volume, with enhancement of liver and vessels. Scan done till maximum arterial enhancement obtained. Probe switched off for ten seconds. Switching on probe, breaks the bubbles, giving the second, interval delay flash of high signal, due to disruption of microbubbles which have accumulated. Second IV injection. High MI (mechanical index) insonation of liver, four minutes after injection. This gives post-vascular phase, due to disruption of bubbles that have accumulated in the sinusoids for 4 min.

113. **A-T, B-F, C-F, D-T, E-T**
FNH—enhancement in three phases. HCC—enhancement in vascular and flash, no enhancement in post-vascular phase. Mets—no enhancement in all phases, occasionally can show focal enhancement in flash. Hemangioma—peripheral nodular enhancement in the flash phase only. Progressive centripetal filling.

114. **A-T, B-T, C-T, D-F, E-F**
Gadolinium—shortens T1, resulting in high signal in T1W images. SPIO—(superparamagnetic iron oxide), taken by reticuloendothelial cells (Kupffer cells) in liver, produce T2 shortening. The liver will appear dark in T2W images, but lesions without Kupffer cells will appear bright against the dark background.

115. **A-F, B-T, C-T, D-T, E-T**
Gadolinium—0.1 mmol/kg. Hypervascular metastasis show arterial enhancement.

116. **A-F, B-T, C-T, D-T, E-T**
Lesions with Kupffer cells will take up SPIO, which produce T2 shortening and hence show low signal in T2W images. FNH and adenoma are such lesions. Occasionally, well-differentiated HCC may have Kupffer cells. Benign and malignant lesions can be

differentiated. HCCs show less SPIO uptake in contrast to benign lesions and show less than 40% drop in signal intensity in delayed images. Benign lesions show more uptake and more than 40% signal drop. Metastasis does not have Kupffer cell and hence does not decrease in signal, standing out. Hemangioma also shows decreased signal, because of slow vascular flow, although it does not have Kupffer cells.

117. **A-T, B-T, C-T, D-T, E-T**
These two agents are also hepatobiliary agents, the selective uptake due to the chelates. The enhancement begins immediately, rises for 20 min and persists for two hours. Lesions without hepatocytes such as metastasis appear dark. But hepatocellular lesions enhance.

118. **A-T, B-T, C-T, D-T, E-T**
USPIO are smaller than SPIO. Unlike SPIO, they are blood pool agents, stay longer in vascular system, shorten T1 and T2, hence normal liver and vessels enhance in T1 and are dark in T2, with good contrast of lesions. More uptake in lymph nodes and bone marrow. Stay for longer time in circulation. So this is useful in both T1 and T2W images.

119. **A-T, B-T, C-T, D-T, E-T**
Cavernomatous malformation is seen in portal venous thrombosis and is due to collateral vessel formation. Bowel wall edema is more common on the right side of the abdomen.

120. **A-F, B-T, C-F, D-T, E-T**
Dilatation of intrahepatic biliary radicles is more sensitive in the setting of liver transplantation. Epithelial casts indicate preservation injury and the liver has to be retransplanted. Strictures are more common in the first two weeks.

121. **A-T, B-T, C-T, D-F, E-T**
Prolonged cold ischemic time is another common cause.

122. **A-F, B-T, C-F, D-F, E-F**
Nonanastomostic strictures indicate bad prognosis as it is usually due to diffuse insult to biliary tree. Majority of bile leak occurs in the first postoperative month. Bilomas have to be aspirated to maintain the graft. Most common cause of leak is anastomostic breakdown followed by T tube leakage and hepatic arterial thrombosis.

123. **A-T, B-T, C-F, D-F, E-T**
Large volume ascites is due to hepatic venous obstruction or infection or renal failure. Haematomas need not be aspirated and

it is difficult to aspirate clotted blood in the first two weeks. Septations is not pathognomonic of abscess.

124. **A-F, B-T, C-T, D-T, E-T**
Garbi classification of hydatid cysts.
I—unilocular simple cyst, II—cyst with floating membrane, III—daugher cysts/septations with predominant fluid component, IV—predominant heterogeneous solid component, with daughter cysts and membranes, V—calcified cyst.
Type I is the most common hepatic type, although II and III are more common in the other parts. Any simple cyst in liver in endemic areas, hydatid is the diagnosis unless proved otherwise.

125. **A-T, B-F, C-F, D-F, E-T**
Manganese DPDP is selectively taken by hepatocytes and produces T1 shortening. So the liver appears bright in T1W images. Lesions without hepatocytes will appear dark against the bright background of liver. This is ideal for metastasis. Only manganese is essential for the signal, DPDP being used to reduce toxicity of manganese.

126. **A-F, B-T, C-T, D-T, E-T**
Lesions without hepatocytes are ideal for evaluation by Mn DPDP, as they will be seen as dark structures against the diffusely enhancing liver. This is ideal for metastasis. Lesions such as FNH, adenoma, well diff HCC have hepatocytes and show uptake similar to liver, which will be seen in delayed images too. Carcinoid metastasis also shows uptake.

127. **A-F, B-F, C-F, E-T, E-F**
Type I cyst occurs in a younger population. Hydatid sand can happen even in type I simple cyst. Biliary dilatation can be either due to pressure effect or due to biliary rupture. Split sign is due to detachment of parasite from the pericyst which is formed due to host response.

128. **A-F, B-T, C-T, D-F, E-T**
Schistosoma mansoni and *japonicum* affect liver, hematobium affects bladder. The larva is shed by snails, penetrates the skin of humans, enters by lymphatics of veins to heart, then to pulmonary circulation, systemic circulation, mesenteric system, portal veins, maturation, periportal fibrosis and perisinusoidal portal hypertension. Turtle back appearance is produced due to pseudoseptation, notching and geographic areas of calcification. Birds claw appearance is seen due to scanning of portal triads perpendicularly.

129. **A-T, B-F, C-F, D-F, E-F**

It is more common in the extrahepatic portion of the hepatic artery, with two-thirds occurring in the common hepatic artery. It is more common in men. Atherosclerosis is the most common cause, inflammation and iatrogenic being the other causes.

130. **A-T, B-F, C-F, D-T, E-T**

Haemobilia, epigastric pain and jaundice form the characteristic triad of clinical features. Rupture occurs equally into the peritoneal cavity and biliary tract. Common hepatic artery can be embolised, because of collateral supply, but is avoided in the postgastro-duodenal arterial segment. However, the aneurysm can be embolised, even if it is in the postgastroduodenal arterial segment.

131. **A-T, B-T, C-F, D-T, E-T**

Hepatic resection is the mainstay in management of hepatic cancers. The survival rates are 55-80% in the first year and 25-50% in five years. Very advanced disease, poor clinical state and unfavourable location are contraindications for hepatic resection. Percutaneous ethanol injection is one of the many percutaneous treatment options, which are used as palliative methods. There is no absolute size limit on the size or number lesions to be treated. But not more than 3 lesions and no lesion more than 3 cm are treated in a single session, because of the limit on the injection volume treated per session and because of greater effectiveness for smaller tumours. The diffusion of ethanol is limited in metastasis than hepatocellular carcinoma, because of the firmer consistency.

132. **A-T, B-T, C-T, D-T, E-T**

There are many minimally invasive treatment options for management of hepatocellular carcinoma. They include intrarterial chemoembolisation, percutaneous injection of substances such as alcohol, acetic acid or hot saline, heating methods such as radio-frequency, electrocautery, interstitial laser therapy, microwave coagulation therapy and high intensity focused ultrasound, and cryotherapy. The commonly used are radiofrequency ablation for hepatic metastasis and percutaneous ethanol injection for hepatocellular carcinoma.

133. **A-F, B-T, C-F, D-T, E-F**

In radiofrequency tumour ablation, alternating current induces ionic agitation, which results in frictional heat production within the tissues. This heat produces immediate coagulation necrosis at temperatures above 50°C. Preferential cytotoxic effect on tumour cells is seen at temperatures between 41-45°C. It takes 15 minutes, for cytotoxicity, at 45°C and for each degree drop, the time doubles, and it takes 240 min at 41°C.

134. **A-F, B-T, C-T, D-T, E-T**
The aim in radiofrequency ablation is to kill the target tumour and a cuff of normal hepatic parenchyma measuring 5-10 mm. The size of necrotic tumour depends on the probe gauge, length of the exposed probe tip, temperature along exposed electrode and duration of therapy. The largest tumor diameter that can be killed by a single electrode is 1.6 cm. The volume of coagulated tissue can be increased by using multiprobe electrodes and by saline enhancement. Cooling the electrode with saline, prevents charring of the liver and reduces impedance of the tissues adjacent to the electrode.

135. **A-F, B-T, C-T, D-T, E-T**

136. **A-T, B-T, C-T, D-F, E-F**
75% of blood supply to liver is from portal vein which is essential when hepatic artery is embolised. Childs Type C is the severe clinical type. Larger lesions are managed first.

137. **A-T, B-F, C-T, D-F, E-F, F-F**
Intra-arterial lignocaine for analgesia. PVA is the embolic agent. Lipiodol, omnipaque and cytotoxic agent are the ingredients. Follow-up CT scan begins at 2 weeks. Antibiotics covering gram positive and negative organisms are essential to prevent sepsis. If more than 50% of tumour shows lipiodol uptake in two weeks, it is a success and procedure repeated. If less than 50% of tumour shows uptake, CT is repeated after two months and a further procedure done if that CT shows reduction in size.

138. **A-F, B-F, C-T, D-F, E-T**
The density of mesenteric fat is increased in comparison to that of retroperitoneal fat. Arterioportal fistulas are seen in cirrhosis itself and do not necessarily indicate a hepatocellular carcinoma. Regenerating nodules and adenomatous hyperplasia have portal venous supply in 96% of cases and hepatic arterial supply in only 4% and is not possible to differentiate. They are hyperdense on CT scans. Hepatocellular carcinomas have hepatic arterial supply in 95% of cases.

139. **A-T, B-T, C-T, D-F, E-T**
SPIO is taken up by normal Kupffer cells in liver and other reticuloendothelial cells. Cirrhosis produces a heterogeneous uptake. In spleen, there is more uptake because of increased iron deposition. Hence, spleen appears darker than normal. Flying bat

appearance is seen in severe cirrhosis due to atrophy of right lobe of liver, lack of uptake in the hilar region due to large portal vein and uptake in spleen. The hepatic arteries are hypervascular and show corkscrew appearance. Normal wedged hepatic venography shows fifth order banches. But these are not visualised in fibrosis. With severe fibrosis, even first and second order branches may not be visualised.

140. **A-T, B-T, C-T, D-T, E-T**

141. **A-F, B-F, C-F, D-F, E-F**
The plain film findings are due to hepatomegaly in early stages, shrunken liver in later stages and due to portal hypertension. Diaphragm is elevated with restriction of movements. Duodenum is displaced inferomedially due to hepatomegaly or displaced anteriorly due to retroperitoneal edema or superiorly due to shrinkage. Stomach displaced inferomedially (H), posteriorly (left lobe) or right and upward (S). Colon displaced caudally and ventrally (H), superiorly (S), chiladitis syndrome (colonic interposition between superior surface of liver and diaphragm (25%). Inferomedial displacement (H) or suprolateral displacement (S) of gallbladder. Kidney displaced downwards (H), medial (right lobe), superiorly (S), bilateral nephromegaly due to hypertrophy. Prominent azygos vein, lateral displacement of left paravertebral line, soft tissue density adjacent to descending aorta due to varix in pulmonary ligament round shadow in fatty tissue anterior and inferior to liver due to umbilical vein. Primary pulmonary hypertension is seen in up to 2% of cirrhotics, producing prominent pulmonary artery and right heart hypertrophy (H—hepatomegaly, S—shrunken).

142. **A-T, B-T, C-T, D-T, E-F**
Agenesis of lobes, accessory lobes, postnecrotic scarred liver, resection and radiation are other causes.

143. **A-T, B-T, C-F, D-F, E-T**
Normal size microbubbles is <10μm, usually 2-7 micrometers, as larger particles cannot pass through capillaries. Ultrasound contrast enhances signal. It is distributed within the blood and extracellular space. It contrasts in the compression part and expands in rarefaction phases of ultrasound cycle can demonstrate vascular pertusion.

144. **A-F, B-T, C-T, D-F, E-T**
Portal vein is usually imaged by midline transverse/oblique approach. Rt. branches are scanned by intercoild approach. Flow

is usually hepatopetal with respiratory variations and no pulsatility. Periodic (variation) with cardiac cycle seen, Helical Flow seen in liver disease.

145. **A-F, B-T, C-T, D-F, E-T**
Pills, pregnancy, polycythemia rubra vera, paroxysmal nocturnal hemoglobinuria and thrombocytosis are most common causes.

146. **A-T, B-T, C-T, D-F, E-T**
Other tumours such as hepatoma, renal carcinoma, metastasis, IVC tumour are causes.
IVC diaphragm is a very common cause.

147. **A-T, B-F, C-T, D-F, E-F**
Type I—IVC, hepatic V; II—major hepatic veins, IVC, III— centrilobular hepatic veins.
Caudate lobe is enlarged, the others are atrophic. The liver and spleen are enlarged in the early stage. The right inferior hepatic vein is enlarged. There is communication of right or middle hepatic vein with the right inferior hepatic vein.

148. **A-F, B-T, C-T, D-T, E-T**

149. **A-F, B-F, C-T, D-F, E-F**
Acute Budd-Chiari syndrome is characterised by sudden onset, hepatomegaly, gross ascites and normal liver function tests.
The caudate lobe is not hypertrophied due to the acute onset. In early phases of contrast enhancement, the caudate lobe enhances and the peripheral portions do not enhance, whereas in the late phase, the caudate lobe is nonenhancing, and peripheral areas show patchy enhancement. This is called flip-flop phenomenon.

150. **A-F, B-T, C-T, D-T, E-T**

151. **A-T, B-T, C-T, D-T, E-T**
Other metabolic conditions include alpha one antitrypsin deficiency, protoprophyria, Gaucher's disesae, tyrosinemia, galactosemia and glycogen storage disease type III.

152. **A-T, B-T, C-F, D-F, E-T**
Common causes are alcoholic liver disease and viral hepatitis. Sarcoidosis, congenital syphilis, hepatitis B, non A non B, D, schistosomiasis, primary biliary cirrhosis, sclerosing cholangitis, secondary biliary cirrhosis, Indian childhood cirrhosis, cryptogenic cirrhosis and toxic injury are other causes.

153. **A-T, B-T, C-F, D-T, E-F**
Nitrofurantoin is another cause.

154. A-T, B-T, C-T, D-T, E-F
Hepatitis and alpha 1 antitrypsin deficiency are other causes.

155. A-F, B-F, C-T, D-T, E-T
Alcoholism is the most common cause of micronodular cirrhosis. Hemochromatosis, venous obstruction, small bowel bypass and biliary obstruction are other causes.
Viral hepatitis is the most common cause of macronodular cirrhosis. Other causes are Wilson's and alpha 1 antitrypsin deficiency.

156. A-F, B-T, C-F, D-T, E-T
Micronodular cirrhosis by definition is less than 3 mm. Dysplastic nodules have adenomatous hyperplasia and dysplastic hepatocytes. Regenerative nodules are characterised by proliferation of hepatocytes with supporting stroma.
Cirrhotic nodules are predominantly regenerative nodules.

157. A-T, B-T, C-T, D-T, E-T
Gallstones are associated and there are many reasons for it. Associated alcoholism, bile stasis due to decreased intake, hypersplenism and hemolysis are the risk factors. Bleeding disorders are also very common.

158. A-T, B-F, C-T, D-F, E-T
Dysplastic nodules are nodular hepatocellular proliferations at least 1 mm in diameter. Can be low/high grade. Contain dysplastic hepatocytes without evidence of malignancy.

159. A-T, B-F, C-T, D-T, E-F
MRI—flow voids from collaterals. Absent hepatic veins.
Doppler—hepatic veins—flow absent or reversed: no respiratory variations. IVC—reversed slow flow.
Portal veins—loss of respiratory variation, slow, hepatofugal, thrombosis, congestion index > 0.1. Hepatic artery—high resistive index.

160. A-F, B-F, C-T, D-F, E-T, F-T
The right lobe and medial segment of left lobe are atrophied. The caudate lobe is not affected. There is compensatory hypertropy of the lateral segments of the left lobe.
Caudate lobe/right lobe >0.65. Quadrate lobe < 3 cm.
Liver enlarged in early stages and atrophied in lateral stages. The surface is nodular. The GB angle is normally more than 40 degrees. It is less than 35 degrees in cirrhosis.

161. **A-F, B-T, C-F, D-T, E-T**
The liver is shrunken and shows coarse increased echotexture. The sound transmission is decreased. The definition of portal venous walls is decreased or normal. Regenerative nodules are isoechoic. Hepatic arteries are dilated due to increased flow.

162. **A-F, B-F, C-F, D-T, E-T, F-F**
In early stage the liver is hypodense due to fatty change and in later stages it is hypo/isodense. Regenerative nodules are·iso/hyperdense. The dysplastic nodules are usually supplied by the portal vein. Peribiliary cysts are produced due to obstructed peribiliary glands and produces periportal hypodensities. The right lobe is atrophied in cirrhosis. The normal ratio is 1: 1.44, in cirrhosis it is less than 1: 1.3.

163. **A-T, B-T, C-T, D-F, E-F**
Portal hypertension, GI bleeding, encephalopathy can be seen.

164. **A-T, B-F, C-T, D-F, E-T**
The hepatic arteries are dilated due to increased flow and are corkscrew shaped.
Shunting between hepatic arteries and portal vein, with delayed entry into the hepatic veins. Hepatic veins are not seen beyond 5th degree branches due to compression by nodules. Parenchymal phase is mottled due to regenerative nodules and fibrosis.

165. **A-T, B-T, C-T, D-T, E-T**

166. **A-F, B-F, C-T, D-T, E-F**

167. **A-T, B-T, C-T, D-T, E-T**
Causes of portal hypertension:
Prehepatic—Increased flow due to idiopathic, tropical spleno-megaly, AV fistula
Portal vein—thrombosis, invasion, compression
Splenic—thrombosis, invasion, compression
Intrahepatic:
Presinudoisal—congenital hepatic fibrosis, primary biliary cirrhosis, chronic active hepatitis, schistosomiasis, sarcoidosis, lymphoma, idiopathic, copper, arsenic.
Sinusoidal—cirrhosis, noncirrhotic, acute alcoholic hepatitis, Vit A, cytotoxic drugs.
Postsinusoidal—veno-occlusive disease, alcoholic central hyaline sclerosis.
Posthepatic:
Hepatic vein—thrombosis, webs tumours, veno-occlusive disease
IVC—tumours, webs, thrombus, invasion

Heart—constrictive pericarditis, congestive cardiac failure.
Extrahepatic—umbilical infections, appendicitis, dehydration, ulcerative colitis, Crohn's, biliary infections, splenectomy, occludal porta systemic shunts, chronic pancreatitis, pancreatic carcinoma, hepatobiliary surgeries, protien C deficiency, myeloproliferative disorders, portal vein thrombosis, HCC in cirrhosis, autoimmune, oral contraceptives, thrombophlebitis migrains and pregnancy.

168. **A-T, B-T, C-F, D-T, E-T**
Polycystic liver disease and liver failure are absolute contraindications. Refractory ascites is an indication. Ideal end portosystemic gradient is <12 mm Hg. Haemoperitoneum is due to capsular laceration.

169. **A-T, B-T, C-T, D-T, E-F**
HIDA scan—Normally tracer should be seen in duodenum by 30-60 mins. In the earlier phases tracer is in liver and hence a focal liver lesion can be assessed. In cholecystitis, there is no uptake in GB after 60 min.

170. **A-T, B-F, C-F, D-T, E-T**
Portal vein > 13, splenic vein > 11, superior mesenteric vein >12, coronary > 7, esophageal > 4.
Gandy gamma bodies are siderotic nodules due to haemorrhage, seen in the spleen and are hyperechoic. There is increased flow in the superior mesenteric and splenic veins with little respiratory variation. The presence of recanalised umbilical vein indicates the hepatofugal portal flow is prominent than hepatofugal umbilical flow and hence extrahepatic portal hypertension is unlikely.

171. **A-T, B-T C-T, D-F, E-T**
The T2 signal is low due to iron deposition.

172. **A-T, B-T, C-T, D-F, E-F**
The liver shows high density due to glycogen, which is 10 HU more than that of spleen.
Dilated intrahepatic ducts are well seen. Ligamentum teres separates two lobes.
It is the iron which causes increased liver density in hemochromatosis.

173. **A-T, B-T, C-T, D-T, E-F**
ALT, GGT, LDL, AST, Anb—Mitochondrial antibody, ESR are elevated. Ursodeoxycholic acid, immunosuppressants, colchicine and antihistaminics are used.

174. **A-T, B-F, C-T, D-F, E-T**
Most of bladder ruptures are extraperitoneal. Minor liver lacerations are managed conservatively.

175. A-F, B-T, C-T, D-T, E-F
The spleen is the most frequently injured organ in abdominal trauma followed by the liver and kidney. Liver is involved in 20% of blunt abdominal trauma, 30% of gunshot wounds and 40% of stab injuries. Although splenic laceration is more common than liver laceration, liver laceration has a higher mortality and morbidity rate.

176. A-F, B-T, C-T, D-T, E-T
In 45% of patients, liver and splenic laceration coexist. The presence of coexisting splenic, CNS or diaphragmatic injuries increases the mortality from 0.4% to 15%. The management of abdominal trauma is conservative in the absence of hemodynamic instability. Presence of hemoperitoneum is not an absolute indication for surgery. Presence of hemodynamic instability secondary to liver or splenic hemorrhage, concurrent presence of significant bowel or mesenteric injury are the indications of early surgery. Adequate control of hepatic hemorrhage is obtained by compressing liver surface with gauze packs and allowing repair by resorption and coalescence of laceration. Surgical resection of liver is avoided.

177. A-T, B-T, C-F, D-T, E-T
The advent of CT has played a major role in conservative management of abdominal trauma, provided the person is hemodynamically stable. Oral contrast increases diagnostic sensitivity of bowel, mesenteric and pancreatic injury. It is avoided if there is arteriography planned as the contrast will obscure field of view. 150 ml of IV contrast is given at the rate of 2-4 ml/sec and images are obtained after 60-70 sec. Arterial phase images are obtained if there is suspicion of aneurysm.

178. A-T, B-T, C-T, D-T, E-T
The right lobe of liver is commonly affected than the left lobe, and it is the posterior segments close to the spine which are commonly affected. Injuries to the left lobe of the liver are usually associated with injuries to retroperitoneum, including pancreas, transverse colon and duodenum. Liver lacerations are common in the perivascular region paralleling the line of right and middle hepatic arteries and posterior segmental divisions of portal vein. 13% of cases have hepatic vein injury and severe hemorrhage is caused when right hepatic vein is avulsed from IVC. Periportal low density is commonly seen in CT scans and indicates either blood or lymph of bile. Gallbladder injury occurs in only 2% of cases and is associated with pericholecystic fluid or blood in

association with an area of focal thickening or disruption of gallbladder.

179. A-T, B-T, C-T, D-F, E-T

Injury to the bile duct is uncommon and occurs either at the porta hepatis or pancreaticobiliary junction and is usually associated with major vascular or pancreaticoduodenal injuries. The CT signs are edema in the hepatoduodenal ligament, free fluid and associated parenchymal or duodenal injury. Although follow-up CT does not have a major impact in the management, it plays a role in reassuring. There is no observable evidence of healing and resolution within the first week. But any continuing hemorrhage and fluid collections can be evaluated. In splenic injuries, only Grade 4 and Grade 5 require urgent surgical intervention. Extravasation of contrast indicates active heamorrhage and requires intervention regardless of grade.

180. A-T, B-F, C-F, D-T, E-T

Segmental bowel wall thickening, more than 4 mm, in the presence of adequate luminal distension is the most sensitive indicator of bowel wall injury. Intramural air is also a sensitive sign. Sentinel clot is seen adjacent to a site of bowel wall injury and is a sensitive marker. Free peritoneal or retroperitoneal air may indicate full thickness injury, but false positive results are seen in barotraumas at resuscitation or peritoneal lavage. Abnormal contrast enhancement due to reduced mucosal perfusion, occurs both in bowel and mesenteric injury. Hemoperitoneum also occurs in either. Mesenteric infiltration is a nonspecific sign unless associated with intrinsic mural changes.

181. A-F, B-T, C-F, D-T, E-T

Hepatofugal flow, biliary obstruction, LDH > 425 U/L are other contraindications.

182. A-T, B-T, C-T, D-T, D-T

Hepatic infarction, liver failure, cholecystitis, pulmonary embolism, aneurysms, perforation of arteries, tumour rupture, variceal bleeding are other complications.

183. A-T, B-F, C-T, D-T, E-F

Postembolisation syndrome is seen in fifteen percent only. Nontarget embolisation is a major complication.

184. A-F, B-T, C-T, D-T, E-F, F-T

Tumours less than 3 cm, are destroyed by 3 cm spread of heat from a triple radiofrequency electrode. Tumours 3-4 cm in diameter require six overlapping ablations, and those more than

4 cm require 12 ablations. During heating, a thermal cylinder is created around the track of the electrode from the deepest to the most superficial portions of the tumor. Only transient elevation of liver function test may be seen. Liver abscess and hemorrhage are recognized infrequent complications. Ultrasound is not very useful for assessing complete necrosis, as echotexture of fibrosis and neoplasia overlap. Contrast enhanced CT, MRI and PET scan are useful for this differentiation.

185. **A-T, B-T, C-T, D-T, E-T**

RF ablation is a quick, safe and highly effective technique for debulking primary and secondary hepatic tumours. Although it offers high promise for local tumour eradication, it is difficult to create an adequate tumour free margin around tumours, because of difficulty in accurate placement of electrode and the differential blood flow existing between the tumour and normal hepatic parenchyma. This results in incomplete ablation and tumour recurrence. It is more effective in debulking tumours than radiation or chemotherapy. It has fewer complications than chemoembolisation. It is minimally invasive and can be used as many times as needed. Unlike percutaneous ethanol injection, it can be used to treat both primary and secondary hepatic tumours and requires fewer sessions to treat HCC.

186. **A-F, B-T, C-T, D-T, E-T**

Chronic granulomatous disease is an inherited (x-linked) disorder in which the phagocytes cannot make the respiratory bout required for killing microorganisms, causing bacterial and fungal infections. Abscesses are seen in lung/liver/spleen/skin. Perianal abscess and fistulae are seen. Osteomyelitis, pneumonia are features.

187. **A-F, B-T, C-F, D-T, E-F**

More than 80% of metastasis to liver from unknown primary are adenocarcinomas. Search for a primary, will be successful in only 10% of these patients. Liver biopsy should be performed in all these patients. If it turns out to be neuroendocrine metastasis, the survival is good. If it is adenocarcinoma, the prognosis is bad even with treatment (median survival: with treatment—49 days, without treatment—52 days), regardless if primary is found. So, no further work up is required.

188. **A-T, B-T, C-F, D-F, E-T**

Bicoloured hepatic veins are due to collateral vessels formation in chronic disease. The caudate lobe and left lobe are enlarged, but the right lobe is atrophied. Enhancement radiates from the center of the liver to the periphery, in early scans.

In delayed images, the liver enhances homogeneously. Fibrotic, atrophic areas do not enhance in early or delayed images.

189. A-F, B-F, C-T, D-F, E-T

The phasic variation is lost in portal hypertension and the typical triphasic pattern is lost, because the liver loses its compliance and cannot accommodate the reversed flow during cardiac cycle. There is increased flow in the superior mesenteric artery and splenic artery. The lesser omentum is thickened and edematous and should be measured in between the origin of celiac axis and the inferior surface of liver in a longitudinal direction. The resistive index in hepatic artery is more than 0. 78. Hepatofugal flow is not seen in splenorenal shunt, but in portacaval and mesocaval shunt.

190. A-T, B-T, C-T, D-F, E-T

CT has 95% accuracy for splenic injuries. Unclotted blood 30-45 HU. Clotted blood 45-60 HU, arterial extravasation 60-150 HU. Lacerations best seen in portal phase.

Miscellaneous

1. Radiation enteritis:
- A. Acute injury is seen in 2-3 weeks after treatment
- B. Acute radiation injury depends on the dose of radiation
- C. Chronic radiation injury affects the mitotically active intestinal crypt cells
- D. Single ulcer is seen in the anterior wall of the rectum
- E. More common in thin elderly females

2. Peliosis hepatis:
- A. Blood filled spaces, which are exclusively seen in liver
- B. Enhancement characteristics mimic hemangioma
- C. Never larger than 10 mm
- D. Tuberculosis is a cause of peliosis hepatis
- E. Hyperechoic in normal liver

3. MRCP is superior to ERCP in the following conditions:
- A. Pancreatic pseudocyst
- B. Biliary cystadenoma
- C. Pancreas divisum
- D. Biliary enteric anastomosis
- E. Assessment before cholecystectomy

4. MRCP:
- A. Not good in the presence of enterobiliary anastomosis
- B. MRCP is better than ERCP for chronic pancreatitis
- C. Intrahepatic ducts are visualised better than extrahepatic ducts
- D. Single shot fast spin echo sequences eliminate motion artefacts
- E. Has better spatial resolution than ERCP

5. Biliary drainage:
- A. Endoscopic drainage is performed only if percutaneous drainage fails
- B. In hilar tumours, both the right and left hepatic ducts should be drained

C. Drainage is best performed in the same duct punctured during PTC
D. In hilar tumours, catheters in left ductal system achieves more drainage than right ductal system
E. Left ductal system is best punctured with ultrasound guidance

6. **Abdominal actinomycosis:**
   A. Left iliac fossa is the most common location
   B. IUCD is a cause of actinomycosis
   C. Chicken bone is a cause of abdominal actinomycosis
   D. Causes ureteric obstruction
   E. The most common site of actinomycosis
   F. Gram negative, aerobic rod

7. **Features of GI amyloidosis:**
   A. Rectal biopsy is positive in 75% of amyloidosis
   B. Gastric ulcers
   C. Submucosal nodules
   D. Calcification
   E. Aphthoid ulcers
   F. Enlarged ileocaecal valve

8. **Causes of secondary amyloidosis:**
   A. Rheumatoid arthritis
   B. Scleroderma
   C. Sarcoidosis
   D. Familial Mediterranean fever
   E. Multiple myeloma

9. **AIDS in gastrointestinal tract:**
   A. Cryptosporidiosis causes thickening of volvulae conniventes
   B. Pseudo Whipple's disease is caused by MAI infection
   C. Increased risk of anorectal carcinoma
   D. Duodenum is the most common site of Kaposi's sarcoma in bowel
   E. Diffuse bowel wall enhancement favours lymphoma than Kaposi's sarcoma

10. **MRCP:**
    A. Distal biliary duct is best assessed in thick collimation coronal reconstruction
    B. Images are acquired in thin and thick collimation
    C. Persistent dilatation of the ducts more than 2 minutes after secretin implies papillary stenosis
    D. Normal and abnormal biliary duct can be differentiated in 90% of·times
    E. Fasting should be avoided before examination, so that there is a good fluid contrast in the duodenum

11. **AIDS in GIT:**
    A. Cytomegalovirus produces acalculous cholecystitis
    B. Necrotic nodes are seen in MAI infection
    C. Lymphadenopathy is a feature of cryptosporidiosis infection
    D. Caecum is the most common bowel location for CMV
    E. Focal hepatic lesions are more common in tuberculosis than MAI

12. **Parasitic infections of GIT:**
    A. Hookworm infection is localised to the distal ileum
    B. Tapeworm infection is best diagnosed by double contrast barium enema
    C. Schistosomiasis is a well known cause of small bowel strictures
    D. Strongyloidosis has a predilection for producing ulcers in the ileum
    E. Clonorchis sinensis produces calculi within intrahepatic bile ducts
    F. Giardiasis produces reactive arthritis and Vit B_{12} malabsorption

13. **The following are associated with schistosomiasis infection:**
    A. Bladder carcinoma
    B. Lymphoma
    C. Glomerulonephritis
    D. Cor pulmonale
    E. Hepatoma

14. **Inflammatory aortic aneurysm:**
    A. Fever is not seen
    B. The incidence of rupture is less than atherosclerotic aneurysm
    C. Obstruction of the left ureter is very common
    D. Calcification is uncommon, unlike atherosclerotic aneurysm
    E. The adventitia is thickened and does not enhance

15. **Inflammatory aortic aneurysm:**
    A. The morbidity after surgery is less than in atherosclerotic aneurysm
    B. Viscosity of blood is increased
    C. Majority are infrarenal
    D. Associated with vertebral changes
    E. Majority are fusiform
    F. Presence of gas is highly suggestive

16. **Pancreas divisum:**
    A. Majority of the ductal secretion of pancreas drains through the ventral pancreatic duct
    B. Pancreatitis is due to stenosed minor papilla
    C. Second commonest congenital pancreatic abnormality after annular pancreas
    D. CT scan shows fat attenuation cleft between head and body of pancreas
    E. Secretin improves diagnosis in ultrasound and MRI

17. **Choledochal cyst:**
    A. High risk of pancreatitis
    B. Complicated by adenocarcinoma
    C. Pain is the most common presentation
    D. The pancreatic duct is inserted into the distal common bile duct
    E. Hepatic abscess is a complication

18. **Brunner gland hypertrophy:**
    A. Associated with chronic renal failure
    B. Associated with cystic fibrosis
    C. Predominantly seen in second part of duodenum
    D. Larger than nodular lymphoid hyperplasia
    E. Associated with peptic ulcer

19. **Bad prognostic factors in abdominal HIV:**
    A. Splenomegaly   B. Gross lymphadenopathy
    C. Ascites   D. Focal hepatic lesion
    E. Hepatomegaly

20. **Radiological features of acute infectious hepatitis:**
    A. Lymph nodes in the hepatogastric ligament
    B. Gallbladder wall thickening in 98%
    C. Sludge within gallbladder
    D. Periportal hyperdensities
    E. Sparing of caudate lobe

21. **Pancreatic transplant:**
    A. Acute graft rejection shows high echogenic areas due to haemorrhage
    B. The graft is enlarged in chronic rejection
    C. Ultrasound is the most sensitive method for diagnosis of rejection
    D. Fluid collection around the graft does not require any treatment
    E. T2 relaxation time is increased in graft rejection

22. **Metallic endoprosthesis for biliary obstruction:**
    A. Second choice after plastic stents for biliary drainage
    B. Contraindicated in presence of a tumour
    C. Introduced through smaller track than plastic stent
    D. Patency rate is more than plastic stent
    E. Migration is a major problem than plastic stent
    F. Can't be used in straight segment of duct

23. **Causes of filling defects within biliary duct in MRCP:**
    A. Surgery
    B. Flow voids
    C. Concentrated bile
    D. Cholesterol stone
    E. Biliary enteric fistula

24. **Biliary strictures:**
    A. 80% of benign strictures are secondary to cholecystectomy
    B. Pancreatic carcinoma is the most common cause of malignant biliary stricture
    C. Ductal ectasia is the most common finding in chronic pancreatitis
    D. In type III hilar stricture, one drain is enough
    E. Absence of pancreatic duct dilatation excludes pancreatic carcinoma

25. **Causes of benign biliary strictures:**
    A. Liver transplantation
    B. Choledochal cyst
    C. Polyarteritis nodosa
    D. Cystic fibrosis
    E. Duodenal diverticulum

26. **Hepatic lesions that enhance centrally:**
    A. Peliosis hepatis
    B. Hemangiomas
    C. Focal nodular hyperplasia
    D. Adenomas
    E. Hepatocellular carcinoma

ANSWERS

1. **A-T, B-F, C-F, D-T, E-T**
Acute injury affects the mitotically active intestinal crypt cells and
is seen in 2-3 weeks. Chronic injury affects mitotically less active
vascular endothelial cells and connective tissue, which are seen
after months to years. Acute injury depends on the type of
radiation, fractionation of dose and frequency of radiation.
Chronic radiation injury depends on the dose of radiation. 45-65
Gy is required for small intestinal damage, 55-80 Gy for rectum.
In thin females, more small bowel loops are seen in the pelvis and
are prone for radiation injury. Hypertension, diabetes, atherosclerosis, previous surgeries, adriamycin, 5 fluorouracil, bleomycin,
methotrexate, hyperbaric oxygen and inflammatory bowel disease
increase the risk of radiation injury.

2. **A-F, B-F, C-F, D-T, E-T**
Peliosis hepatis is blood filled cystic spaces seen in liver, which
are formed due to lysis of reticulin fibrils which support the
hepatocytes and sinusoids. Can measure upto 4-5 cm. Anabolic
steroids, oral contraceptives, tamoxifen, azathioprine, polyvinyl
chloride, thorium, arsenic, tuberculosis, HIV, hepatocellular
tumours are the recognised causes. It is also seen in spleen, lymph
nodes, bone marrow, lung, pleura, adrenals, kidneys and small
bowel. It is hypoechoic in fatty liver, hyperechoic in normal liver
and can be heterogeneous if there is haemorrhage. Central
enhancement is seen with Levovist administration. CT is
hypodense in fatty liver. It is hypodense in normal liver,
hyperdense in fatty liver. In arterial phase, there can be central
enhancement with peripheral filling or homogeneous enhancement.
In equilibrium phase, it is isodense and it can be hyperdense in
delayed scans due to contrast retention. Variable signal intensity
is seen in T1 and high signal is seen in T2. Angiography shows
multiple vascular nodules. It is common in the right lobe.

3. **A-T, B-T, C-T, D-T, E-T**
Fifty percent of pancreatic pseudocysts do not fill with dye during
ERCP. Biliary cystadenomas and cystadenocarcinomas do not fill
with contrast due to mucinous secretion. MRCP is very useful for
any pancreaticobiliary disease. Aberrant ductal anatomy is best
assessed with MRCP. It is a non invasive, accurate, no radiation,
cheap, not operator dependent, good assessment of ductal and
extraductal system.

4. **A-F, B-F, C-T, D-T, E-F**

MRCP is the preferred modality for evaluation of enterobiliary anastomosis. MRCP has less spatial resolution than ERCP and it is not useful for evaluation of small pancreatic ducts in chronic pancreatitis and intrahepatic ducts in sclerosing cholangitis. Proximal intrahepatic ducts beyond the right and left hepatic duct are difficult to visualise because of the low spatial resolution and imaging in non distended state. Fast spin echo or single shot fast spin echo sequences are used with torso phase arrayed coil. Single shot fast spin echo sequence is very fast, eliminates motion artefacts, increases signal to noise ratio, but has lesser spatial resolution.

5. **A-F, B-F, C-F, D-F, E-T**

For mid and lower duct strictures, endoprosthesis is usually placed using endoscopic techniques. Only in technically difficult cases, hilar tumours and upper biliary strictures, percutaneous drainage is preferred. Drainage is usually performed using a second puncture into a horizontally oriented ductal system, after PTC. In hilar tumours, it is enough to drain one system. The other system is drained only if there is inadequate drainage or cholangitis. Right side is more often drained due to larger volume and ease of technique. Left system can also be easily punctured using ultrasound guidance.

6. **A-F, B-T, C-T, D-T, E-F, F-F**

Right iliac fossa is the most common site of abdominal actinomycosis. It is usually acquired secondary to abdominal surgeries or ingestion of foreign body. Pelvic actinomycosis is associated with IUCD use for at least 8 years duration. Cervicofacial actinomycosis accounts for 50-70% of cases, thoracic in 15-20% of cases. Abdominal location is less common. It is a gram positive, anaerobic rod. Ureteric obstruction can be caused by retroperitoneal fibrosis. Mass and sinuses are seen in the right iliac fossa.

7. **A-T, B-T, C-T, D-T, E-F, F-T**

Motor dysfunction, nodular and thickened folds, ulcers, mucosal atrophy, malabsorption, hepatosplenomegaly, intraluminal and intramural masses, obstruction and calcified deposits are other features.

8. **A-T, B-F, C-F, D-T, E-T**

Tuberculosis, chronic osteomyelitis and granulomatous ileitis are other causes of secondary amyloidosis. Unlike primary amyloidosis, treatment of the underlying chronic condition halts or even cures the secondary amyloidosis.

9. **A-T, B-T, C-T, D-T, E-T**
   Cryptosporidiosis also causes cholangitis.*Mycobacterium avium intracellulare* produces clinical and histological findings resembling Whipple's disease and is seen in proximal small bowel. Increased incidence of squamous cell carcinoma of anus, which is very aggressive and invasive. Kaposi's sarcoma is usually seen as submucosal nodules with enhancing lymph nodes. Lymphoma shows diffuse bowel wall thickening and enhancement.

10. **A-F, B-T, C-T, D-T, E-T**
    The MRCP images in coronal plane, reconstructed with 3D MIP resemble a conventional ERCP, but with lesser spatial resolution. The ducts are normally in non distended state. Secretin distends the ducts for 2 minutes after injection. Persistent dilatation can also be due to chronic pancreatitis. The main biliary and pancreatic ducts are visualised in more than 95% of time. Fasting for 3 hours is preferred, so that there are no unwanted signals from gastrointestinal tract. There is enough fluid at 3 hours to just outline the main papilla.

11. **A-T, B-F, C-F, D-T, E-T**
    Cytomegalovirus and cryptosporidiosis cause acalculous cholecystitis and cholangitis. Necrotic nodes are seen in MTB not in MAI. Hepatomegaly is more common in MAI. Splenomegaly is even in both. Focal hepatic and splenic lesions are more common in MTB.

12. **A-F, B-F, C-F, D-F, E-T, F-T**
    Hookworm infection is caused by Ankylostoma duodenale or Necator americanus which are mainly seen in the duodenum and proximal jejunum and produce iron deficiency anemia and pulmonary infiltrates with eosinophilia(PIE). Tapeworm infection is seen in the small bowel. Schistosomiasis produces inflammation and strictures in the large bowel. Strongyloides stercoralis affects the stomach, duodenum and jejunum. In early stages, the mucosal folds are thickened and edematous, with dilatation and absence of peristalsis. Later stages show ulceration, thickened, rigid, fibrosed wall and obliteration of folds. Schistosomiasis japonicum and mansoni produce granulomatous colitis or terminal ileitis and bloody diarrhoea. Giardiasis is a protozoan which is seen in stomach, duodenum and small bowel. It produces acute diarrhoea in 90%. Malabsorption, reactive arthritis, urticaria are other manifestations.

13. **A-T, B-F, C-T, D-T, E-F**
    Schistosomiasis of bladder(Schistosomiasis haematobium) is a predisposing factor for squamous carcinoma of bladder. Hepatosplenic schistosomiasis (S. japonicum and mansoni) produces

periportal fibrosis, portal hypertension, cirrhosis, variceal bleeding, pulmonary hypertension, cor pulmonale, granulomatous colitis, glomerulonephritis and renal failure.

14. **A-F, B-F, C-T, D-F, E-T, F-F**
Inflammatory aneurysms comprise 10% of abdominal aneurysms. Fever and weight loss are noted in addition to the normal features of AAA. The aneurysm has thick wall and there is perianeurysmal soft tissue stranding.Ultrasound shows thick echogenic wall which is surrounded by hypoechoic inflammatory mass. CT scan shows thick, calcified aortic wall with periaortic inflammatory soft tissue/ stranding/ fluid. Contrast scan shows intense enhancement of the lumen, with delayed enhancement of inflammatory mass and no enhancement of thickened fibrous adventitia. Inflammatory mass can cause adhesion to adjacent structures such as bowel, ureter and IVC. Contrary to popular belief, calcification is present in these aneurysms.

15. **A-F, B-T, C-F, D-T, E-F, F-T**
Surgical morbidity is higher than atherosclerotic aneurysm, due to sepsis and renal failure. Leucocytosis and raised ESR are lab findings. 70% are in suprarenal location either in thoracic or abdominal aorta. Vertebral osteomyelitis and gas are associated findings. Majority are saccular. Rapid expansion is a salient features. High uptake is seen in WBC and Gallium scans.

16. **A-F, B-T, C-F, D-T, E-T**
In normal pancreas, the main pancreatic duct (Wirsung) is formed by dorsal pancreatic duct in the tail and boy and ventral pancreatic duct in head . Accessory pancreatic duct (Santorini) is formed by remaining portion of duct in dorsal pancreas and drains proximally by accessory papilla in the duodenal loop. Pancreas divisum is the most common congenital abnormality of pancreas due to failure of fusion of ventral and dorsal pancreatic ducts resulting in drainage of pancreatic juice via the Santorini duct through the minor papilla. This increased flow through a small duct produces functional stenosis and overdistension of duct, resulting in recurrent acute pancreatitis.ERCP shows large accessory duct. CT shows an accessory duct that does not join the bile duct and the normal vertical segment of main pancreatic duct caudal to accessory duct is not seen. Fat attenuation oblique cleft is seen separating the pancreatic head and body. Secretin increases bicarbonate and pancreatic fluid secretion, distending the duct and hence leading to better visualisation. (Twice)

17. **A-T, B-T, C-T, D-T, E-T**

Cholelithiasis, cirrhosis, portal hypertension, cholangiocarcinoma are other complications. Epigastric or right upper quadrant pain, jaundice and right upper quadrant mass are the typical findings, which are not always present. Because of the anomalous insertion of pancreatic duct into distal bile duct, reflux of pancreatic juice into bile duct damages the duct and results in cyst formation. It is more common in females and there are five types.

18. **A-T, B-T, C-F, D-T, E-T**

Brunner gland hypertrophy is hypertophy of tubuloalveolar glands in the submucosa of duodenum, usually in response to peptic ulcer. It is usually seen in the duodenal bulb. It is seen as nodular filling defects and thickened folds, which are less numerous and larger than lymphoid hyperplasia. Also associated with Zollinger-Ellison syndrome.

19. **A-F, B-T, C-T, D-T, E-F**

Gross lymphadenopathy, focal hepatic masses and ascites indicate severe immunosuppression and indicate bad prognosis.

20. **A-T, B-T, C-T, D-F, E-F**

The findings in acute hepatitis are nonspecific. In ultrasound, hepatomegaly, diffuse low echogenicity, periportal hyperechogenicity, thick gallbladder wall, contacted gallbladder with sludge are seen. In CT scan, hepatomegaly, inhomogenous density, periportal hypodensity due to fluid collection, thickened GB wall and lymphadenopathy in hilum and hepatogastric ligament are seen.

21. **A-F, B-F, C-F, D-F, E-T**

MRI is the most sensitive and specific method for diagnosing pancreatic graft rejection. Low signal in T1 and high signal in T2(T2 relaxation time more than 86 ms, normal 59 ms)is seen. Ultrasound shows large, hypoechoic pancreas in acute rejection and small, bright pancreas in chronic rejection. Decreased perfusion is seen in blood pool imaging. Perigraft fluid is secondary to post-transplant pancreatitis and requires percutaneous drainage.

22. **A-F, B-T, C-T, D-T, E-F, F-F**

Metallic stents are preferred than plastic stents because of longer patency rates and decreased need for reintevention. Plastic stent should be used if there is duodenal tumour infiltration. The introducer systems are smaller than plastic stents.

23. **A-T, B-T, C-T, D-T, E-T**

    Surgical clips, pneumobilia(secondary to fistula or instrumentation), stones, clots, tumours are the causes of biliary filling defects.

24. **A-T, B-T, C-T, D-F, E-F**

    Bismuth Corlette classification of malignant hilar obstruction. I—distal to primary confluence of right and left hepatic duct, II— involvement of primary but not secondary confluence, III—involvement of one secondary confluence a—right, b—left, IV— involvement of both secondary confluences. In I and II, one drain is enough. In III and IV, right anterior and posterior or right anterior and left drains are necessary. Cholangiocarcinoma, hepatoma, metastasis and lymphadenopathy are other causes. Although double duct sign is seen in pancreatic duct carcinoma, in 20%, there is no pancreatic ductal dilatation.

25. **A-T, B-T, C-T, D-T, E-T**

    Postcholecystectomy, trauma, pancreatitis, stones, HIV, tuberculosis, radiation, chemotherapy, liver transplantation, idiopathic, choledochal cyst, Mirizzi syndrome, instrumentation, papillary dysfunction, PAN, SLE, Crohn's disease, duodenal diverticulum, hepatic artery aneurysm, cystic fibrosis with liver involvement, eosinophilic cholecystitis, and cholangitis are other causes of benign biliary stricture.

26. **A-T, B-T, C-T, D-F, E-T**

    Seen in high flow hemangiomas.

Bibliography

1. American Journal of Roentgenology, American Roentgen Ray Society.
2. Carol M Rumack, Diagnostic Ultrasound, Mosby.
3. Clinical Radiology, The Royal College of Radiologists, UK.
4. David Cosgrove, Hylton Meire, Keith Dewbury, Clinical Ultrasound, A Comprehensive Text, Churchill Livingstone.
5. David Sutton, Textbook of Radiology and Imaging, 7th edn, Churchill Livingstone.
6. Friedman AC, Radiology of the Liver, Biliary Tract, Pancreas and Spleen, Williams & Wilkins.
7. GH Whitehouse, Brian S Worthington, Graham H Whitehouse, BS Worthington, Techniques in Diagnostic Imaging, Blackwell.
8. Grainger and Allison's Diagnostic Radiology, 4th edn, A Textbook of Medical Imaging, Churchill Livingstone Publishers.
9. Jamie Wier, Peter H Abrahams, Imaging Atlas of Human Anatomy, Mosby.
10. KC Clark, E Naylor, EJ Roebuck, AS Whitley, RA Swallow, Positioning in Radiography, Butterworth Heinemann.
11. Michael Federle, Pocket Radiologist, Abdomen Top 100 Diagnoses, Saunders.
12. Pablo Ros, Dean Bidgood Jr, Abdominal Magnetic Resonance Imaging, Mosby.
13. Patrick C Freeny, Giles W Stevenson, Margulis and Burhenne's Alimentary Tract Radiology, 5th edn, Mosby.
14. PF Butler, Applied Radiological Anatomy, Cambridge University Press.
15. Radiographics Journal, Radiological Society of North America.
16. Radiological Clinics of North America, Saunders.
17. Radiology, Radiological Society of North America.
18. Richard M Gore, Textbook of Gastrointestinal Radiology, Elsevier.
19. Robert Halpert, Gastrointestinal Radiology, The Requisites, Mosby.
20. Ronald Eisenberg, Gastrointestinal Radiology, A Pattern Approach, Lippincott, Williams & Wilkins.
21. Ryan S, Nichols MC, Anatomy for Diagnostic Imaging, Saunders.
22. Seminars in Roentgenology. Saunders.
23. Stephen Chapman, Richard Nakielny, A Guide to Radiological Procedures, Saunders.
24. Stephen Chapman, Richard Nakielny, AIDS Radiological Differential Diagnosis, Saunders.
25. Theodore E Keats, Mark W Anderson, Atlas of Normal Roentgen Variants that may Stimulate Disease, Mosby.
26. Wolfgang H Dahnert, Radiology Review Manual, 5th edn, Lippincott Williams & Wilkins.